Management of Cumulative Trauma Disorders

Management of Cumulative Trauma Disorders

Edited by

Martha J. Sanders, M.A., OTR/L

Assistant Professor of Occupational Therapy,
Quinnipiac College, Hamden; President,
Prevention Works, Madison, Connecticut

With 11 Contributing Authors

Butterworth–Heinemann
Boston   Oxford   Johannesburg   Melbourne   New Delhi   Singapore

Library of Congress Cataloging-in-Publication Data

Management of cumulative trauma disorders / edited by Martha J.
    Sanders.
        p. cm.
    Includes bibliographical references and index.
    ISBN 0-7506-9561-7
    1. Overuse injuries.   I. Sanders, Martha J.
    [DNLM: 1. Repetition Strain Injury--therapy.   2. Occupational
Health.   3. Risk Factors.   WE 175 M2655 1997]
RD97.6.M36   1997
617.1--dc21
DNLM/DLC
for Library of Congress   96-50459
                                                                              CIP

British Library Cataloguing-in-Publication Data
A catalogue record for this book is available from the British Library.

The publisher offers special discounts on bulk orders of this book.
For information, please contact:

Manager of Special Sales
Butterworth–Heinemann
313 Washington Street
Newton, MA 02158-1626
Tel: 617-928-2500
Fax: 617-928-2620

For information on all B-H medical publications available, contact our World Wide Web home page
at: http://www.bh.com/med

10 9 8 7 6 5 4 3 2 1

Printed in the United States of America

To my father, who taught me the self-fulfilling nature of work; to my mother, whose strong soul has inspired us all; and to my friend and husband, Paul, whose words and actions demonstrate that knowledge creates a world of possibilities

Contents

Contributing Authors

Donald L. Clark, P.T., B.A., B.S.
Private practice, Willimantic, Connecticut

Susan V. Duff, M.S., P.T., OTR/L, CHT
Instructor in Anatomy and Biomechanics, Department of Biobehavioral Studies,
Teacher's College, Columbia University, New York; private practice, hand
therapy and pediatrics, New York

Dorothy Farrar Edwards, Ph.D., OTR
Assistant Professor of Occupational Therapy and Neurology, Washington University
School of Medicine, St. Louis

Melanie T. Ellexson, M.B.A., OTR, F.A.O.T.A.
AVP/Executive Director, STEPS Industrial Rehabiliation Clinics, Schwab Rehabilitation Hospital, Chicago

Barbara J. Headley, M.S., P.T.
President, Innovative Systems for Rehabilitation Inc., Boulder, Colorado

Caryl D. Johnson, OTR, CHT
Private practice, New York

James W. King, M.A., OTR, CHT
Certified Hand Therapist, HealthSouth Sports Medicine and Rehabilitation Center,
Waco, Texas

Michael S. Melnik, M.S., OTR
President, Prevention*Plus*, Inc., Minneapolis, Minnesota

Claudia Michalak-Turcotte, C.D.A., R.D.H., M.S.
Associate Professor, Department of Allied Dental, Tunxis Community-Technical College, Farmington; Department of Allied Dental—Dental Hygiene, University of Connecticut School of Dental Medicine, Farmington

Martha J. Sanders, M.A., OTR/L
Assistant Professor of Occupational Therapy, Quinnipiac College, Hamden;
President, Prevention Works, Madison, Connecticut

Richard K. Schwartz, M.S., OTR, F.S.R.
President, Richard K. Schwartz Consulting Services, Inc., San Antonio, Texas

Judith Pelletier Sehnal, M.S., OTR/L, CPE
Senior Technical Consultant, Human Factors Engineering, Loss Control Department,
The Hartford, Hartford, Connecticut

Preface

The management of cumulative trauma disorders (CTDs) is becoming a part of mainstream practice for many health care practitioners. Clinicians, both new and experienced, are expected not only to treat these conditions but to understand the perspectives of all individuals involved and anticipate the potential problems when returning workers to the job.

This book was developed to provide health care practitioners with a resource for understanding the nature of CTDs and the various aspects of their management. The information is presented in a logical, practical manner with a strong emphasis on theory as a basis for understanding.

Management of Cumulative Trauma Disorders first presents the history of CTDs and discusses CTDs from the perspectives of the individual worker, industrial supervisor, and medical professional. These perspectives highlight the need for an interdisciplinary approach and enable health care practitioners to formulate their roles in dealing with CTDs.

The book then introduces the specific conditions associated with CTDs and discusses the risk factors for developing these conditions. The job analysis provides a practical approach to identifying the risks and demands of a given job. Workplace recommendations are then made, with commentaries from real-life experiences. A discussion of the current trends in screening and monitoring workplace CTDs, as well as preventing CTDs, serves as an overview of the broad array of issues involved in managing these disorders. Specific programs for high-risk populations are discussed and outlined for video display terminal operators, dental hygienists, and performing musicians. Finally, the chapter on outcome assessment provides the tools to determine the cost-effectiveness of CTD programming.

Throughout the book, our goal is to promote a healthy, happy, and productive workplace for the future.

M.J.S.

Acknowledgments

Many individuals gave unselfishly to the creation of this book. I wish to thank all authors for the time they took from their personal lives to contribute to this book. I very much appreciate the patience and dedication of Karen Oberheim, Medical Editor at Butterworth–Heinemann, without whom this book would not be possible. I also wish to thank Lynn Dorsey, Quinnipiac College Audiovisual Specialist, for her time and expertise; Norma Keegan, Quinnipiac College Interlibrary Loan Clerk, for her perseverance in locating reference materials; and Roberta Solimene, OTR/L CHT, for her ideas on work design.

Finally, I am grateful to Cheryl Atwood and Claudia Michalak-Turcotte for providing the photographs.

M.J.S.

PART I

Perspectives from the Individual Worker, Medicine, Insurance, and Industry

Chapter 1

Cumulative Trauma Disorders: A Worldwide Dilemma

Martha J. Sanders

Our society prides itself on the belief that technical advancements in information processing, manufacturing technology, and medical science will enhance the quality of life for all individuals. Logic dictates that if we work more efficiently, we will be more productive and, therefore, more satisfied with our personal work, our wages, and the use of our leisure time. Unfortunately, the basic assumptions that underlie this logic are gradually being undermined by the hidden costs of doing business in today's highly technical society. The hidden costs that we address are the escalating incidents of stress-related and cumulative trauma disorders (CTDs) for the thousands of workers responsible for our soaring productivity.

Today, we are witnessing what has been termed an *industrial epidemic* (Schenck 1989)—that is, an overwhelming increase in reports of work-related disorders that affect not only industry productivity and labor costs but also the quality of workers' lives both inside and outside the workplace. The problem has dramatic repercussions. As employment positions become less secure, workers are less willing to perform jobs that jeopardize their health and limit future earning potential. As businesses become increasingly competitive, employers complain that the cost of CTDs reduces profits by increasing worker's compensation costs and decreasing productivity. The cost of managing these disorders reverberates from the factory or office floor to the medical and often legal arenas, all of which remove the employee farther from work and drive our health care costs even higher.

The differences in focus among industrial, medical, insurance, and legal systems exacerbates the problem. Each system possesses a unique set of goals, language, and procedures that can alienate other provider systems. Though each provider contributes a valuable perspective, one provider cannot effectively remedy CTDs to the exclusion of other systems. Clearly, in the management of CTDs, the whole is truly greater than the sum of the parts.

The perspective of the authors of this book is that effective prevention and management programs for CTDs must integrate all perspectives thoroughly. The values of individual workers and worker cultures must be integrated with the medical, industrial, and insurance systems so that long-term solutions can be reached. Although health care practitioners will enter the arena of CTD management from medical, industrial, or even educational systems, all practitioners will need to appreciate the contribution of other systems and be prepared to work with representatives from those systems toward a thorough, comprehensive CTD management plan.

In this book, we systematically examine the means by which health care practitioners can effect change to facilitate safer, more productive workplaces. Contextual background from the individual worker, medical, and industrial perspectives are presented to sensitize health care practitioners to the concerns of each participant.

From all perspectives, worker health is a priority in our efforts. If companies are to survive, managers need to maximize productivity and minimize medical costs. If workers are to maintain quality of work and home life, workers need to take responsibility for protecting their health. If medicine is to alleviate disability, health professionals must step beyond the clinics into the "real world" of industry and business. Cooperatively, we must balance productivity with health, consider long-term gains versus short-term profit, and re-examine the value of work for today's worker.

From the high-speed assembly lines to the propagating computer terminals, modern tools of the trade certainly have improved our standard of living. But what about our quality of work life? Are we any better off than we were at the turn of the century? As Eli Ginzberg (1982, p. 75) eloquently stated, "It remains to be seen whether or not the potential of modern technology will turn out to be a blessing."

History of Cumulative Trauma Disorders

The occurrence of CTDs in industry is not new. In 1717, Bernardo Ramazzini, the father of occupational medicine, in his treatise *De Morbis Artificum Diatriba* ("The Diseases of Workers") (translated by Wright 1940), first introduced to physicians the common musculoskeletal disorders that arose from eighteenth-century occupations. Ramazzini observed that many diseases or conditions appeared to be related to patients' exposures to hazardous work environments. At that time, however, physicians rarely asked patients about their work. Ramazzini, therefore, began one of the first systematic attempts to attribute specific diseases or conditions to factors in workers' environments. Ramazzini documented the musculoskeletal, respiratory, dermatologic, and emotional problems exhibited by his patients; he then observed workers at their jobs and related specific aspects of the environment (such as hazardous materials, airborne toxins, and excessive physical demands) to these medical conditions. In essence, Ramazzini laid the foundation for occupational health practices today. Ramazzini opens his treatise with the following overview:

Various and manifold is the harvest of diseases reaped by certain workers from the crafts and trades that they pursue; all the profit that they get is fatal injury to their health. That crop germinates mostly, I think, from two causes. The first and most potent is the harmful character of the materials that they handle for these emit noxious vapors and very fine particles inimical to human beings and in-

duce particular diseases; the second cause I ascribe to certain violent and irregular motions and unnatural postures of the body, by reason of which the natural structure of the vital machine is so impaired that serious diseases gradually develop therefrom (Ramazzini 1717, p. 15).

Ramazzini (1717) poignantly describes the morbidity of many acquired conditions and the futile reward of illnesses that many workers suffered as a result of enduring hazardous work environments. He describes the following conditions that resulted from specific occupations:

Of sedentary workers, he observes, "[M]en and women who sit while they work at their jobs, become bent, hump-backed and hold their heads like people looking for something on the ground; this is the effect of their sedentary life and the bent posture as they sit . . . and sew . . ." (p. 282).

Regarding scribes and notaries, he states:

[T]he maladies that afflict the clerks afore said arise from three causes: First, constant sitting, secondly the incessant movement of the hand and always in the same direction, thirdly the strain on the mind from the effort not to disfigure the books by errors or cause loss to their employers when they add, subtract, or do sums of arithmetic . . . Furthermore, incessant driving of the pen over paper causes intense fatigue of the hand and the whole arm because of the continuous and almost tonic strain on the muscles and tendons, which in course of time results in failure of power of the right hand (Ramazzini 1717, pp. 421, 423).

Regarding painters, he found that "their sedentary life and melancholic temperament may be partly to blame, for they are almost entirely cut off from intercourse with other men and constantly absorbed in the creations of their imagination" (Ramazzini 1717, p. 67). He noted of bakers, "[N]ow and again, I have noticed bakers with swelled hands, and painful, too; in fact, the hands of all such workers become thickened by the constant pressure of kneading the dough" (p. 229).

Ramazzini identified hazards in workers' environments that we have come to associate with the risk factors for CTDs today. He recognized not only the physical demands such as "violent and irregular motions," "bent posture," "incessant use of the hands," and "tonic strain on the muscles," but also the emotional or mental demands that contribute to work-related fatigue, such as "melancholic temperament," "sedentary life," and "strain on the mind." Still, disorders of workers were treated on an individual basis, and workers had relatively few choices about whether or not to work in the face of disorders.

Cumulative Trauma Disorders in the Twentieth Century

As the Industrial Revolution gained momentum and assembly-line pacing, predetermined motion and time standards, long hours at work, and the performance of repetitive tasks became the norm, the serious and problematic nature of work-related diseases was increasingly recognized. When worker's compensation laws were amended and expanded to cover conditions such as tenosynovitis, insurance companies began to record and further examine these injuries as related to their clients' occupations (Conn 1931).

Physicians became instrumental in determining whether these disorders were actually related to work. Physicians therefore began to compile data that equated musculoskeletal symptoms with workplace factors. Conn (1931) examined rubber company workers who had tenosynovitis and determined that new "high-speed hand operations," "increased intensity of effort," and being new to the job clearly predisposed individuals to disorders such as tenosynovitis. Hammer (1934), who attempted to delineate the "tolerances" or number of repetitions that human tendons could withstand before tenosynovitis developed, concluded that tenosynovitis would occur in human tendons if repetitions exceeded 30–40 per minute, or 1,500–2,000 manipulations per hour. Hammer noted certain hand symptoms consistent with carpal tunnel syndrome, but this condition was not explored further until 1947 by Phalen (1947).

Flowerdew and Bode (1942) raised the issue of improper training and physical conditioning as a cause of tenosynovitis in some workers. Among a group of 52 military personnel assigned to farm work in Great Britain, 16 developed tenosynovitis of the wrist and finger extensors shortly after starting intensive manual work. Fourteen of these 16 individuals had no previous manual labor experience. Blood (1942), a medical officer at a company in Great Britain, agreed that "newcomers to a repetitive stereotyped job are particularly vulnerable, but . . . cases crop up among employees who have had years of experience at these jobs, particularly after

returning to work following a holiday or sick leave" (p 468). Blood attributed a 50% increase in cases of tenosynovitis from 1940 to 1941 to an influx of new workers in his industry.

As automation progressed and manual work became lighter and more efficient, musculoskeletal problems related specifically to office work became apparent. In the 1950s, new office equipment such as high-speed typewriters and keypunch operations streamlined tasks by eliminating movements not directly related to the job (such as retrieving the typewriter carriage after each line). Automation eliminated both the "mini–rest breaks" inherent in operating the old machinery and the need for workers to use several different muscle groups to accomplish a task. Physically, jobs became sedentary, static, and, unvarying; localized muscles were relied on to perform the work. Mentally, the work routines became highly monotonous, although detailed work demanded high levels of concentration. Workers lost a sense of the overall task to which they were contributing (Giuliano 1982).

By the mid-1950s, the musculoskeletal and mental fatigue problems associated with operating new and repetitive machines were clear. The Fifth Session of the International Labor Organization Advisory Committee on Salaried Employees and Professional Workers reported the serious physical consequences created by mechanized work (ILO Advisory Committee 1960). Clerical workers complained of low-back and neck pain; keypunch operators complained of "painful nerves" in the hands; accounting-machine operators complained of fatigue, eye strain, pain and stiffness in cervical and lumbar regions, and numbness in the right hand (Maeda et al. 1980). Although these disorders crossed national boundaries, peaks in reporting occurred at different times for each country.

Occupational Cervicobrachial Disorder in Japan

In Japan, a dramatic increase in musculoskeletal disorders was reported between 1960 and 1980. Complaints first were reported in keypunch operators (17%). Later, typists (13%), telephone operators (16%), office keyboard operators (14%), and assembly-line workers (16%) reported pain in the hands and arms that interfered with their abilities to perform their jobs (Maeda 1977; Ohara et al. 1982). The claims rose to such a proportion that, in 1964, the Japanese Ministry of Labor issued guidelines for keyboard operators, demanding that workers spend no more than 5 hours per day on the keyboard, take a 10-minute rest break every hour, and perform fewer than 40,000 keystrokes per day. In companies that implemented these preventive measures, the incidence of arm and hand disorders decreased from an overall prevalence of 10–20% to 2–5% (Ohara et al. 1982). However, the overall number of individuals who received compensation for hand and arm disorders in the private sector in Japan increased from 90 in 1970 to 546 in 1975 (Maeda 1977).

In 1971, Japan formed the Japanese Committee on Cervicobrachial Syndrome to define the syndrome and fully identify contributing factors. The committee proposed the name *occupational cervicobrachial disorder* (OCD) and defined the problem as a functional or organic disorder (or both) resulting from mental strain or neuromuscular fatigue due to performing jobs in a fixed position or with repetitive movements of the upper extremity (Keikenenwan Shokogun Iinkai [Japanese Association of Industrial Health] 1973).

The Japanese committee then conducted a mass screening of individuals in private industry to further delineate the causative factors for OCD. Researchers concluded that "how the workers use their muscular and nervous systems at work" and "how the task is organized into the work system as a whole" underlie the condition (Maeda 1977, p. 200). Researchers specifically identified static loading of the postural muscles, dynamic loading of localized arm and hand muscles, and lack of "active" rest breaks during the day as factors contributing to OCD. The condition was found to advance with excessive workload and insufficient recovery from fatigue.

The Japanese committee astutely regarded visual eye strain and mental fatigue as being related to OCD. It urged physicians to further investigate the relationship between sleep disturbance, or "chronic fatigue," and symptoms of OCD (Maeda 1977). A 20-year review of the disorder by Maeda analyzed the progression of the disease in Japan and posed questions about exposure or dose-effect relationships. Maeda et al. (1982) found that OCD first peaked in individuals within 6–12 months of starting a new job (possibly due to overwork of untrained individuals) and then peaked again between

2 and 3 years (due to chronic fatigue of muscles). Maeda identified the fundamental controversy that exists today—namely, whether OCD is caused by factors solely within the workplace or whether psychological factors such as personal anxiety or workplace stress are the core problem that becomes magnified by the physical aspects of the workplace.

Other countries subsequently began to examine the incidence of musculoskeletal disorders related to office work. In each country, a gross rise in worker's compensation claims for musculoskeletal disorders served as the catalyst for research of the problem. Specific task forces were established in each country to study CTDs within the socioeconomic context of that country. Most countries followed a similar chronologic pattern of first recognizing acute hand and arm pain in workers, then identifying problems related to static posturing of the shoulder and cervical regions, and finally relating specific medical problems to workplace factors.

Repetitive Strain Injury in Australia

In the 1970s and 1980s, Australia observed a dramatic increase in the number of telecommunications workers who reported symptoms of arm pain or muscular fatigue (Ferguson 1971a; Chatterjee 1978; McDermott 1986). Ferguson (1971a) first investigated the prevalence of "telegraphists' cramp" in 517 male workers in the Australian telegraph service and found that 20% of the workers complained of an "occupational cramp" or "occupational myalgias." Ferguson reported that 75% of these workers had a history of "neurosis" and complained of work overload or job dissatisfaction. Ferguson therefore attributed the "cramp" more to psychological and social factors within the workplace than to the physical performance of the job.

In a later study of 77 female workers in an electronics assembly plant in whom tendinitis was diagnosed, Ferguson (1971b) acknowledged the awkward and repetitive nature of electronics jobs as contributing to workers' symptoms. However, Ferguson questioned the validity of the initial diagnosis of tendinitis and the necessity for the "excessive" medical leave (more than 4 months) for workers with this condition. Ferguson (1971b) advocated early return to work and medical surveillance in addition to ergonomic changes.

The term *repetitive strain injury* (RSI) was adopted among Australian medical investigators in the early 1980s, although most did not believe that the term adequately described the condition (Stone 1983; McDermott 1986; Ireland 1992). Within years, RSI had "spread" in Australia from telegraphists and typists to "tradesmen" and production-line, clerical, data-processing, and postal workers. McDermott (1986) explained that the number of occupational claims for RSI in Australia increased generally from 300 to 400% in data-processing, accounting, and postal services from the mid-1970s to the early 1980s. The Commonwealth Government of Australia, in response to the spiraling cost of RSI in that country, set up a task force on RSI, seeking input from the National Occupational Health and Safety Commission. This task force concluded that a combination of ergonomic and psychological factors contributed to the problem (McDermott 1986).

Clearly investigators in Australia resisted relating RSI to biomechanical factors within the workplace and struggled with the definition of RSI as a separate disease entity as opposed to a grouping of conditions with similar occupational etiologies. Ireland (1992), a researcher from Australia, still contends that musculoskeletal pain relates only to workers' psychological stress, because no objective medical tests (e.g., nerve conduction or electromyography) can diagnose the condition definitively. Despite the strong association of RSI with psychological factors, few studies attempted to evaluate the psychological aspects of RSI.

Occupational Disorders in Sweden, Finland, and Norway

The Nordic countries have long been involved in industrial health care. However, most of the research in musculoskeletal problems has been related to low-back pain. Swedish researchers began to examine upper-extremity musculoskeletal disorders related to work in the 1980s in response to increasing complaints of neck and shoulder pain among blue-collar workers (Bjelle et al. 1981; Kvarnstrom 1983; Dimberg et al. 1989).

Kvarnstrom (1983) and Bjelle et al. (1981), examined the records of workers on long-term sick leave in large industrial plants in Sweden, and noted the increasing magnitude of neck and shoul-

der problems. Kvarnstrom found that 48% of all workers on long-term sick leave had musculoskeletal conditions; neck and shoulder problems were the most common disorders among light-manufacturing workers. When Kvarnstrom (1983) studied the demographic, work task, and social factors related to shoulder problems in 112 workers, the risk factors related to the presence of shoulder pain were as follows:

- *Age:* Older workers were affected more often
- *Gender:* Female workers were 10 times more likely than male workers to suffer shoulder pain
- *Type of work:* Light-manufacturing jobs were most often associated with shoulder pain
- *Salary:* Piece-rate incentives were positively correlated with shoulder pain
- *Nationality:* Immigrants were at higher risk than other workers for developing shoulder pain

Some factors could be explained by the relationship among variables. For example, women tended to be clustered in the higher-risk jobs, and immigrant workers, because of their limited language skills, did not have the opportunity for proper training or job rotation.

When cases were matched with controls, Kvarnstrom (1983) found that a group piece-rate system, shift work, and regard for the work as repetitive, monotonous, and stressful were significant among case subjects. Significantly more case subjects than controls cited a poor relationship with their supervisors, although no difference in relationships with their peers was seen between groups. Finally, Kvarnstrom noted a significant association of shoulder pain with social factors, including being married, having a sick spouse, having children at home, working alternate shifts from one's spouse, and having few leisure activities. Researchers discussed the heavy burden placed on workers with both job and home responsibilities (see Chapter 2).

Recommendations from this study were to promote analysis of the work environment by both medical and technical personnel and to implement both routine medical checkups and education for workers (Kvarnstrom 1983).

Nordic researchers recognized the difficulty in comparing studies from country to country because of a lack of uniform terminology and criteria for diagnosis (Kvarnstrom 1983; Kuorinka et al. 1987). The Nordic Council of Ministers therefore supported a project to develop a standardized Nordic questionnaire for the purposes of collectively recording and compiling information. Using this questionnaire, the estimated prevalence of hand and wrist disorders in Sweden ranged from 18% among Swedish scissor makers to 56% among Swedish packers (Luopajärvi et al. 1979).

Cumulative Trauma Disorders in North America

The United States witnessed a gradual rise in CTDs from 1980 to 1986. The incidence then rose tremendously from 50,000 in 1985 to 281,800 in 1992 (Bureau of Labor Statistics 1992).

In the United States, carpal tunnel syndrome (CTS) was the initial focus of investigation. The occupational causes of CTS were first investigated by Armstrong and Chaffin (1979). Researchers compared the hand size and work method in two groups of female seamstresses, one with a known history of CTS and one with no previous history. Researchers found that women with a history of CTS used more force and wrist deviation when performing the task than those with no history of CTS. Researchers questioned whether the differences in work method between the groups was the cause or the effect of CTS in the affected women.

In an effort to delineate risk factors in an industrial population, researchers investigated the relationship between force and repetition in a job task and the prevalence of CTS in 652 industrial workers (Silverstein et al. 1987). Workers were classified into four job categories based on daily exposures to force and repetition. Results of a physical examination and interview indicated that workers in high-force, high-repetition jobs were 15 times more likely to have CTS than workers in low-force, low-repetition jobs. High repetitiveness appeared to be a greater risk factor than force; vibration was a confounding variable in this study.

As the reported incidence of CTDs skyrocketed, researchers began to document and examine the prevalence of CTD in specific high-risk occupations. Self-reported studies indicated upper-extremity symptoms among the following occupational samples: 62.5% of female supermarket checkers (Margolis & Kraus 1987), 63–87% of dental hygienists (McDonald et al. 1988; Atwood & Michalak 1992), and 82% of electricians (Hunting et al.

1994). Researchers attributed the increased incidence to newly introduced job technology combined with postural loads and long hours of repetitive, static, and highly detailed work.

Researchers are currently identifying methods both to record and analyze accurately the upper-extremity motions of individual workers (Harber et al. 1993). In addition, researchers are seeking methods of evaluating the relative contribution of workplace stressors to the development of CTDs (Putz-Anderson et al. 1992; Bernard et al. 1992; Carayon 1994).

Overall, studies regarding the incidence and etiologies of CTDs have come full circle in terms of recognizing the relative contribution of biomechanical factors and workplace stressors that affect the individual worker. Although each research team has highlighted an important perspective, Kvarnstrom (1983) notes that epidemiologic studies between countries and occupational groups are difficult to compare, citing the following reasons:

1. Studies from different time periods are difficult to compare because of differences in the social role of health and illness.
2. Socioeconomic differences between study groups may invalidate comparisons.
3. The gender bias in different populations and occupations affects results (e.g., women tend to be clustered in high-risk jobs).
4. Reporting systems for epidemiologic studies differ among countries.
5. Inclusion criteria for diagnostic categories and the quantification of risk factors differ among studies.

Nevertheless, all contributions add depth and perspective to the complete picture of CTDs.

Chapter 2 focuses on the various perspectives involved in managing this condition.

References

Armstrong TJ & Chaffin DB (1979). Carpal tunnel syndrome and selected attributes. *J Occup Med*, 2,481–486.

Atwood MJ & Michalak C (1992). The occurrence of cumulative trauma disorders in dental hygienists. *Work*, 2(4),17–31.

Bernard B, Sauter SL, Fine LJ, Petersen MR, & Hales TR (1992). Psychosocial and work organization risk factors for cumulative trauma disorders in the hands and wrists of newspaper employees. *Scand J Work Environ Health*, 18(Suppl 2),119–120.

Blood W (1942). Tenosynovitis in industrial workers. *Br Med J*, 2,468.

Bjelle A, Hagberg M, & Michaelson G (1981). Occupational and individual factors in acute shoulder-neck disorders among industrial workers. *Br J Industrial Med*, 38,356–363.

Bureau of Labor Statistics, Department of Labor (1992). *Survey of Occupational Injuries and Illnesses*. Washington, DC: Department of Labor.

Carayon P (1994). A systems approach to reducing physical and psychological stress: application in automated offices. In GE Bradley & HW Hendrick (Eds). *Human Factors in Organizational Design and Management—IV*. Amsterdam: Elsevier.

Chatterjee DE (1978). Repetition strain injury—a recent review. *J Soc Occup Med*, 37,100–105.

Conn HR (1931). Tenosynovitis. *Ohio State Med J*, 27,713–716.

Dimberg L, Olaffsson A, Stefansson E, Aagaard H, Oden A, Andersson G, Hansson T, & Hagert C (1989). The correlation between work environment and the occurrence of cervicobrachial symptoms. *J Occup Med*, 31,447–453.

Ferguson D (1971a). An Australian study of telegraphists' cramp. *Br J Industrial Med*, 28,280–285.

Ferguson D (1971b). Repetition injuries in process workers. *Med J Aust*, 2,408–412.

Flowerdew RE & Bode OB (1942). Tenosynovitis in untrained farm-workers. *Br Med J*, 2,367.

Ginzberg E (1982). The mechanization of work. *Sci Am*, 247(3),67–75.

Giuliano VE (1982). The mechanization of office work. *Sci Am*, 247(3),149–164.

Hammer A (1934). Tenosynovitis. *Medical Record*, 140,353–355.

Harber P, Bloswick D, Beck J, Pena L, Baker D, & Lee J (1993). Supermarket checker motions and cumulative trauma risk. *J Occup Med*, 35,805–811.

Hunting KL, Welch LS, Cuccerini BA, & Seiger LA (1994). Musculoskeletal symptoms among electricians. *Am J Ind Med*, 25,149–163.

The International Labour Organization Advisory Committee (1960). Effects of mechanisation and automation in officers, III. *Int Labour Rev*, 81,350.

Ireland DCR (1992). The Australian experience with cumulative trauma disorders. In LH Millender, D Louis, & BP Simmons (Eds). *Occupational Disorders of the Upper Extremities*. New York: Churchill Livingstone.

Keikenenwan Shokogun Iinkai (1973). Nihon sangyo-eisei gakkai keikenenwan shokogun iinkai hokokusho (Report of the committee on occupational cervicobrachial syndrome of the Japanese Association of Industrial Health). *Jpn J Ind Health*, 15,304–311.

Kuorinka B, Jonsson B, Kilbom A, Vinterberg H, Biering-Sorensen F, Andersson G, & Jorgensen K (1987). Standardised Nordic questionnaires for the analysis of musculoskeletal symptoms. *Appl Ergonom*, 18,233–237.

Kvarnstrom S (1983). Occurrence of musculoskeletal disorders in a manufacturing industry with special attention to occupational shoulder disorders. *Scand J Rehabil Med*, 8,1–61.

Luopajärvi T, Kuorinka I, Virolainen M, & Holmberg M (1979). Prevalence of tenosynovitis and other injuries of the upper extremities in repetitive work. *Scand J Work Environ Health*, 5(Suppl 3),48–55.

Maeda K (1977). Occupational cervicobrachial disorder and its causative factors. *J Hum Ergol*, 6,193–202.

Maeda K, Hunting W, & Grandjean E (1980). Localized fatigue in accounting machine operators. *J Occup Med*, 22,810–816.

Maeda K, Horiguchi S, & Hosokawa M (1982). History of the studies on occupational cervicobrachial disorder in Japan and remaining problems. *J Hum Ergol*, 11,17–29.

Margolis W & Kraus JF (1987). The prevalence of carpal tunnel symptoms in female supermarket checkers. *J Occup Med*, 29,953–956.

McDermott FT (1986). Repetition strain injury: a review of current understanding. *Med J Aust*, 144,196–200.

McDonald G, Robertson MM, & Erickson JA (1988). Carpal tunnel syndrome among Minnesota dental hygienists. *J Dent Hygiene*, 63,79–85.

Ohara H, Itani T, & Aoyama H (1982). Prevalence of occupational cervicobrachial disorder among different occupational groups in Japan. *J Hum Ergol*, 11,55–63.

Phalen GS (1947). The carpal-tunnel syndrome. *J Bone Joint Surg Am*, 48(2),211–228.

Putz-Anderson V, Doyle GT, & Hales TR (1992). Ergonomic analysis to characterize task constraint and repetitiveness as risk factors for musculoskeletal disorders in telecommunication office work. *Scand J Work Environ Health*, 18(Suppl 2),123–126.

Ramazzini B (1717). *De Morbis Artificum Diatriba*. In W Wright (Trans, 1940). *The Diseases of Workers*. Chicago: University of Chicago Press.

Schenck RR (1989). Carpal tunnel syndrome: the new "industrial epidemic." *AAOHN J*, 37(6),226–231.

Silverstein BA, Fine LJ, & Armstrong TJ (1987). Occupational factors and carpal tunnel syndrome. *Am J Indust Med*, 11,343–358.

Stone WE (1983). Repetitive strain injuries. *Med J Aust*, 2,616–618.

Chapter 2

The Individual Worker Perspective

Martha J. Sanders

How can you explain why one guy gets carpal tunnel syndrome and one doesn't, when they're both doing the same job, using the same tools, working the same hours, and getting the same pay? It doesn't make sense.

—Shift supervisor to therapist

A multitude of variables exists in the search to identify factors involved in a cumulative trauma disorder (CTD). Is the worker too short, or is the work positioned too high? Does the worker sit for hours at a time with no stretch break? Was the worker properly trained to perform the job? Factors in workplace design or administrative procedures, for example, may be an obvious and reasonable starting point for investigation. However, workers' attitudes, values, and routines regarding the job may determine whether a person will comply with recommendations provided by the health care practitioner. To facilitate the appropriate recommendations, health care practitioners must understand workers' jobs from the perspective of the individual worker. The following discussion addresses workers' perspectives of their jobs.

Personal Values

The meaning or value that workers attribute to their jobs figures consciously or unconsciously into workers' motivation to prevent injury or even to return to work. That is, some individuals view work as a means for survival and have little concern for which job they perform. Other individuals view

work as a central aspect of their lives contributing to their self-worth or identity.

The beliefs that guide one's actions toward goals are called *values*. Kielhofner and Burke (1985, pp. 17–18) explain that "as individuals interact with various environments, they generally assimilate the values of those environments, acquiring convictions about what actions are good, right, and important." Values, therefore, determine the relative worth that individuals give to an object or phenomenon and also serve as the basis for making decisions. Although the actual number of a person's values is relatively small, these values drive one's actions toward future goals and guide the manner in which one behaves on a daily basis (Rokeach 1973).

Vocational theorists believe that workers will be more satisfied with their jobs if personal values are congruent with work values (Rokeach 1973). For example, a worker who values a comfortable life and who makes a good salary may be more satisfied with a job than a worker who values control or creativity and works on a machine-paced assembly line (notwithstanding other aspects of the job).

Although health care practitioners do not always focus on matching workers' personal and work values, understanding these concepts may lend insight into workers' attitudes toward changing behaviors. The following case illustrates the powerful influence of personal values on work behavior.

Nick is a 47-year-old meat cutter who developed a chronic lateral epicondylitis after cutting meat for 25 years. After 3 years of intermittent therapy that brought little relief, Nick finally underwent surgery and embarked on a gradual return-to-work program. Within 3 months, the pain had returned. When the therapist revisited Nick at his job, the therapist advised Nick to stretch periodically and to "slow down." Nick stated, "I can't. That's what I'm known for. I'm the best because I'm fast, with or without a bum elbow. We'll have to think of something different."

Nick was respected among his fellow workers because he was the speediest, most efficient meat cutter. Although pacing himself at work may have decreased his elbow pain, admiration from his fellow workers was more important to his self-esteem and identity as a meat cutter.

Work Values

The concept of values relates not only to individual workers but to groups of workers in the same job or profession (referred to as *work groups*). Work groups share similar values or ideas about the "right way to do the job." These ideas may relate to the quality of the job, to priorities for performing tasks, or even to the unspoken rules of conduct that govern how and when workers ask each other for help or complain about pain. Social networks between workers are believed to have a significant impact on individuals' attitudes toward work and on their tendency to report symptoms or painful conditions arising from work-related tasks (Finholt 1994).

In addition to sharing similar values, work groups share similar tools, daily routines, language, and symbols that reflect their jobs. In other words, work groups are "minicultures" that develop from shared work experiences among their members. The culture of the work group influences and gradually shapes workers' perspectives on performing or modifying their jobs.

Work Culture

This concept of culture is relevant to our understanding of workers' jobs and behaviors. Overall, *culture* refers to the behaviors, rules, and social values that individuals learn through experiences within such social institutions as family, school, peer groups, and church. Individuals learn values relevant to work (e.g., perseverance, honesty, and responsibility) as children long before these values are realized in the workplace. In the workplace,

these early values are integrated into vocational readiness and technical skills that contribute to the adult work role (Ginsberg 1957).

Individuals become assimilated into a work culture through various channels, including technical training, formal orientations, and informal experiences. New workers learn technical skills through educational programs, vocational training, on-the-job training, and trial and error. Workers learn such formal workplace rules as punctuality, work quality, and productivity standards through company orientations, policy and procedure manuals, and yearly performance reviews. Finally, new workers learn the important, yet unspoken, informal "do's and don'ts" of the job through conversation with seasoned workers, by modeling others, and by observing usual and unusual events. These informal channels may exert the greatest impact on work attitudes (Van Maanen 1976).

Initially, new workers are concerned with performing and complying with work role expectations. However, over time, individuals contribute their own talents and perspectives to both the task and to interactional aspects of the job, so that the work culture subtly changes with the input of new workers (Van Maanen 1976; Jablin 1987). (For further reading about organizational socialization, see Van Maanen 1976; Jablin 1987; Ginsberg 1957.)

Cultural assimilation is so insidious that individuals are generally unaware of the elements of their own culture (Hall 1973). However, it is clear that workers' attitudes toward injury prevention can be affected at every step of the assimilation process by positive feedback and support from management and peers. The better we understand work role assimilation, workers' routines, daily priorities, and relationships with other work groups, the better will we understand workers' attitudes toward accepting or rejecting our intervention strategies.

The ethnographic interview is a means to learn about workers' cultures, including their environments, daily routines, and tools. The ethnographic interview enables health care practitioners to answer such questions as the following:

- Can one worker realistically ask another worker for help, or is this considered to be a "cop-out"?
- Can workers be expected to slow down or pace themselves if pay depends on piece-rate incentives?

- What determines *quality* for certain work groups?
- What aspects of a particular job should not be changed?

These seemingly simple questions offer much information about how workers perceive their work role.

Appendix 2.1 offers a semistructured interview that seeks to understand workers' cultures on the basis of the interview techniques described by Spradley (1979). The interview begins with a "grand tour" of the worker's physical environment; then scope narrows to the worker's specific work area and work tasks. Next the interview addresses such job assimilation issues as training and "learning the ropes," and ends with a discussion of the worker's social relationships and work values. The goal of the interview is to provide a context for understanding the workplace demands. Ultimately, health care practitioners seek to understand aspects of the job that are important to the worker.

Spradley advocates that interviewers use the technical words or jargon particular to a work group to encourage workers to explain their jobs more vividly. Although the interview was designed for an individual worker, it can be adapted for a group interview format.

Ethnic Culture

Health care practitioners have learned the necessity of integrating clients' ethnic cultures into clinical programs so that goals are mutual, focused, and relevant. Regarding work, health care practitioners are also beginning to appreciate the range of ethnic values that have an impact on work performance, return-to-work issues, social interactions, and participation in prevention programs.

The following examples underscore the need to appreciate cultural mores. Lange (1988) explores the treatment implications for alcohol rehabilitation with Alaskan Natives and Native Americans. Lange stresses that health care practitioners must understand the natives' social structure and exercise care not to impose authority or control on treatment situations. Further, the values (such as leadership and independence) that health care practitioners traditionally promote in clients are not those valued in natives' society.

Table 2.1. Dominant Values Relative to Work Programming

Japanese
  Deference
  Ability to conform
  Interdependence
  Obligation
  Group achievement
Native American
  Cooperation
  Community service
  Family
  Respect for nature
  Self-productivity
Appalachian
  Kinship ties
  Subsistence living
  Fatalistic
  Present time focus
  Relaxed pace
  Person-oriented
Hispanic
  Aesthetic beauty
  Family
  Fatalistic
  Present time focus
  Spiritual
Anglo-American
  Achievement
  Independence
  Material- or object-oriented
  Control of nature
  Future time focus
  Self-respect

Sources: Compiled from Kluckhohn 1977; Cherrington 1980; Yankelovitch 1981; Kanemoto 1987; Lange 1988; Yelton & Nielson 1991.

Kanemoto (1987) reminds us that individuals' responses to praise also are often culturally based. For example, most American workers thrive on individual recognition for excellence in job performance. However, Japanese workers are humiliated by receiving individual praise. The Japanese culture values group contribution toward a common goal and prefers acknowledgment of all group members involved in a project. Therefore, incentive programs dependent on personal recognition may not be effective with Japanese workers.

Table 2.1 outlines work-related values common to specific ethnic cultures. The list provided is not inclusive of all values and may not be relevant to all individuals from each ethnic culture. Although knowledge of ethnic values may benefit program planning, as always, health care practitioners must resist stereotyping individuals according to these common characteristics. Nonetheless, occupational therapists have incorporated these values into successful work programs for specific groups of workers.

Finally, Krefting (1991) reminds us that personal and professional values may unconsciously bias our attitudes toward workers, particularly when the health care practitioner's values are distinct from those of the workers with whom they interact. Occupational therapists, for example, share the professional values of personal responsibility, competency, mastery over one's environment, and working to one's potential (Yerxa 1983). Many workers who do not share these values must not be stigmatized by health care practitioners.

The Changing Social Context of Work

The social context of work refers to the social and historic events that frame a worker's career. In this book, the social context reflects not only the attitudes or values of society toward work during a certain period but also the worker demographics, the industry or technology trends that shape employees' jobs, and the public policy mandates that affect managing work-related conditions. Together, these factors form the backdrop for working in industry. Health care practitioners should acknowledge the impact of the following factors on injury prevention.

Aging Work Force

Older workers are a growing percentage of the work force. Older workers contribute a strong work ethic, good judgment, and valuable insights about job safety and training. However, industry must acknowledge that older workers may need modifications to maintain productivity (e.g., brighter lighting, less background noise, a temperature-controlled atmosphere, and flexible working parameters (Connolly 1991; Coy & Davenport 1991).

Industry must also realize that although older workers as a group have fewer injuries, they pre-

sent a higher *risk* for injuries, due to repeated exposure over time and changes in the body's resilience and reaction time. Isernhagen (1991) suggests ergonomic modifications for older workers that demand less lifting and impact on joints and slower reaction times.

Culturally Diverse Work Force

As we approach a global economy, a greater number of companies own foreign subsidiaries, and a greater percentage of workers come from diverse ethnic backgrounds (Naisbitt & Aburdene 1990). This diversity brings creativity and manpower to a company. However, technical training and safety standards present a challenge to management due to language differences and cultural mores. For example, managers may be faced with the following challenge in training Japanese workers: When managers request that workers ask questions during training, many do not realize that traditional Japanese culture promotes deference to authority or abstinence from asking questions (Kanemoto 1987). Managers may have to find other ways to elicit feedback, such as written responses. Health care practitioners must also be creative in promoting prevention programs to a traditional Hispanic population, because many individuals in this culture uphold a fatalistic view of the future and may view little association between today's actions and tomorrow's outcomes (Kluckhohn 1977). Health care practitioners must integrate such cultural mores into CTD programming.

Health as a Right, Not a Privilege

Workers once believed that pain was a part of the job and that "you learn to live with it." Workers today understand Occupational Safety and Health Administration laws and their rights to a safe and healthy work environment. Accordingly, workers are more willing to report illnesses and injuries earlier with less concern about their status as a weak or injured worker. Although companies initially may not welcome the increase in reports or claims, this practice will save companies from expensive long-term medical problems.

Job Security

Today, workers are rightfully skeptical about their job futures. Few organizations are insulated from economic pressures and the potential for layoffs is real in many companies. Health care practitioners must realize that workers may be hesitant to return to the job for fear of inability to meet productivity standards and the potential for being fired. Further, workers are reluctant to expend the energy to change or expand their jobs if the possibility for layoffs exists.

Downsizing

The process of downsizing companies has affected workers from high-performing, high-salaried executives to loyal, skilled machinists. For those remaining on the job, downsizing has created a grossly overworked and stressed work force. Production workers are forced to increase the speed of their tasks without sacrificing quality; managers are responsible for a multitude of departmental responsibilities and tasks. Health care practitioners should acknowledge that both white-collar and blue-collar workers are at risk of developing a stress-related disorder or CTD.

Work Ethic

The *work ethic*, a term originally associated with the virtues of working diligently, is being questioned by millions of workers whose compensation for hard work is stressful jobs and little compensation. Whereas work once was basic to an individual's identity, many individuals now value leisure as equal to or more important than work (Cherrington 1980; Yankelovitch 1981). Workers are less eager to work overtime, to stay late for work-related lectures, or to prioritize work over personal lives. Health care practitioners must realize the role and value of work in workers' lives.

Management Trends

The buzzword in management is *teaming*. Teaming refers broadly to developing an interdisciplinary approach to solving problems that encourages all de-

partments to participate in company decisions (Cunningham 1995). "Cell manufacturing" transfers the concept of teaming to the factory floor, where production workers as a team fabricate, test, and package a complete product. Health care practitioners need to take the team approach to industry and must include all team members in the execution and planning of company-wide programs.

Americans with Disabilities Act

The Americans with Disabilities Act (ADA) has presented enormous opportunity for qualified workers with disabilities to enter or return to workplaces provided with the necessary job accommodations. The ADA's focus is on providing "reasonable accommodations" and making public buildings accessible for workers with physical or emotional disabilities (US Department of Justice 1991). Although critics were initially concerned about the ADA's cost to companies, 68% of all job accommodations cost $500 or less and 84% cost $1,500 or less. Health care practitioners should familiarize themselves with the ADA and advocate implementation of the law for qualified workers. (See Chapter 13 for a complete discussion of the ADA.)

In summary, individuals' values regarding their work are influenced by personal and work group cultural norms. For effective intervention, health care practitioners must acknowledge the perspective of workers in the changing dynamics of the workplace.

References

Cherrington DJ (1980). *The Work Ethic*. New York: Amacom.

Connolly JK (1991). Consideration for the visually impaired older worker. *Work*, 2(1),19–28.

Coy JA & Davenport M (1991). Age changes in the older adult worker: implications for injury prevention. *Work*, 2(1),38–46.

Cunningham R (1995). Focal point: trends collide, many injured? *Lasers Optronics*, 14(2),4.

Finholt T (Dec 2, 1994). Psychosocial factors of upper extremity limb disorders. Proceedings from the International Conference on Occupational Disorders of the Upper Extremity, San Francisco, CA.

Ginsberg E (1957). *Occupational Choice: An Approach to a General Theory*. New York: Columbia University Press.

Hall E (1973). *The Silent Language*. Garden City, NJ: Anchor Books.

Isernhagen SJ (1991). An aging challenge for the nineties: balancing the aging process against experience. *Work*, 2(1),10–18.

Jablin F M (1987). Organizational entry, assimilation and exit. In FM Jablin (Ed). *Handbook of Organizational Communication.* Newbury Park, CA: Sage Publications.

Kanemoto JS (1987). Cultural implications in treatment of Japanese American patients. *Occup Therapy Health Care*, 4(1),115–125.

Kielhofner G & Burke JP (1985). Components and determinants of human occupation. In G Kielhofner (Ed). *A Model of Human Occupation: Theory and Application.* Los Angeles: Williams & Wilkins.

Kluckhohn FR (1977). Dominant and variant value orientations. In FR Kluckhohn & E Strodeck (Eds). *Personality in Nature, Society and Culture.* New York: Knopf.

Krefting L (1991). The culture concept in the everyday practice of occupational and physical therapy. *Occup Physical Therapy Ped*, 11(4),1–16.

Lange BK (1988). Ethnographic interview: an occupational therapy needs assessment tool for American Indian and Alaska Native Alcoholics. *Occup Therapy Ment Health*, 8(2),61–80.

Naisbitt J & Aburdene P (1990). *Megatrends 2000: Ten New Directions for the 1990s.* New York: Avon Books.

Rokeach M (1973). *The Nature of Human Values.* New York: Free Press.

Spradley J (1979). *The Ethnographic Interview.* New York: Harcourt Brace Jovanovich.

U.S. Department of Justice, Civil Rights Division, Office of the Americans with Disabilities Act (1991). *ADA Highlights: Title II State and Local Government Services.* Washington, DC: Government Printing Office.

Van Maanen J (1976). Breaking in: socialization to work. In E Dublin (Ed). *Handbook of Work, Socialization and Society.* Chicago: Rand McNally.

Yankelovitch D (1981). The meaning of work. In J O'Toole, JL Scheiber, & LC Wood (Eds). *Working, Changes and Choices.* New York: Human Sciences Press.

Yerxa E (1983). Audacious values: the energy source of occupational therapy practice. In G Kielhofner (Ed). *Health Through Occupation: Theory and Practice in Occupational Therapy.* Philadelphia: Davis.

Appendix 2.1
Worker Role Interview

Name: _____ Date: _____

Job Title: _____

Employer: _____

I am interested in learning about your job.

Where do you work?_____

How long have you worked there? _____

What are your hours? Your shift? _____

What do you do on your job? _____

_____

I am (am not) familiar with your company; can you give me a minitour of the inside of your plant (building)?

_____

Draw the facility if possible.

How is your work area organized (set up)? Are there other people who share your desk (machine, work-station, platform)?_____

_____

Although your job probably varies from day to day, can you describe a *typical* day, beginning with the time at which you arrive at work and ending with the time at which you leave?_____

_____

_____

Now, I would like to ask you a few questions about the specific tasks (jobs, duties) that you do.

After you have punched in (checked in), checked your schedule (requisition sheet, assignment list) and have gone to your work area, what are the steps for each task that you do? _____

_____

Can you estimate what percentage of your time you spend in each part of your job? _____

_____

Is that everything you do, or are there tasks that people *expect* you to do to help others or to fill in?

_____

Now, I want you to think back to when you first began the job.

Why did you want (or what attracted you to) this job?_____

_____

How did you get the job? _____

_____

What was the first day like? _____

_____

Did you feel ready for the job? What skills did you already have for the job; what skills did you need to learn?

_____

_____

How did you learn the job as a whole (e.g., your responsibilities, the schedules, the work flow)?

_____

_____

How do you know if you are doing a good job?_____

_____

You said that initially you were attracted to the job because _____

_____

Is that still why you are working here? Are there other reasons for staying?_____

_____

Can you tell me about a time (incident) at work when you felt especially proud of something that you did? Was there a time when someone tested you and you were right?_____

_____

Can you tell me about an incident that made you so frustrated that you wanted to quit? _____

_____

Other than (refer to previous question), what are the aspects of your job that you do not like? _____

_____

What do you like about your job?_____

_____

Do you find that the workers support each other, or are they really out for themselves? Please explain.

_____

I am interested in how you get along with your boss (bosses). Do your bosses seem concerned with how much work you do, how well you like your job, how comfortable you are, or your chances for a raise or promotion? Tell me about your boss. _____

_____

_____

_____

I would like to understand how you manage your job and home responsibilities. How does work fit with your personal life?

What types of responsibilities or obligations do you have at home? _____

_____

How do you organize your schedule to manage all your responsibilities? Are there other people on whom you can rely for help? _____

_____

How do other people in your occupation (job) manage their responsibilities? _____

_____

Finally, I'm curious about how your parents or other people influenced your job.

What type of work do (did) your parents (caregivers) do? _____

_____

Did you watch or observe them at their jobs?_____

_____

Was there anything that you learned from your parents (caregivers) that you always will remember about work?

_____

_____

Chapter 3
The Medical Context

Martha J. Sanders

Cumulative trauma disorders (CTDs) have long presented an enigma to the medical profession in terms of accurate diagnosis and treatment. CTDs are difficult to diagnose, given that they develop insidiously and are characterized by nonlocalized pain. Conservative treatment often yields to surgery, because many patients do not visit a hand or orthopedic surgeon until the symptoms are severe and function is compromised. Further, physicians are realizing that surgery may not be preferable to conservative treatment, due to the multifactorial nature of the problem (Dobyns 1991; Millender 1992). Medical professionals are reappraising their approaches to CTDs and are reinventing their roles as case managers and advocates for individuals with CTDs (Louis 1987; Dobyns 1991). This chapter presents a medical perspective on CTDs, the various terms and conditions associated with CTDs, and the criteria for identifying a CTD.

Medical Perspective

The traditional medical approach to treating a disorder is problem oriented: The medical model seeks to identify the problem or disorder, treat the disorder, reduce the symptoms, and examine the causative agents. The goal is to remedy the disorder; the assumption is that individuals will comply with recommendations and participate in efforts toward this end. The medical approach proceeds in a linear fashion from problem to solution.

The primary concern of the medical provider is physiologic processes that interfere with an individual's health. When other psychological or socioeconomic problems are involved, these issues are treated as separate and distinct. Dobyns (1991) states that "from the beginning of medical interaction with these problems [CTDs], it has been more difficult than usual to separate the physiologic problems from the psychologic problems and this ambivalence continues . . ." (p. 558). In fact, the physiologic problem with CTDs vies with myriad other issues (e.g., union agreements, unpaid bills, arranging for light-duty work, and unraveling the maze of worker's compensation laws) for the spotlight of concern. The traditional medical model falls short of identifying the problem of CTDs accurately because these work-related disorders are not straightforward, physiologic problems.

The treatment of CTDs similarly involves not only medical intervention but also communicating and arranging for follow-through in industry, insurance, and rehabilitation (Dobyns 1987; Millender 1992). Finally, the reduction of symptoms is often temporary, reoccurring when the worker returns to work or when the worker is overwhelmed by personal or workplace stress. Dobyns states, "The welter of psychologic miasma and socioeconomic motivation attending workplace illness is all too easy to perceive, and the remedies seldom fall within usual medical measures" (Dobyns 1991, p. 588). Clearly, in addressing CTDs, the problem and treatment of tissue pathology cannot be separated from other workplace, social, and legal issues.

Dobyns (1991) explained that physicians must make a cognitive shift in examining workers with

CTDs by addressing physical and socioeconomic issues with equal regard and by developing the patience to deal with these issues. He notes that the role is "tedious, frustrating, and poorly compensated" (p. 590) but that this is the only approach that will serve patients realistically and prevent them from being exploited. Selected issues regarding CTDs from the medical perspective are discussed.

Pressure for Early Return to Work

Although they view their role as managers for CTD cases, many orthopedic physicians note discord within this role. Physicians feel responsible for "healing" workers, yet many workers are never healed; physicians sense pressure to return workers to the job as soon as possible, a process that may satisfy employers but jeopardizes the safety of the workers. Furthermore, physicians are responsible for providing employers with specific functional limitations for injured workers, yet, they rarely perform objective, functional testing; they are largely dependent on health care practitioners to supply this data. In all decisions regarding CTDs, medical, legal and ethical issues weigh heavily (Dobyns 1987; Millender 1992).

Surgery as Treatment

Dobyns (1991) and Louis (1987) raise the inquiry as to whether surgery actually enhances the overall capacity of the worker. A successful outcome for surgery, in terms of tissue repair, does not necessarily ensure a better return-to-work status for the individual worker. The expected goals of surgery must be discussed with the client, employer, and third-party (insurance) payer, with the understanding that the worker may still be limited in full work functioning.

Millender (1992) explained that in his clinical experience, many unskilled workers did not return to work despite long, painful, and complicated rehabilitation efforts, especially when the injuries are compounded by adverse psychosocial conditions. In these cases, job modification or vocational retraining is often preferable to surgery using work-hardening, educational, and vocational programming.

Determining the Source of Cumulative Trauma Disorders

Physicians usually make the initial determination of whether a CTD is work related so that a worker may begin to receive worker's compensation benefits. Unfortunately, the exact contribution of work-related, non-work-related, and personal factors to the development of CTDs is not clear (McDermott 1986).

Although it is generally agreed that environmental, ergonomic, and personal factors combine to produce the resulting conditions, some physicians have contested the notion that CTDs are actually work related. One group of physicians believes that CTDs are an iatrogenic disorder heavily influenced by personal issues (Hadler 1989); others believe that CTDs are related to the psychological stress of the work task rather than to the physical components of the work activity (Ireland 1992). Other nonoccupational factors associated with CTDs are personality, pregnancy, gynecologic conditions, size, obesity, and medical history (Armstrong 1990).

The Medical, Social, and Legal Maze

CTDs begin as workplace problems and quickly become medical problems when medical professionals become involved. The problems further evolve into a tangled web of medical, social, and legal issues that escalate into exorbitant costs for the worker, employer, and insurance systems.

Louis (1987) describes the scenario of a long-term worker who develops carpal tunnel syndrome on the job. The worker notices pain, numbness, and tingling in the fingers, which become worse at night and after hand-intensive work. The worker reports the symptoms to the occupational health nurse (or to the company owner), who gives the worker a splint and dismisses the worker from the job for a week. The following week, the worker, now wearing a splint, returns to the same job and attempts to perform the work. The symptoms develop once again, and the worker is referred to the company physician. The company physician recognizes the pattern of symptoms and sends the worker to an orthopedic surgeon. When electromyography tests or nerve conduction tests are positive, the worker undergoes carpal tunnel surgery, short-term rehabilitation, and returns to the same job 2–3 months later, only to endure a recurrence of symptoms.

At this point, the worker is trapped by a real dilemma. If the worker cannot do the work and the employer has no "light duty," the worker may lose the job. If the worker applies for worker's compensation a second time and is denied, the worker must find a lawyer to contest the case before the worker's compensation board. Finally, if the worker is eligible for job modification under the Americans with Disabilities Act, the employer may resent the extra moneys needed to modify the work environment and may resist such efforts.

When the insurance company becomes aware of the large sums of money appropriated to this case, a rehabilitation nurse is assigned. The nurse requests another impartial, medical examination (called an *independent medical examination*), and so the cycle continues. In this scenario, the only players who benefit are the legal and (to a lesser degree) medical professionals; the worker and employer are still at a loss. Much coordination needs to be done between the medical, industrial, and legal systems, so that the focus remains returning the worker to the job.

Definitions and Terms Associated with Cumulative Trauma Disorders

CTDs is an umbrella term that describes a variety of diagnostic conditions characterized by pain and discomfort that develop gradually in such soft-tissue structures as tendons, tendon sheaths, nerves, muscles, or blood vessels. These conditions are caused, accelerated, or aggravated by repeated stresses or awkward movements in a particular part of the body. Usually CTDs are associated with occupational causes, although nonoccupational activities certainly contribute to the problem (Putz-Anderson 1988; Armstrong 1991).

CTDs are distinct from sprains or strains in that CTDs are not caused from a single incident. Putz-Anderson (1988) explains that each cycle of a work activity has the potential to cause microtears in the involved soft-tissue structures. One repetition may not produce inflammation or pain; however, if adequate time is not allowed for tissue recovery, over a period of time, these microtears can accumulate to produce trauma to a specific area of the body. Thus, a worker on the job may be asymptomatic for years, all the while accruing job-related microtraumas.

Although a CTD may develop anywhere in the body, disorders of the upper extremity are the most frequently reported (Armstrong 1990). The specific diagnoses for identifying a CTD are discussed later in this chapter.

As discussed in Chapter 1, a variety of names have been attributed to this cluster of disorders, depending on the geographic location or the pattern of symptoms first acknowledged. Presently, there is no agreement as to the term used to describe these disorders. Each term has certain advantages and disadvantages regarding some aspect of this type of disorder. Among the more commonly used terms are the following:

- Repetitive strain injury (RSI)
- Occupational cervicobrachial disorder (OCD)
- Overuse syndrome
- Work-related disorders
- Repetitive trauma disorders
- Regional musculoskeletal disorders

The term *repetitive strain injury* was adopted in Australia in reference to soft-tissue conditions, with specific reference to stress as a contributory factor (Chatterjee 1987). The term *overuse syndrome* is used most widely in relation to sports injuries or hobby-related activities rather than to activities relating to work (Herring & Nilson 1987). *Occupational cervicobrachial disorder* is used widely throughout Japan, Germany, and Scandinavia and refers specifically to constrained postures as the causal factor (Maeda et al. 1982).

Common Characteristics of Cumulative Trauma Disorders

Despite the variety of their names, common CTD characteristics have been described in worldwide epidemiologic studies. These characteristics are based on the natures and predominantly occupational causes of the problem. These characteristics promote a common focus on the design of the job, work environment, and on the pattern by which these conditions occur. Characteristics include the following (Kvarnstrom 1983; Putz-Anderson 1988; Armstrong 1991):

1. The causes of CTDs are multifactorial, involving personal, work-related, and non-work-related factors.

Table 3.1. Criteria to Determine the Presence of a Cumulative Trauma Disorder

Interview
  Symptoms of pain, numbness, or tingling
  Symptoms lasting more than 1 week and/or occurring
    more than 20 times in the last year
  No evidence of acute traumatic onset
  No evidence of systemic disease
  Onset of symptoms occurring with present job
Physical examination
  Characteristic signs of specific muscle, tendon, or nerve
    disorders
  Rule out other conditions with referred symptoms

Sources: Adapted from BA Silverstein, LJ Fine, & TJ Armstrong (1986). Hand wrist cumulative trauma disorders in industry. *Br J Indust Med,* 43,779; and BA Silverstein, L Fine, & D Stetson, (1987). Hand-wrist disorders among investment casting plant workers. *J Hand Surg [Am],* 12,838.

2. CTDs involve both mechanical and physiologic mechanisms.
3. CTDs are related to the intensity and duration of work.
4. CTDs may be related to a short, repetitive work cycle, to static work performed in uncomfortable positions, or to a stressful work environment.
5. Symptoms tend to be poorly localized, nonspecific, and episodic.
6. CTDs develop insidiously; they may occur after weeks, months, or years on the job.
7. CTDs recuperate slowly; they may require weeks, months, or years for recovery.

These characteristics have been helpful for understanding the broad implication for CTDs in the workplace. However, specific criteria for CTDs are needed for detecting and treating specific conditions.

Criteria for Determining the Presence of a Cumulative Trauma Disorder

Various criteria have been developed for detecting the presence of a CTD. These criteria are useful in medical and industrial research studies, in the Occupational Safety and Health Administration (OSHA) reporting procedures, and for tracking CTDs in industry. These criteria vary as to specificity of physical symptoms, duration of time with symptoms, and use of provocative tests to determine specific diagnoses.

OSHA (1990) uses broad criteria to document the number of CTDs in industry. OSHA states that if a worker's exposure to the job has caused an onset or aggravation of symptoms, the case is considered a work-related CTD. To qualify as an OSHA-recordable CTD, condition 1 *or* 2 and condition 3 must be met, as follows:

1. One or more physical findings: redness, loss of motion, deformity, swelling, a Tinel's sign, a positive Phalen's test, or other positive provocative tests.

   OR

2. One or more subjective findings: pain, paresthesias, numbness, tingling, aching, stiffness, or burning.

   AND

3. Action taken as a result of this condition: medical treatment at the workplace—self-administered or delivered by medical personnel; lost workdays, less than full-duty status, or transfer to another job.

Once a condition is judged an occupational CTD illness, it must be recorded on the OSHA 200 Log (see Chapter 4).

Other researchers have developed more specific criteria that delineate the specific CTD diagnoses and define a period or frequency within which symptoms must manifest. In their follow-up study of the risk factors for wrist and hand disorders, Silverstein, Fine, and Stetson (1987) used a combined interview and clinical examination format for the designation of a positive CTD. Table 3.1 denotes the criteria for their study. These criteria determine not only the presence of a CTD but also the determination of a specific diagnosis in the physical examination, such as a tendinitis or nerve entrapment.

Specific Diagnoses Associated with Cumulative Trauma Disorders

As stated, a CTD is not a diagnosis but rather a cluster of conditions with similar characteristics. Although a specific diagnosis is key to managing these conditions, the diagnostic processes for chronic

Table 3.2. Conditions Commonly Associated with Cumulative Trauma Disorders

Shoulder and neck
    Supraspinatus tendinitis
    Bicipital tendinitis
    Thoracic outlet syndrome
    Tension neck syndrome
Elbow and forearm
    Lateral and medial epicondylitis
    Pronator teres syndrome
    Radial tunnel syndrome
    Cubital tunnel syndrome
    Tenosynovitis of the forearm flexor and extensor
        muscles
Wrist and hand
    de Quervain's disease
    Carpal tunnel syndrome
    Trigger finger
    Guyon's tunnel syndrome
    Ganglion
    Gamekeeper's thumb
    Hand-arm vibration syndrome
    Hypothenar hammer syndrome

Sources: Compiled from DS Chatterjee (1987). Repetition strain injury—a recent review. *J Soc Occup Med,* 37,100; and TJ Armstrong (1991). Cumulative trauma work place factors. Paper presented at Occupational Orthopedics, American Academy of Orthopedic Surgeons. Dec 10, 1991. New York, NY.

work-related CTDs involve more than a patient history, clinical examination, and routine laboratory tests. Additionally, medical professionals must understand the long-standing problems, the pattern of recurring symptoms, and the differential diagnoses for specific conditions. For example, Bleeker (1987) notes the various conditions that mimic the signs and symptoms of carpal tunnel syndrome: thoracic outlet syndrome, double crush syndrome, polyneuropathies, and cervical rib compression of the median nerve. Medical professionals must be familiar with the clinical tests to rule out these diagnoses.

The specific condition that will develop depends on what part of the body is involved and on the type of work performed. In a review of numerous studies involving CTDs, Moore (1994) found that the majority of conditions associated with CTDs involved the muscle-tendon unit. Disorders typically associated with CTDs involve tendon, nerve, and neurovascular structures. However, given the broad definitions of CTD, a wide range of conditions also may be considered CTDs. Among those conditions

are ganglia, myalgias, and myofascial pain syndrome (see Chapter 5). Table 3.2 presents CTDs common to the hand, wrist, elbow, and shoulder regions.

Finally, medical and allied health professionals alike are recognizing that not all CTDs are alike even after the diagnosis is made (Ireland 1992; Millender 1992). Some clinicians find that pain and psychosocial and emotional issues play a larger role in the treatment of CTDs for some clients than do the actual physical concerns.

For the purposes of understanding and treating the underlying condition appropriately, Millender (1992) has developed four categories of client presentations of CTDs. These categories are not used routinely or accepted globally in the literature; however, they are presented here to provide health care practitioners with the range of perspectives on this topic.

- *Category 1*: The diagnosis is easily established and methods are readily available for treating the condition. The prognosis appears good because the condition is correctable and the client appears highly motivated. There appear to be no extenuating issues.
- *Category 2*: The diagnosis has been established, but neither surgical nor nonsurgical treatment may help return the worker to the job. Job modification or vocational retraining may be more realistic than surgery.
- *Category 3*: Musculoskeletal and nonmedical issues are manifested in this group. Clients typically display chronic pain associated with anger, frustration, and depression toward both the injury and the services that they are receiving. Complications with the legal system and resentment of employers may undermine attempts for treatment.
- *Category 4*: The diagnosis is unclear. Symptoms include generalized, vague discomfort that may extend from the neck and shoulders to the forearm. No overt inflammatory process is evident, but clients report weakness and tenderness. Psychological issues must be addressed.

Future Research Efforts

For future research, Dobyns (1991) proposes that researchers continue to address the tolerances of human tissues and the body's means of adaptation.

This information will enable health care practitioners to develop training programs that will improve and protect the performance of workers. Parameters for physiologic and psychological factors that place individuals at risk must be further identified. A majority of physicians still voice the need for communication and resolution between medical, social, and legal systems. The present arrangement robs every player of time, energy, and dollars.

In summary, Millender (1992) noted that the treatment of workers with CTDs is anything but a linear process:

> [Medical professionals and] . . . physicians who evaluate and treat patients with occupational disorders of the upper extremity must use more than traditional medical methods. They must strive to understand the myriad of physical, psychological, and social problems that affect patients and impede their ability to manage a work-related disorder. (p. 1)

Millender proposed that physicians and medical personnel consider the following four areas in their assessments of CTDs and resolve each area before a worker can return to work successfully:

1. Establish the specific diagnosis, determine the treatment methods, ascertain the prognosis for returning to work.
2. Evaluate the general medical and psychiatric issues that also influence the treatment.
3. Uncover the job, company, industrial, and union factors that will influence treatment process and outcome.
4. Understand the legal issues that influence worker's return to work.

References

Armstrong TJ (1990). Ergonomics and cumulative trauma disorders of the hand and wrist. In JM Hunter, LH Schneider, EJ Mackin, & AD Callahan (Eds). *Rehabilitation and Surgery of the Hand* (3rd ed). Philadelphia: Mosby.

Armstrong TJ (Dec 10, 1991). Cumulative trauma work place factors. Presented at the Occupational Orthopedics meeting, American Academy of Orthopedic Surgeons, New York, NY.

Bleecker MJ (1987). Medical surveillance for carpal tunnel syndrome in workers. *J Hand Surg [Am]*, 12,845–848.

Chatterjee DS (1987). Repetition strain injury—a recent review. *J Soc Occup Med*, 37,100–105.

Dobyns JH (1987). Role of the physician in worker's compensation injuries. *J Hand Surg [Am]*, 12,826–829.

Dobyns JH (1991). Cumulative trauma disorder of the upper limb. *Hand Clin*, 7,587–595.

Hadler NM (1989). Work-related disorders of the upper extremity: I. Cumulative trauma disorders—a critical review. *Occup Probl Med Pract*, 4,1–8.

Herring SA & Nilson KL (1987). Introduction to overuse injuries. *Clin Sports Med*, 6,225–239.

Ireland DCR (1992). The Australian experience with cumulative trauma disorders. In LH Millender, DH Louis, & BP Simmons (Eds). *Occupational Disorders of the Upper Extremity*. London: Churchill Livingstone.

Kvarnstrom S (1983). Occurrence of musculoskeletal disorders in a manufacturing industry with special attention to occupational shoulder disorders. *Scand J Rehabil Med*, 8,1–61.

Louis DS (1987). Cumulative trauma disorders. *J Hand Surg [Am]*, 12,823–825.

Maeda K, Horiguchi S, & Hosokawa M (1982). History of the studies on occupational cervicobrachial disorder in Japan and remaining problems. *J Hum Ergol*, 11,17–29.

McDermott FY (1986). Repetition strain injury: a review of current understanding. *Med J Aust*, 144,196–200.

Millender LH (1992). Occupational disorders of the upper extremity: orthopedic, psychosocial and legal implications. In LH Millender, DH Louis, & BP Simmons (Eds). *Occupational Disorders of the Upper Extremity*. London: Churchill Livingstone.

Moore JS (Dec 1, 1994). The epidemiological context of upper extremity disorders associated with work. Presented at the International Conference on Occupational Disorders of the Upper Extremities, University of California Center for Occupational and Environmental Health and University of Michigan Center for Occupational Health and Safety Engineering, San Francisco, CA.

Occupational Safety and Health Administration, US Department of Labor (1990). *Ergonomic Program Management Guidelines for Meatpacking Plants*. Washington, DC: US Department of Labor/OSHA 3123.

Putz-Anderson V (1988). *Cumulative Trauma Disorders: A Manual for Musculoskeletal Diseases of the Upper Limbs*. Philadelphia: Taylor & Francis.

Silverstein BA, Fine L, & Stetson D (1987). Hand-wrist disorders among investment casting plant workers. *J Hand Surg [Am]*, 12,838–844.

Chapter 4

The Industrial Perspective

Martha J. Sanders

As the incidence of cumulative trauma disorders (CTDs) rises at an alarming rate, the financial costs of CTDs have taken many businesses and industries by surprise. The Occupational Safety and Health Administration (OSHA) estimates the average cost of one disabling condition to be at least $26,000, including estimated wage losses, medical expenses, disability insurance, and administration costs. This figure does not represent the decrease in worker productivity and quality or the increases in worker's compensation premiums for the company. Although some workers hesitate to report early symptoms of CTDs for fear of losing a promotion, the long-term costs of CTDs to industry are clearly significant. In this chapter, we provide a perspective on industry's concerns about CTDs, procedures for reporting CTDs, and the occupational trends in CTDs today.

Industrial Perspective

In industry, managers or supervisors have the primary responsibility of delivering a product or service to customers within a predetermined time and quality standard. Any obstacle to this process competes with a company's ability to remain profitable.

Today, there are multiple regulations and concerns that compete with doing business. For example, personnel and safety regulations protect worker health but interfere with the company's short-term profits; environmental regulations "save the planet," yet often cost huge sums of money for compliance; the American with Disabilities Act promotes equal access to job opportunities for individuals with disabilities, yet may require substantial effort to comply with architectural and interviewing regulations. Each regulation seeks to protect some aspect of the right of employed workers to a healthy work environment.

CTDs represent one more impediment to smooth business operations. From an industry perspective, CTDs are entities that interrupt production and drive worker's compensation and medical costs higher. CTDs further represent a scheduling nightmare for supervisors who must replace injured workers but still deliver a product on time.

Interestingly, when the business climate is good (i.e., the company is busy but not overextended—the "just-right challenge"), the worker tends to be of little concern to the company. When companies are under financial constraints, excessive demands are placed on the worker in the form of longer working hours and higher productivity goals. Workers become stressed, fatigued, and injured; morale becomes progressively apathetic. As businesses struggle to meet deadlines, they are faced with skyrocketing worker's compensation costs, poor quality control, and a shortage of workers to complete the products. Ironically, in such difficult economic times, businesses often eliminate the very programs that enable good workers (e.g., training programs, wellness programs, and employee perks for safe work habits). Although many managers understand in theory that a healthy worker is a productive worker, companies tend to focus on the worker only when there is a problem.

From this bottom-line perspective, one can recognize that the individual worker often becomes lost in the organizational shuffle as industry managers grapple to balance external regulations with business concerns. Clearly, the foci of health care and business are different. In business, the focus is the product; in health care, the focus is the worker. Health care practitioners challenge companies to invest in their workers and thereby increase long-term productivity and profitability.

Presented here is a brief summary of institutions that now regulate worker rights. The summary provides health care practitioners with insight into business's regulatory overhead.

- *The Occupational Safety and Health Administration (OSHA)*: A part of the U.S. Department of Labor, this body is the government agency responsible for developing, implementing, and enforcing safety and health standards for workers in business and industry. OSHA works with industry representatives, employers, and employees to develop safety programs that will reduce workplace injury. OSHA is subsidized by both state and federal funding.
- *The Bureau of Labor Statistics*: Also under the jurisdiction of the U.S. Department of Labor, this agency administers and maintains the OSHA record-keeping system and compiles work-injury statistics (Bureau of Labor Statistics 1986). The National Institute of Occupational Safety and Health is the research branch of OSHA.
- *The Americans with Disabilities Act (ADA)*: This federal law sponsored by the Equal Employment Opportunity Commission strives to ensure equal access to jobs for individuals with disabilities (US Department of Justice 1991; see Chapter 13).
- *Worker's compensation insurance*: This type of insurance, carried by the employer, provides coverage for employees who are injured in the course of a workday. The bulk of industries' insurance dollars are spent on worker's compensation (Manning 1994).
- *Trade unions*: These formal organizations of workers negotiate with management for health insurance, good working conditions, and benefits for workers.

Although each regulating body serves to better the work environment for the employee, industries are accountable for the cost and personnel necessary for compliance. The personnel responsible for implementing and monitoring procedures will vary according to the company. Designated professionals may include occupational health nurses or physicians, safety engineers, human resource personnel, insurance representative, or even the president of the company.

Industry Reporting of Cumulative Trauma Disorders

Increasingly, government and private industries are focusing efforts on reducing worker's compensation and medical costs. To monitor the number and types of injuries, lost workdays, and medical costs, OSHA requires all public- and private-sector employers with more than 10 employees (except those in certain low-hazard industries) to maintain a record of worker injuries. Two forms are necessary for OSHA record keeping: the Log and Summary of Occupational Illnesses and Injuries (OSHA No. 200) and the Supplementary Record of Occupational Illnesses and Injuries (OSHA No. 101).

The OSHA 200 Log documents the date, occupation of the worker, department, and description of the injury. The form further classifies the type of worker injury and records the days lost from work or permanent duties (Bureau of Labor Statistics 1986; Figure 4.1).

The Supplementary Record of Occupational Illnesses and Injuries is an expanded survey sent to a random sample of industries. Implemented in 1992, this survey records additional information about the case characteristics of each injury or illness. The case characteristics include worker demographics (age, gender, and length of service), occupation, nature of the disabling condition, body part affected, and the objects or substances that produced the condition. This revised survey permits comparisons between industries and a specific analysis of the variables that result in disabling conditions (Bureau of Labor Statistics 1995).

According to federal injury-reporting procedures, an OSHA "recordable" includes all fatal injuries, all nonfatal illnesses, and only those nonfatal injuries that involve one or more of the following: loss of consciousness, restriction of work or motion, transfer to another job, or medical treatment. It is not necessary to record injuries that require such first aid as adhesive bandages, antiseptic, or one-time use of a nonprescription medication (Bureau of Labor Statistics 1986).

To use and complete the form effectively, an employer should understand the terminology as defined by OSHA. The publication, *A Brief Guide to Record-Keeping Requirements of Occupational Illnesses and Injuries* (Bureau of Labor Statistics 1986) assists employers in defining and discussing specific details of the reporting process. Employers and health care practitioners should be aware of the important distinctions between occupational illnesses and occupational injuries on the OSHA 200 form. Occupational illnesses and injuries are classified according to the nature of the event that caused the injury, not the resulting condition of the employee. The following definitions will assist health care practitioners in understanding the OSHA reporting terminology.

- *Occupational injury*: an injury resulting from a single, isolated accident or exposure in the work environment. Examples of injuries are cuts, sprains, fractures, insect bites, and amputations.
- *Occupational illness*: any abnormal condition or disorder caused by exposure to environmental factors associated with employment. For the purpose of classifying illnesses, seven categories of occupational illnesses are used: occupational skin diseases, dust disease of the lungs, respiratory conditions due to toxins, poisoning, disorders due to physical agents, disorders associated with repeated trauma, and other ailments.

The expanded category of "repeated traumas" includes conditions associated with CTDs (e.g., synovitis, bursitis, tenosynovitis, Raynaud's phenomenon, and carpal tunnel syndrome) and other conditions due to repeated motion, pressure, and vibration. Noise-induced hearing loss is also included in this category.

Lost workdays can be categorized in two ways (Bureau of Labor Statistics 1986):

- *Days away from work* refers to those days on which an employee would have worked but was prohibited by occupational illness or injury.
- *Days of restricted work activity* are those days wherein an employee was assigned another temporary job, did not work full-time in the

permanent job, or did not perform all the duties of the permanent job owing to illness or injury.

The OSHA 200 Log is a valuable tool for monitoring workplace injuries in a company. For example, the total number of injuries or illnesses in a company can be compared from year to year; the specific categories of illnesses can be examined by department or by time period to elucidate the jobs or events that may have produced the conditions; or the company can determine the number of lost workdays per department or illness, thereby helping the company to prioritize prevention efforts.

Health care practitioners and safety personnel can monitor the patterns and incidence of CTDs in a company by reviewing the medical records, workers' compensation records, and safety and accident records. Putz-Anderson (1988) notes that many CTDs are not reported and suggests that formal records do not provide an accurate assessment of the present situation. Companies should survey workers as to the location, frequency, and duration of painful symptoms and should conduct medical screening examinations when feasible (Putz-Anderson 1988; see Chapter 13).

Industry Comparisons of Cumulative Trauma Disorders

Once the CTDs are reported, comparisons in occupational injuries and illnesses can be made across industries, occupations, gender, age, and length of time working. These comparisons may be made in terms of prevalence, incidence, and incidence rate.

Prevalence

Prevalence is a measure of the frequency of a disorder at one point in time. Prevalence is often expressed as a percentage of a population. For example, if 12 of 200 workers in an insurance claims office showed signs and symptoms of carpal tunnel syndrome during a physical examination, the prevalence of carpal tunnel syndrome in that population would be computed as 12/200, or 0.06, for that specific point in time (Putz-Anderson 1988).

Figure 4.1. A. Page 1 of the log and summary of occupational illnesses and injuries (OSHA 200 Log) records the date, employee's name, occupation, department, and a description of the injury or illness. **B.** Page 2 of the OSHA 200 Log records the extent and outcome of workplace injuries or illnesses. Documentation includes the number of lost workdays and types of illnesses. (Reprinted from Bureau of Labor Statistics, US Department of Labor [1986]. *A Brief Guide to Record-Keeping Requirements for Occupational Injuries and Illness.* O.M.B. 1220-0029. Washington, DC: US Department of Labor.)

Bureau of Labor Statistics
Log and Summary of Occupational
Injuries and Illnesses

NOTE: **This form is required by Public Law 91-596 and must be kept in the establishment for 5 years. Failure to maintain and post can result in the issuance of citations and assessment of penalties.** *(See posting requirements on the other side of form.)*

RECORDABLE CASES: You are required to record information about every occupational **death;** every nonfatal occupational **illness;** and those nonfatal occupational **injuries** which involve one or more of the following: loss of consciousness, restriction of work or motion, transfer to another job, or medical treatment (other than first aid). *(See definitions on the other side of form.)*

Case or File Number	Date of Injury or Onset of Illness	Employee's Name	Occupation	Department	Description of Injury or Illness
Enter a nonduplicating number which will facilitate comparisons with supplementary records.	Enter Mo./day	Enter first name or initial, middle initial, last name.	Enter regular job title, not activity employee was performing when injured or at onset of illness. In the absence of a formal title, enter a brief description of the employee's duties.	Enter department in which the employee is regularly employed or a description of normal workplace to which employee is assigned, even though temporarily working in another department at the time of injury or illness	Enter a brief description of the injury or illness and indicate the part or parts of body affected. Typical entries for this column might be: Amputation of 1st joint right forefinger; Strain of lower back; Contact dermatitis on both hands; Electrocution—body.
(A)	(B)	(C)	(D)	(E)	(F)
					PREVIOUS PAGE TOTALS ↑
					TOTALS (Instructions on other side of form.) ↑

OSHA No. 200

A

U.S. Department of Labor

For Calendar Year 19 _____   Page _____ of _____

Form Approved
O.M.B. No. 1220-0029
See OMB Disclosure
Statement on reverse.

Company Name _____
Establishment Name _____
Establishment Address _____

Extent of and Outcome of INJURY

Fatalities	Nonfatal Injuries				
Injury Related	Injuries With Lost Workdays				Injuries Without Lost Workdays
Enter DATE of death. Mo./day/yr.	Enter a CHECK if injury involves days away from work, or days of restricted work activity, or both.	Enter a CHECK if injury involves days away from work.	Enter number of DAYS away from work.	Enter number of DAYS of restricted work activity.	Enter a CHECK if no entry was made in columns 1 or 2 but the injury is recordable as defined above.
(1)	(2)	(3)	(4)	(5)	(6)

Type, Extent of, and Outcome of ILLNESS

Type of Illness

CHECK Only One Column for Each Illness
(See other side of form for terminations or permanent transfers.)

(a) Occupational skin diseases or disorders	(b) Dust diseases of the lungs	(c) Respiratory conditions due to toxic agents	(d) Poisoning (systemic effects of toxic materials)	(e) Disorders due to physical agents	(f) Disorders associated with repeated trauma	(g) All other occupational illnesses
			(7)			

Fatalities	Nonfatal Illnesses				
Illness Related	Illness With Lost Workdays				Illness Without Lost Workdays
Enter DATE of death. Mo./day/yr.	Enter a CHECK if illness involves days away from work, or days of restricted work activity, or both.	Enter a CHECK if illness involves days away from work.	Enter number of DAYS away from work.	Enter number of DAYS of restricted work activity.	Enter a CHECK if no entry was made in columns 8 or 9.
(8)	(9)	(10)	(11)	(12)	(13)

Certification of Annual Summary Totals By _____ Title _____ Date _____

OSHA No. 200

POST ONLY THIS PORTION OF THE LAST PAGE NO LATER THAN FEBRUARY 1.

B

Incidence

Incidence is the number of new cases recorded during a specific period. Occupational injuries and illnesses are recorded according to hours of worker exposure during a calendar year (Putz-Anderson 1988).

Incidence Rate

The incidence rate is the number of injuries, illness, or lost workdays of a group of workers per a specific unit of exposure time. OSHA bases incidence rates on a common exposure base of 100 full-time workers in order to allow comparisons between companies or industries regardless of size.

Incidence rates are calculated in the following manner:

$$N/EH \times 200,000 = \text{incidence rate}$$

where N = number of injuries, illnesses, or lost days, and EH = employee hours, total hours worked by all employees during the calendar year.

The total number of recordable injuries or illness for the calendar year (N; taken from the OSHA 200 Log) is multiplied by 200,000, representing a base of 100 full-time workers. (A full-time worker is considered to be employed 40 hours per week, 50 weeks per year, for a total of 2,000 hours per year.) This number is divided by the total number of hours worked by all full-time employees during that calendar year (EH; determined by the number of employees multiplied by 2,000 hours) for the final rate (Putz-Anderson 1988; Connecticut Department of Labor 1995).

The following case illustrates computation of incidence rates. An electronics assembly plant employed 152 full-time workers for the calendar year of 1990. During that year, five new cases of carpal tunnel syndrome were reported among the assembly-line workers. The incidence rate is calculated as follows:

$$\frac{\text{Cases (N)}}{\text{Hours worked (EH)}}$$

$$\frac{5}{152 \times 2,000} \times 200,000 = 3.3$$

This incidence rate may be regarded as moderate to low, compared to the industry standard. However, the company may decide to perform an ergonomic work-site analysis to determine a potential problem (see Chapter 10).

The incidence rate is the standard used to compare the company incidence rate against the industry average. The industry averages for the total number of cases, lost workday cases, and lost workdays are listed in the National Safety Council's *Accident Facts* (National Safety Council 1995) according to Standard Industrial Classification codes and are summarized in the Annual Survey of Occupational Illnesses and Injuries (Bureau of Labor Statistics 1995).

Trends in Occupational Injuries and Illnesses

All the information is compiled to identify current trends in occupational injuries and illnesses. Health care practitioners should be knowledgeable about the trends in occupational illnesses for dialogue with industry and program planning. This section reviews illnesses and injury statistics from the 1993 Annual Survey of Occupational Illnesses and Injuries and discusses the worker and case demographics relevant to CTDs.

General Trends in Occupational Incidents

Although the number of work-related fatalities has declined steadily over the last decade, the number of occupational illnesses has risen consistently since 1982. This rise has been dramatic, representing over a fourfold increase in total illnesses from 1986 to 1992. The increase in reported cases of repetitive trauma is largely responsible for this pattern (Figure 4.2).

In 1993, the Bureau of Labor Statistics considered the three most hazardous occupations to be truck driver, nonconstruction laborer, and nursing aide and orderly. Each of these occupations reported more than 1 million cases in 1993, which represented a much higher share of illnesses and injuries than their share of total employment. Men incurred approximately two-thirds of all workplace injuries and illnesses (which is also a larger share than their 55% of total employment). However,

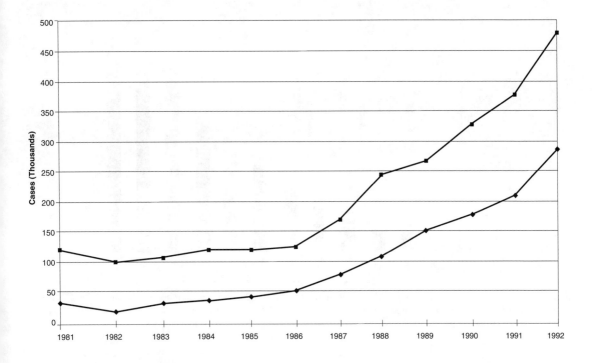

Figure 4.2. Occupational illnesses and cumulative trauma disorders (CTDs). The rise in occupational illnesses since 1982 reflects the increasing incidents of CTDs in industry. (■ = occupational illnesses; ♦ = CTDs.) (Reprinted with permission from *CTD News* [1992]. CTDs have jumped 26% BLS says. *CTD News*, 3[2],3.)

women accounted for almost 65% of all repetitive motion injuries (Bureau of Labor Statistics 1995).

Incidents Related to
Cumulative Trauma Disorders

Although injuries from repetitive trauma accounted for only 5% of the total occupational illnesses and injuries, these injuries accounted for nearly 66% of the total occupational illnesses. Figure 4.3 demonstrates that injuries from repetitive trauma have risen every year since 1982, with increases of 20% in 1991, 26% in 1992, and 7% in 1993 (CTD News 1994).

The Bureau of Labor Statistics delineates the percentage of CTDs contributed per general category of industry (Table 4.1). Manufacturing continues to lead, with the highest proportion of CTD cases. However, the percentage of CTDs in the service sector has risen steadily in the last 3 years.

With regard to the number of cases with CTDs involving lost workdays, the service industry vies with manufacturing for 23.8% and 25.9% of all CTD cases, respectively.

In 1993, the Annual Survey of Occupational Illnesses and Injuries (Bureau of Labor Statistics) reported the following industries with the highest *number* of CTDs:

- Motor vehicle and equipment manufacturing (42,600)
- Meat packing (38,300)
- Aircraft and parts assembly (9,500)
- Men's and boys' clothing manufacturing (7,900)
- Grocery store (6,400)

The incident rates in these industries varies from 145.3 per 10,000 workers in men's and boys' clothing manufacturing to 109.0 in the meat-packing industry and 66.8 in motor vehicle

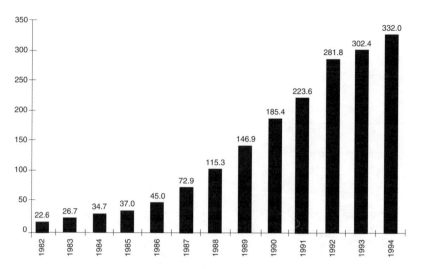

Figure 4.3. Cumulative trauma disorder (CTD) cases (in thousands), 1982–1993. The number of cases involving CTDs has risen dramatically since 1986. (Reprinted with permission from *CTD News* (1994). Number of CTD cases continues to rise. *CTD News*, 3[condensed issue].)

Table 4.1. Characteristics of Cases Involving Repetitive Motion

Case Characteristic	Percentage of Case Total for Repetitive Motion
Men	35
Women	64
Manufacturing	53
Retail, trade	14
Services	18
Health care	6
Other	15

Note: Gender and industry characteristics indicate that the majority of illnesses involving repetitive motion occur in women and in manufacturing industries.
Source: Bureau of Labor, US Department of Labor (1995). Survey of Occupational Injuries and Illnesses, 1993. Washington, DC: US Department of Labor.

and equipment manufacturing (Bureau of Labor Statistics 1995).

The occupations reporting the highest number of cases were operators, fabricators and laborers; machine operators, including sewing machine operators; and technical-sales and administrative support,

including secretaries, typists, and data-entry keyers (Bureau of Labor Statistics 1995).

Workdays Lost Due to Cumulative Trauma Disorders

One of the most telling statistics for health care practitioners' consideration is the average number of lost workdays per injury and illness category. Although the average number of lost workdays for all injuries and illnesses is 6 days, the average number of lost workdays for repetitive motion or CTDs is 20 days (Figure 4.4); the average jumps to 30 days for carpal tunnel syndrome specifically (Figure 4.5). Clearly, although CTDs do not represent the highest percentage of total cases, CTDs do represent one of the highest cost categories, due to the high number of lost workdays.

Further trends in occupational illnesses and injuries from the 1993 annual survey are highlighted in the following statistics:

- The majority of workers who sustain occupational injuries and illnesses are between the ages of 25 and 44.

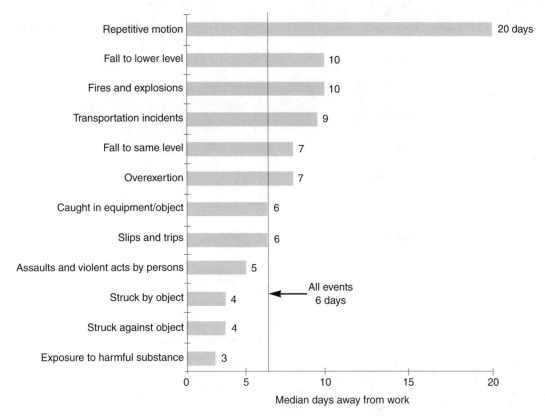

Figure 4.4. Median days away from work, characterized by event or exposure, 1993. Incidents due to repetitive motion averaged 20 lost workdays per case; the average for all incidents was 6 days per incident. (Reprinted from Bureau of Labor Statistics, US Department of Labor [1995]. *Survey of Occupational Injuries and Illnesses, 1993.* Washington, DC: US Department of Labor.)

- The duration of injury and illness increases with worker age. Workers aged 16–35 averaged 4 lost workdays per incident; workers older than 55 averaged 10 lost workdays per incident.
- The length of service before incurring an illness or injury was 1–5 years for 34% of injured workers and more than 5 years for 27% of injured workers.
- The occupations with the highest median days away from work due to injuries or illnesses were timber loggers and drywall installers (11 days) and data-entry keyers, operating engineers, millwrights, postal workers, electrical installers, and bus drivers (10 days).
- The upper extremities, including the wrist, hand, and fingers, were involved in 23% of all worker illnesses or injuries (Figure 4.6). The

wrist was involved in more than 50% of all CTD cases (Bureau of Labor Statistics 1995).

Cumulative Trauma Disorders Associated with Occupational Groupings

Certain occupations have come to be associated with certain CTDs, due to the nature of the tasks. Typically, occupations that involve repetitive or forceful pinching, grasping, and awkward postures have been associated with such CTDs as carpal tunnel syndrome, de Quervain's disease, lateral epicondylitis, Guyon's canal syndrome, and tendinitis of the shoulder and wrist. Occupations commonly associated with these conditions include electrical assembly, meat cutting, bench work, and carpentry.

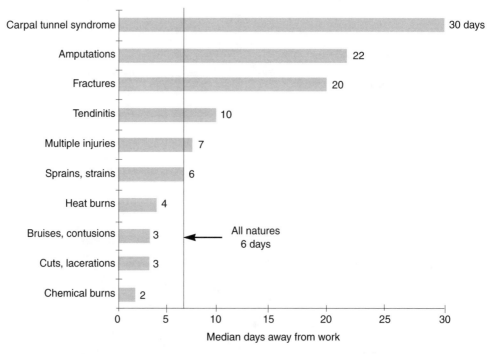

Figure 4.5. Median days away from work, characterized by nature of injury or illness. Cases involving carpal tunnel syndrome incurred a median of 30 days away from work, as compared to 6 days for all other types of injuries or illnesses. (Reprinted from Bureau of Labor Statistics, US Department of Labor [1995]. *Survey of Occupational Injuries and Illnesses, 1993.* Washington, DC: US Department of Labor.)

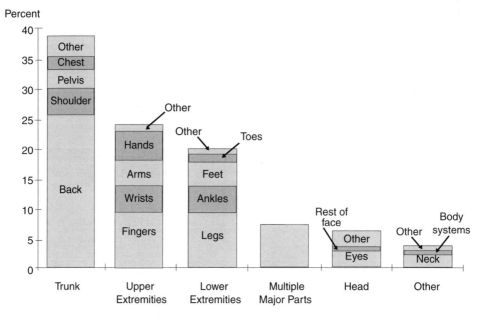

Figure 4.6. Part of the body affected. The upper extremities, including the hands, arms, wrist, and fingers, were involved in almost one-fourth of all injuries and illnesses that resulted in lost workdays. (Reprinted from Bureau of Labor Statistics, US Department of Labor [1995]. *Survey of Occupational Injuries and Illnesses, 1993.* Washington, DC: US Department of Labor.)

Table 4.2. Occupations Commonly Associated with Cumulative Trauma Disorders

Occupation	Cumulative Trauma Disorder
Manufacturing	
Buffing and grinding worker	CTS, pronator teres, ganglion, de Quervain's disease, HAVS, TOS
Assembly worker	CTS, lateral epicondylitis, TOS, shoulder or wrist tendinitis
Overhead assembly worker	Shoulder tendinitis, TOS
Small-parts assembly worker	CTS, de Quervain's disease, lateral epicondylitis, TOS
Machinist (punch or drill press)	de Quervain's disease, lateral epicondylitis, shoulder or wrist tendinitis
Packer	CTS, de Quervain's disease, shoulder or wrist tendinitis
Materials handler	Shoulder tendinitis, TOS
Service	
Typist, data-entry clerk	CTS, de Quervain's disease, lateral epicondylitis, TOS
Housekeeper, cook	CTS, de Quervain's disease
Grocery checker	CTS, wrist tendinitis, TOS
Telecommunications	CTS, Guyon's canal, cervical pain
Postal worker	CTS, lateral epicondylitis, TOS
Retail, trade	
Meatcutter, meatpacker	de Quervain's disease, lateral epicondylitis, shoulder or wrist tendinitis
Construction worker	CTS, lateral epicondylitis, shoulder tendinitis, HAVS
Musician	CTS, ganglion, lateral epicondylitis, cervical pain, TOS
Carpenter	CTS, ganglion, de Quervain's disease, lateral epicondylitis, Guyon's canal
Sewer, cutter	CTS, de Quervain's disease, TOS
Health services	
Nursing, allied health, dentistry personnel	CTS, lateral epicondylitis, TOS
Operating room personnel	CTS, de Quervain's disease

CTS = carpal tunnel syndrome; HAVS = hand-arm vibration syndrome; TOS = thoracic outlet syndrome.
Sources: Compiled from the author's experience and from V Putz-Anderson (Ed) (1988). *Cumulative Trauma Disorders: A Manual of Musculoskeletal Diseases for the Upper Limbs.* Philadelphia: Taylor & Francis; KHE Kroemer (1992). Avoiding cumulative trauma disorders in shops and offices. *Am Indust Hyg Assoc J*, 53,596–604; and BA Silverstein, LJ Fine, & TJ Armstrong (1987). Occupational factors and carpal tunnel syndrome. *Am J Indust Med*, 11,343–358.

Table 4.2 is a compilation of information on the common CTDs that may develop as a result of prolonged exposure to certain occupations. The chart is not a complete listing of the occupations or CTDs occurring in industry, nor does it indicate the frequency of certain conditions (Silverstein et al. 1987; Kroemer 1992).

More recently, investigators have focused attention on CTDs that develop as a result of the technologic changes in managing information and services. For example, Margolis and Krause (1987) found that up to 63% of all grocery checkers reported musculoskeletal pain. The problem developed with the inception of the laser scanner, which completely changed the biomechanics of the checker's job. Whereas grocery checkers once pushed items off a conveyor belt, they now pass each item over a scanner screen, which demands frequent flexion and extension of a wrist weighted with groceries. The telecommunications industry also continues to report a high rate of CTDs caused by the repetitive nature of office work and stress inherent in the job (Putz-Anderson et al. 1992). Although the work is not strenuous, it involves similar repeated motions throughout the task in a potentially stressful work environment (see Chapter 7).

Researchers are also acknowledging to a greater extent the effects of work exposure on shoulder and other upper-extremity disorders. Whereas carpal tunnel syndrome was initially the focus of study, in reviewing numerous investigations, Moore (1994) found that the prevalence of carpal tunnel syndrome was only approximately 4–6% across numerous high-risk occupations. Moore concluded that research should examine the more prevalent disorders of the muscle-tendon unit (such as tendinitis) and the associated job tasks.

In summary, the manufacturing industry continues to demonstrate the highest percentage of CTD cases. However, the service and retail trade industry show gradual increases in the number of cases reported. Although typically ranked among the lowest injury industries, the fields of finance and real estate doubled their number of occupational illnesses and injuries in the last 3 years in the state of Connecticut (Connecticut Department of Labor 1995). The high cost of CTDs to industry is reflected in the average of 20 lost workdays per CTD case. The industrial perspective is intertwined with financial and business considerations. Supervisors and managers realize that industry must work with other health care systems to maintain healthy, productive workers.

References

Bureau of Labor Statistics, US Department of Labor (1986). *A Brief Guide to Record-Keeping Requirements for Occupational Injuries and Illness*. O.M.B. 1220-0029. Washington, DC: US Department of Labor.

Bureau of Labor Statistics, US Department of Labor (1995). *Annual Survey of Occupational Illnesses and Injuries, 1993*, Washington, DC: US Department of Labor.

Bureau of Labor Statistics, US Department of Labor (1995). *Worker Injuries and Illnesses by Selected Characteristics, 1993*. Washington, DC: US Department of Labor, 95-142.

Connecticut Department of Labor, Division of Occupational Safety and Health (1995). *Connecticut Occupational Injuries and Illness 1993 and Census of Fatal Occupational Injuries 1994*. Wethersfield, CT: Connecticut Department of Labor.

CTD News (1992). First national figures on CTDs. *CTD News*, 1(9),8.

CTD News (1994). Number of CTD cases continues to rise. *CTD News*, 3(9),1.

Kroemer KHE (1992). Avoiding cumulative trauma disorders in shops and offices. *Am Indust Hyg Assoc J*, 53,596–604.

Manning MV (1994). *So You're the Safety Director! A Guide to the Formulation and Implementation of a Safety Program*. Minneapolis: Prevention Plus.

Margolis W & Kraus JF (1987). The prevalence of carpal tunnel syndrome symptoms in female supermarket checkers. *J Occup Med*, 29,953–957.

Moore JS (Dec 1994). The epidemiological context of upper-extremity disorders associated with work. Presented at the International Conference on Occupational Disorders of the Upper Extremities, University of California Center for Occupational and Environmental Health and University of Michigan Center for Occupational Health and Safety Engineering, San Francisco, CA.

National Safety Council (1995). *Accident Facts*. Itasca, IL: National Safety Council.

Putz-Anderson V (Ed) (1988). *Cumulative Trauma Disorders: A Manual of Musculoskeletal Diseases for the Upper Limbs*. Philadelphia: Taylor & Francis.

Putz-Anderson V, Doyle GT, & Hales TR (1992). Ergonomic analysis to characterize task constraint and repetitiveness of risk factors for musculoskeletal disorders in telecommunication office work. *Scand J Work Environ Health*, 18(Suppl 2),123–126.

Silverstein BA, Fine LJ, & Armstrong TJ (1987). Occupational factors and carpal tunnel syndrome. *Am J Indust Med*, 11,343–358.

US Department of Justice, Civil Rights Division, Office of the Americans with Disabilities Act (1991). *ADA Highlights: Title 1 and Title 2*. Washington, DC: Government Printing Office.

PART II
Neuromuscular Conditions

Chapter 5

Tendinitis, Entrapment Neuropathies, and Related Conditions

Susan V. Duff

The neuromuscular system is uniquely designed to withstand the stresses and strains of everyday life. Occasionally, the demands placed on select structures exceed physiologic limits. The body's response to extrinsic and intrinsic demands can significantly influence one's participation in work, recreation, and self-care tasks.

Cumulative trauma disorders (CTDs) or repetitive strain injuries are neuromuscular conditions that evolve secondary to low-intensity stresses applied gradually or repetitively. Disorders frequently attributed to cumulative trauma include tendinitis and nerve compressions or entrapments. Related conditions include myofascial trigger points and bursitis. CTDs are explored in this chapter in terms of the mechanism of occurrence and rehabilitation.

Neuromuscular Disorders

Tendinitis

Tendinitis is a common neuromuscular disorder that has been linked to repetitive activity in vulnerable structures. Although it is regarded as an inflammatory condition of the muscle-tendon unit, if the involved tissues are not allowed to heal, degenerative changes ensue. To ensure full comprehension of this tendon pathology, the anatomy is reviewed here.

Regional Anatomy

Muscles attach to bone via tendons, and tendons attach to muscle at the myotendinous junction. Tension produced in skeletal muscle is transmitted through the myotendinous junction to the tendon and results in joint motion. Both the myotendinous junction and the tendon are uniquely designed to handle the forces encountered during contraction and resultant movement (Garrett & Tidball 1988; Carlstedt & Nordin 1989). Defining tendinitis completely requires a review of tendon anatomy and associated structures.

Tendon. The unique structure of tendons is well documented and is pictured in Figure 5.1. Tendons are composed of 30% collagen and 2% elastin embedded within an extracellular matrix, 68% of which is water (Borynsenko & Beringer 1989). Collagen resists tensile forces, whereas elastin increases tendon extensibility. Collagen fibrils, formed from fibroblasts, combine via cross-links to form microfibrils. The microfibrils are arranged in parallel, which enhances the tendon's ability to manage high unidirectional loads (O'Brien 1992; Birk & Zycband 1994). A sheath, called the *endotenon,* surrounds each myofibril bundle or fascicle. Nerves and blood vessels travel within this endotenon. Groups of fascicles are held together by a loose areolar tissue that has elastic and tensile properties and is called the *paratenon* or tenosyn-

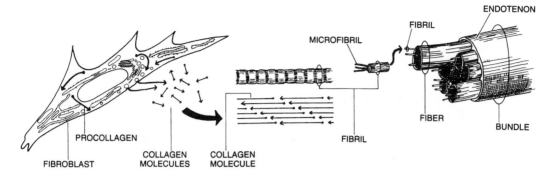

Figure 5.1. Schematic representation of collagen fibrils, fibers, and bundles in tendons and collagenous ligaments (not drawn to scale). Collagen molecules, triple helices of coiled polypeptide chains, are synthesized and secreted by the fibroblasts. These molecules (depicted with heads and tails to represent positive and negative polar charges) aggregate in the extracellular matrix in a parallel arrangement to form microfibrils and then fibrils. The staggered array of the molecules, in which each overlaps the other, gives a banded appearance to the collagen fibrils under the electron microscope. The fibrils aggregate further into fibers, which come together into densely packed bundles. (Reprinted with permission from CA Carlstedt & M Nordin [1989]. Biomechanics of tendons and ligaments. In M Nordin & VH Frankel [Eds]. *Basic Biomechanics of the Musculoskeletal System* [2nd ed]. Philadelphia: Lea & Febiger.)

ovium. The paratenon, which forms a protective sheath around the tendon and enhances gliding, may become inflamed secondary to repetitive movement across bony prominences or other structures (Thorson & Szabo 1989). In regions of low friction, only the paratenon surrounds the tendon. In select areas of high friction, such as the long flexor tendons, a synovia-like membrane, called the *epitenon,* lies beneath the paratenon. This thin layer of epitenon surrounds several fiber bundles and adheres to the tendon surface. Lubricating fluid lies between the paratenon and epitenon in these select regions (Kastelic et al. 1978). At the insertion into bone, the endotenon continues as *Sharpey's fibers* and becomes continuous with the periosteum. Tendon composition at the insertion site is bonier and much less fibrous (Carlstedt & Nordin 1989).

Myotendinous Junction. The myotendinous junction can be differentiated from tendon by its highly folded tissue. The multiple folds are set at extremely low angles to the force vectors that cross them. This unique structure increases the surface area for tension transfer ten- to twentyfold, enhancing the adhesive strength of the junction (Tidball 1983; O'Brien 1992). The sarcomeres near the myotendinous region are stiffer than are other muscle fibers, as evidenced by their shorter lengths when the muscle is loaded or stretched (Gordon et al.

1966). Despite its complex structure, the myotendinous junction is still viewed by some as the weakest link in the muscle-tendon unit.

Vascularity. Most tendons have extrinsic and intrinsic sources of vascularity (Gelberman 1991). *Extrinsic* vascularity refers to blood supplied from an external source, whereas *intrinsic* vascularity refers to nutrition made available within the tendon. The extrinsic blood supply is divided among three tendon regions: (1) the musculotendinous junction, (2) the tendon length, and (3) the tendon-bone junction. Tendon vessels that insert into cartilaginous regions are separated from those of bone (Woo et al. 1987). Tendons that insert into periosteum or the diaphysis have an anastomosis between the tendon and bone (O'Brien 1992; Curwin & Stanish 1984). Small feeder vessels may branch from larger vessels, as exemplified by the vincula of the long finger flexor tendons. Despite the reported extrinsic blood supply, tendons are relatively avascular, especially near the insertion sites, which is why they appear white (Benjamin et al. 1986; Borynsenko & Beringer 1989). In regions of excess force and pressure, the blood supply to tendons is variable. For instance, vessels are absent in regions in which the tendon must travel around a pulley. Because of this variable blood supply, the tendon must also rely on intrinsic blood flow. Diffusion of nutrients during movement is one form of intrinsic blood supply. Tendons with a synovial sheath of epitenon, such as the long flexor tendons, receive some intrinsic nutrition in this manner (Lundborg & Rank 1978). Although tendon injuries typically occur in regions with a reduced blood supply, Backman et al. (1991) conclude that tendon degeneration cannot be attributed primarily to circulatory impairment. Thus, other factors such as tolerance to loads, friction, and repetitive motion contribute to tendon degeneration.

Nerve Innervation.   Proprioceptive information from tendons is transduced by muscle spindles and Golgi tendon organs (GTOs), whereas pain information is picked up by nociceptors. Muscle spindles within the muscle belly and myotendinous junction are responsive to changes in muscle length and velocity. The spindles have both an afferent and efferent nerve supply. Variations in active muscle force (tension) are picked up by GTOs embedded in the myotendinous junction. Passive force, previously considered to be transduced through the GTOs, is now known to be transmitted primarily through surrounding connective tissue. The nerve fibers supplying the GTO receptors invaginate themselves between collagen fibers. As muscle tension is transferred to the tendon, collagen fibers compress the underlying nerve endings, thereby inducing a stream of nerve conduction. Although muscle spindles respond to alterations in muscle length and GTOs respond to muscle tension, they both provide feedback and feed-forward information necessary for adequate neuromotor control (Rothwell 1995). Myelinated and unmyelinated sensory nerve endings pick up noxious stimuli in the region of the tendon and myotendinous junction and carry them along either an A delta or C fiber to the spinal cord (Wolf 1984). Pain information reaching the spinal cord connects with other regions of the central nervous system (CNS) and reaches a perceptual level once it makes a cortical connection.

Biomechanics of Tendons

Tendons are one type of connective tissue that responds to alterations in tensile load (stress) and length (strain). The strength of the tendon is correlated with its thickness and collagen content versus the maximal tension that its associated muscle can

exert (Elliott 1967; Noyes et al. 1974; O'Brien 1992). Both the size of the tendon and the demands placed on it will effect its biomechanical properties.

Stress-Strain Curve.   As seen in Figure 7.1, the stress-strain curve demonstrates how loading affects tendons (Curwin & Stanish 1984; Carlstedt 1987). *Stress,* or load magnitude per unit area, is determined by dividing tensile load by the cross-sectional area perpendicular to the direction of the load. *Strain* is the percentage of tendon elongation (deformation) under a load relative to its resting length. The initial slow rise of the stress-strain curve refers to the initial response to loading or stretch, during which time the wavy collagen fibers straighten out. The linear rise in the curve represents the stiffening of the tendon in response to loading, which indicates that it takes a progressively greater force to induce elongation. The peak in the curve refers to the maximum strength of the tendon. The normal range of length-tension in mammalian tendon is 49–98 N/m^2. If a tendon is loaded past this maximum point, usually it undergoes rapid failure. According to Elliott (1967), the maximum strength of a tendon is approximately twice the maximum isometric tension that can be generated in a tendon's muscle.

Viscoelasticity.   Tendons display viscoelastic or rate-dependent (time-dependent) behavior with loads. At high rates of strain, tendons store more energy, require more force to rupture, and undergo greater elongation (Kennedy & Baxter-Willis 1976). At high stress rates, tendons absorb less energy and are capable of moving heavy loads. At low stress rates, tendons absorb more energy and are less effective at moving heavy loads (Fyfe & Stanish 1992). The creep test and the stress-relaxation test are two ways of measuring tendon viscoelasticity. *Creep* refers to the gradual lengthening of a tendon in response to a constant stress or load. During the creep test, the load is held safely below the linear portion of the stress-strain curve, and stress is held constant. If the load is altered cyclically instead of being held at a constant rate, the change in length is less pronounced. During the *stress-relaxation test,* strain (length) is held constant while the load is held below the linear region of the stress-strain curve. At a constant level of strain, tension in the tendon gradually decreases. Given cyclic alterations in strain, the reduction in stress is less significant (Carlstedt & Nordin 1989).

Factors Affecting the Integrity of Tendons

Age and drugs can have a tremendous impact on the mechanical behavior of a tendon. The level of exercise and activity can also affect its integrity.

Aging.   During early tendon maturation, collagen fibril diameter increases along with the number of cross-links, leading to maximum tendon strength between the third and sixth decade (Yamada 1970). With aging, collagen stiffens, and the fibers shrink, thereby reducing tensile strength and increasing the potential for tearing (O'Brien 1992). By the seventh decade, strength has declined rapidly. However, Riley et al. (1994a) found no significant difference in content of the supraspinous tendon in persons from 11 to 95 years of age. Instead, they postulated that changes in collagen content could be attributed to years of repeated injury that resulted in microtears, weakening of the tendon structure, and predisposition to injury.

Anti-Inflammatory Medications.   The effect of anti-inflammatory medications depends on whether they contain steroids. Nonsteroidal anti-inflammatory drugs (NSAIDs) such as aspirin and indomethacin have been found to increase the rate of biomechanical restoration of tissue. Side effects from NSAIDs are minimal. Corticosteroid injections are also intended to reduce pain and inflammation. Despite their value, corticosteroids do have significant side effects that include a reduction in collagen and ground substance production. This reduction may lead to tendon atrophy and subsequent rupture after excessive physical activity (Kennedy & Baxter-Willis 1976; Vogel 1977; Ohkawa 1982; Carlstedt et al. 1986a, b; Nirschl 1992).

Mechanical Demands.   Tendons remodel in response to mechanical demands, undergoing a continual process of resorption and repair. Despite this ability, they are less metabolically active than other human tissues. The rate of collagen turnover in tendons is between 50 and 100 days and is altered by exercise and disuse (Gerber et al. 1960). On the basis of animal studies, consistent exercise has been found to increase tendon tensile strength. This gain is accomplished through increases in the number of collagen cross-links, water and ground substance content, and the size and number of collagen fibers (Noyes et al. 1974; Woo et al. 1975). In contrast, disuse or immobilization results in decreased water and ground substance concentration and a decrease in metabolic enzymes. Inactivity also contributes to collagen degradation and resorption (Woo 1982). These changes lead to a reduction in tensile strength.

Tendon Pathology

Disruptive Forces.   Tension, compression, and shear are three forces that can disrupt the structure of normal tendons. Injury can occur when a force or load magnitude is too high, too frequent in occurrence, or both. Kastelic and Baer (1980) have suggested that tendons elongate secondary to slippage of the transverse bonds between collagen fibrils. Although these bonds are quite strong, after excessive or frequent force the proteoglycan matrix cannot hold them, resulting in inflammation and small microtears in the tendinous region. Individual collagen fibrils in tendons do lengthen in response to tensile stress, yet damage can occur even after an 8.5% elongation. Fast eccentric contractions in weak or fatigued muscles may lead to injury (Noonan & Garrett 1992). Muscles with a higher percentage of fast-twitch fibers are more likely to be involved in quick movements, which is why they may be the first muscles injured.

Vulnerable Anatomic Sites.   Vulnerable sites for tendon injury include tendon attachment sites, the myotendinous junction, and segments in which the tendon must traverse a tunnel. Attachment sites are vulnerable because of their limited blood supply, which varies depending on whether the tendon inserts into bone or cartilage. The myotendinous junction is susceptible to injury because of its reduced sarcomere extensibility. This junction has been determined to be the most common place for rupture (Garrett et al. 1988). Given its two vulnerable conditions, the common extensor tendon near the elbow, which has a poor blood supply and whose attachment site lies close to the myotendinous junction, is highly susceptible to repetitive strain injury. Tunnels are a third vulnerable site. Gliding through tunnels may be restricted if the tendons or surrounding tissue have undergone partial trauma. For

Table 5.1. Definitions of Tendon Injuries

Tendinitis	Vascular disruption and small micro-tears to the tendon, induced by a high rate of stress or strain, resulting in an acute inflammation
Paratendinitis	An inflammation and thickening of the paratenon
Tenosynovitis	An inflammation of the synovial lining
Tendinosis	Chronic degenerative pathology of the tendon, caused by repetitive, low load, stress, and strain

Sources: Modified from WB Leadbetter (1992). Cell-matrix response in tendon injury. *Clin Sports Med*, 11,533–578; and RP Nirschl (1992). Elbow tendinosis/tennis elbow. *Clin Sports Med*, 11,851–869.

example, if, as a result of frequent high forces, the synovial sheaths of the long flexor tendons become inflamed within the carpal tunnel, the tendons and sheath may swell. The swollen tendons may not be able to glide freely and eventually could put undo pressure on the median nerve because of lack of space within the carpal canal (Pratt 1991). When these vulnerable sites combine with conditions of risk, injury results.

Tendon Response to Injury

Terminology. A few key terms associated with tendon injuries are reviewed here and summarized in Table 5.1. *Tendinitis* is a general term that implies there has been a vascular disruption resulting in an acute inflammation induced by small tendon microtears. Acute tendinitis typically involves a high rate of elongation or strain that may resolve within a few months. *Paratendinitis* refers to an inflammation and thickening of the paratenon. *Tenosynovitis* is used to describe an inflammation of the synovial lining; however, that term now falls under the category of paratendinitis. *Tendinosis* refers to chronic degenerative pathology of the tendon, caused by repetitive, low-load stress and strain (Leadbetter 1992; Nirschl 1992).

Pathology. Tendon pathology can be divided into two general categories: macrotraumatic (i.e., acute tissue destruction) and microtraumatic (i.e., chronic abuse or load). A subacute phase represents the stage in which the acute injury begins to subside and healing begins (Leadbetter 1992). The pathology of these different forms of tendon injury differs in terms of histology and mechanism of occurrence.

Acute Conditions. Acute tendon injury results from quick eccentric movements made under heavy loads or high strain (Leadbetter 1992). An acute injury sets up a cycle of regeneration and repair that begins with inflammation and progresses to collagen formation. If the stresses and strain on the tendon are alleviated and wound healing is allowed to progress, an acute injury should resolve quickly. Unfortunately, the typical sites for tendinitis are those vulnerable regions most subjected to repetitive forces by the light and heavy activities of daily living. As a result, many acute injuries go unresolved and may become chronic injuries affecting the integrity of the tissue itself.

Chronic Conditions. In chronic conditions, the signs and symptoms of tendon injury last months or years without resolution. Unlike the acute stage, typical chronic injuries have an insidious onset caused by subthreshold, repetitive stresses or strains to vulnerable tendon regions (Leadbetter 1992). If immature scar or unconditioned muscle tendon units are subjected to dynamic and cyclic overloading, degeneration results (Markison 1992). Degenerative tendon pathology may stem from hypoxia, which eliminates the sequential progression of wound repair seen in acute injuries (Jozsa et al. 1990).

Chronic tendinitis has been referred to as *tendinosis* because histologic examination of chronic injuries often reveals the presence of atypical granulationlike tissue called *angiofibroblastic tendinosis* (Leadbetter 1991; Nirschl 1992). Tendons afflicted with tendinosis experience fiber disorganization, scattered vascular ingrowth, and occasional local necrosis or calcification (Puddu et al. 1976; Clancey 1990). In surgical cases of chronically injured tendons, tissue degeneration has been reported on the basis of reduced collagen content; a gray, frail appearance of tendons; fibrosis at the insertion sites; and tendon calcification (Riley et al. 1994a, b). There is disagreement regarding the presence or absence of inflammatory cells in chronic degenerative tissue (Backman et al. 1990; Jozsa et al. 1990; Leadbetter 1992; Nirschl 1992).

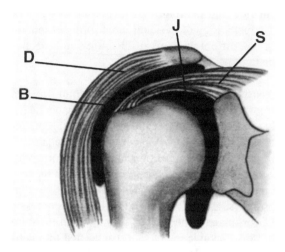

Figure 5.2. Subacromial bursa frontal view. (B = subacromial bursa; D = deltoid muscle; J = glenohumeral joint cavity; S = supraspinatous tendon.) (Reprinted with permission from LR Mercier [1995]. *Practical Orthopedics* [4th ed, p. 55]. Philadelphia: Mosby.)

Conditions Related to Tendinitis

Myofascial Trigger Points.   A trigger point is a palpable, hyperirritable spot within a nodule or taut band of muscle or its fascia (Travell & Simons 1983). A twitch response may be produced on contraction of the taut band. Compression to the trigger point may induce local tenderness and *referred pain*, or pain perceived away from the site of origin.

It has been suggested that acute muscular strain may overload the contractile elements of a muscle (Travell & Simons 1983, p. 36). This strain may damage such muscle constituents as the sarcoplasmic reticulum and may cause release of calcium. If the sarcoplasmic reticulum is damaged, calcium cannot be restored to its original location postcontraction. The normal energy source of adenosine triphosphate in combination with the excess calcium will cause a sustained contraction of the exposed muscle fibers. Uncontrolled metabolism in this region may cause local vasoconstriction and may lead to a trigger point–mediated reflex response via local sensory and sympathetic nerve fiber activation. As a result of local changes, muscle fibers in this region typically become shortened. In summary, a trigger point induced by excess stress or strain becomes the site of increased metabolism, reduced circulation, sensitized nerves,

and shortened muscle fibers. Once established, the trigger point can be palpated as a taut band or nodule. Excess fatigue during repetitive contractions or repetitive contraction of a damaged region may exacerbate the condition and lead to chronic trigger points within a muscle region.

The primary characteristic of trigger points is a typical referral pattern of pain induced by the trigger itself. In addition, local tenderness with a palpable band of fibers will be noted on physical examination, and the muscle will be shortened and weak (Moran 1994).

Bursitis.   Bursitis is an inflammatory condition of the bursal lining or the synovial fluid encased within the bursa (Cyriax 1982). Inflammation of any bursa can limit activity significantly. Inflammation of the synovial fluid may cause the bursa to enlarge. In the upper limb, the most commonly occurring bursitis is associated with the glenohumeral joint. The second most frequently occurring bursitis is associated with the olecranon bursa of the elbow.

The glenohumeral joint bursa has two connected parts, the subdeltoid and the subacromial bursae; the terms are used interchangeably (Pratt 1991). From this point on, the term *subacromial bursa* will be used (Figure 5.2). This bursa can be palpated with the humerus in passive extension, inferior to the acromion, and lateral to the bicipital groove. Because the inner wall of the subacromial bursa is the outer wall of the supraspinous tendon, bursitis often occurs in combination with supraspinous tendinitis (Cailliet 1991). Bursitis in this region is also associated with impingement syndrome described later under Rotator Cuff Tendinitis. Acute subacromial bursitis presents with a sudden onset of limited active abduction without any precipitating injury and with tenderness on palpation. Typically, there is no capsular pattern or associated muscle spasm. In addition, pain is not elicited on resisted abduction. As the acute bursitis resolves, a painful arc emerges. Recurrence is likely at intervals of 2–5 years. Typically, chronic bursitis has a gradual onset without a specific cause. With this condition, there is a painful arc of abduction but no pain with resisted movement. A calcified deposit may develop within the bursa (Cyriax 1982).

Olecranon bursitis also may present as either an acute or chronic condition. With acute bursitis, the olecranon region is enlarged, limiting elbow extension and elbow weight bearing. The region is often tender to palpation. As the acute condition progresses to chronic, the olecranon region may remain engorged even though tenderness to touch is reduced. If elbow range of motion (ROM) is not preserved, limitations may persist after the initial inflammatory condition subsides (Cyriax 1982).

Peripheral Neurovascular Compressions and Entrapment Syndromes

Peripheral compression neuropathies and neurovascular entrapment syndromes frequently are linked to cumulative trauma. Typically, compressions are caused by anatomic abnormalities or adaptive shortening of tissues, which reduces the potential space in which the nerve travels. Over time, the nerve may become compromised because of inadequate space (Walsh 1994). Entrapments are frequently caused by repetitive trauma to a nerve or its interfacing tissue, resulting in early inflammation and later fibrosis (Sunderland 1978). Compressions and entrapments may occur in combination. For example, a nerve may be vulnerable to compressive forces secondary to a reduction in travel space. Repetitive trauma within this reduced space may inflame the nerve or its surrounding tissue, leading to entrapment. A complete understanding of the implications of compressive neuropathies and entrapment conditions requires a review of physiology and pathology.

Nerve Anatomy and Physiology

Stimuli picked up by sensory receptors are coded by transducers into neural activity. Once transduced, the information is carried through peripheral nerves to the CNS, where it eventually registers in the somatosensory cortex. Because processing of somatosensory and motor information occurs distributively throughout the nervous system, both the peripheral nervous system (PNS) and the CNS (with their associated connective tissues) are affected by nerve compressions.

Connective Tissues.   Continuity between the PNS and CNS is maintained through supportive connective tissues (Figure 5.3) (Sunderland 1978; Matloub & Yousif 1992). The central axon is surrounded by endoneurium. Groups of four or five axons, which form fascicles, are covered by a strong layer of perineurium. A bundle of fascicles is enveloped further in a loose layer of epineurium. The mesoneurium surrounds the entire nerve in a meshlike fashion, connecting it to nearby interfacing tissues. Most regions of the peripheral nerve contain all connective tissue layers, except for the nerve roots, which lie near the spinal cord. The lack of epineurium, in particular, significantly reduces the regeneration potential of nerve roots despite their close proximity to the cell bodies.

Vascularity.   Nerves depend on an ongoing supply of oxygen and nutrients provided by a well-developed vascular network. Each connective tissue layer contains blood vessels with extensive anastomoses (Lundborg 1979; Matloub & Yousif 1992). A bidirectional perineurial diffusion barrier is the most external protective zone for the nerve. This perineurial barrier protects the endoneurium from the effects of proteins and edema. Epineurial blood vessels allow passage of small amounts of proteins, whereas the walls of the internal endoneurial capillaries provide a blood-nerve barrier. This endoneurial blood-nerve barrier, maintained by tight junctions of endothelial cells, protects the axon against the invasion of all proteins and from the ischemic effects of short-lasting epineurial edema (Olsson & Kristensson 1971).

Transport of Axoplasm.   The axon contains a viscouslike substance, axoplasm, which assists in the bidirectional flow of materials to and from the cell body. Axoplasm is considered thixotropic; therefore, movement is required to keep the viscosity low and to prevent gelling (Haak et al. 1976; Baker et al. 1977). Essential neural substances manufactured in the cell body are transported down the axon to the nerve terminal (synapse) via antegrade transport of axoplasm (Figure 5.4) (Droz et al. 1975; Grafstein & Forman 1980; Dahlin & Lundborg 1990). Translocation of materials from the nerve terminal is passed back through the axoplasm to the cell body via retrograde transport. Retrograde transport also informs the cell's body of the status of the axon, its terminals, and the nearby environment (Bisby & Keen 1986).

The rate or velocity of axoplasmic flow is related to function (Grafstein & Forman 1980). Slow antegrade transport replaces axoplasm along the

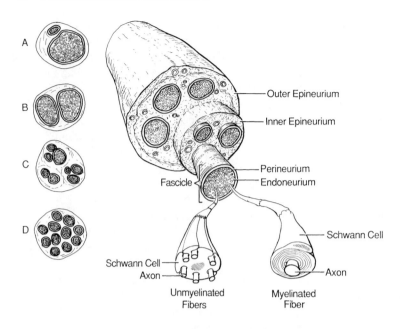

Figure 5.3. Connective tissues of peripheral nerves. Connective tissue elements consist of the endoneurium, the perineurium, and the inner and outer epineurium. Individual fascicles contain a heterogeneous mix of myelinated and unmyelinated fibers, but some fascicles demonstrate a preponderance of one type. Basic patterns of intraneural structure are demonstrated. A peripheral nerve is considered monofascicular if it holds one large fascicle (*A*) or oligofascicular for a few large fascicles (*B*). Polyfascicular nerves consist of many fascicles, which may be grouped (*C*) or may exhibit no identifiable group patterns (*D*). (Reprinted with permission from JK Terzis & KL Smith [1990]. *The Peripheral Nerve: Structure, Function and Reconstruction* [p. 16]. New York: Raven Press.)

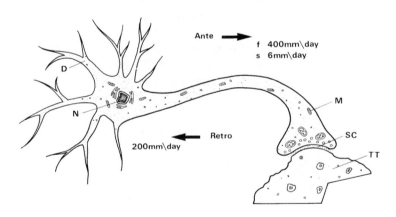

Figure 5.4. Axoplasmic flow within a single neuron. (D = dendrite; N = nucleus; M = mitochondria; SC = synaptic cleft; TT = target tissue.) (Reprinted with permission from DS Butler [1991]. *Mobilisation of the Nervous System* [p. 25]. New York: Churchill Livingstone.)

length of the axon at a rate of 1–30 mm per day. Fast antegrade transport moves enzymes, neurotransmitters, vesicles, lipids, and glycoproteins at a velocity of 400 mm per day. Retrograde transport recycles vesicles from the nerve terminal and transports nerve growth factors to the cell body at a velocity ranging from 1–2 mm per day to 300 mm per day. One role of nerve growth factors is to regulate select neuropeptides, such as substance P (Otten 1984; Dahlin & Lundborg 1990). Because axoplasmic flow enhances communication between the cell body, its axon, and its terminals, injury at

one segment of the nerve may have an indirect impact on function at another segment (Upton & McComas 1973).

Biomechanics of Peripheral Nerves

Response to Tension.   Peripheral nerves initially respond to tension by straightening out fascicles. As a particular load increases, the nerve will elongate because of the elastic properties of its connective tissues (Bora et al. 1980). It has been suggested that collagen, not elastin, may be re-

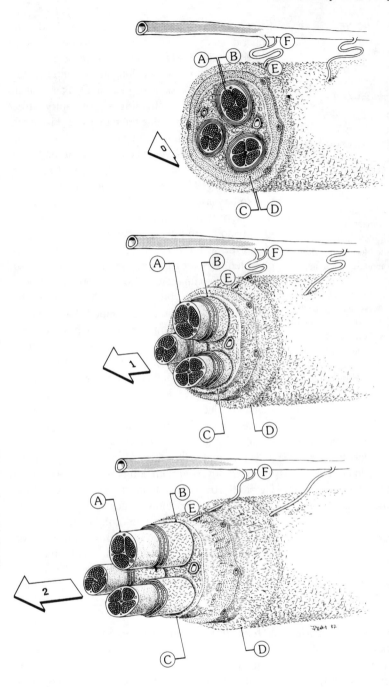

Figure 5.5. Gliding of inner connective tissues of peripheral nerves. (A = fascicle; B = perineurium; C = epineurium; D = adventitia; E = regional feeding vessel; F = extrinsic vessel.) (Reprinted with permission from G Lundborg [1988]. *Nerve Injury and Repair* [p. 92]. New York: Churchill Livingstone.)

sponsible for the viscoelastic properties of the peripheral nerve, because elastin makes up only a small portion of the three connective tissues, being in greatest abundance within the perineurium (Tassler et al. 1994). If mechanical deformation exceeds the nerve's ability to withstand a particular load, deterioration results.

Nerve Gliding. Peripheral nerves move in relation to their interfacing soft tissue (Figure 5.5). For example, during active motion, the median nerve glides 7–14 mm at the wrist level and 5–7 mm at the elbow level (Wilgis & Murphy 1986). Internally, the interfascicular epineurium allows the nerve fascicles to glide against one another (Millesi et al. 1990; Rath &

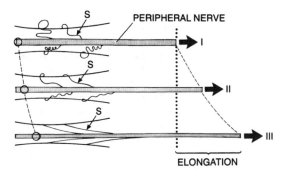

Figure 5.6. Nerve elongation and associated ischemia. Stage I: The segmental blood vessels (*S*) are normally coiled to allow for the physiologic movements of the nerve. Stage II: Under gradually increasing elongation, these regional vessels become stretched, and the blood flow within is impaired. Stage III: The cross-sectional area of the nerve (represented within the circle) is reduced during stretching, and the intraneural blood flow is impaired further. Complete cessation of all blood flow in the nerve usually occurs at approximately 15% elongation. (Reprinted with permission from B Rydevik, G Lundborg, & R Skalak [1989]. Biomechanics of peripheral nerves. In M Nordin & VH Frankel [Eds]. *Basic Biomechanics of the Musculoskeletal System* [2nd ed, p. 81]. Philadelphia: Lea & Febiger.)

Millesi 1990). Because peripheral nerves must have the ability to adapt passively and actively to different positions of the body, damage to the interfacing tissues or any nerve component will likely have a negative impact on nerve function (Millesi et al. 1990).

Pathology of Nerve Compressions

Disruptive Factors. Nerve compressions may arise from either ischemia, direct mechanical injury, or both. The initial cause of injury is often mechanical because of chronic low-pressure shear forces and excessive stretching (Dyck et al. 1990). Mechanical factors may induce ischemia and may affect microcirculation and vascular permeability. Mechanical factors include abnormal anatomy, postural deficits, trauma, and iatrogenic factors. Following repetitive injury, the nerve may become entrapped (Walsh 1994). After entrapment, the presence of edema and the formation of fibrosis begin to limit intraneural (internal) and extraneural (external) nerve mobility (Millesi et al. 1990; Butler 1991). If the interfacing tissues become affected, nerve gliding may be reduced significantly.

Effect on Blood Flow. The maximum load a peripheral nerve can withstand depends on its course and composition. Although the connective tissues associated with a nerve can elongate, its blood vessels do not adapt to the same degree. Small alterations in length, pressure, or loading significantly affect nerves, and overstretching them may cause ischemia (Figure 5.6). The human median nerve can tolerate loads from 73 to 220 N, whereas the ulnar nerve can tolerate loads from 65 to 155 N without damage. Sunderland (1978) found the limit of nerve elongation to be between 11 and 17%, with structural failure occurring between 15 and 23% of resting length. Ogata and Naito (1986) found that average stretching of the sciatic nerve of more than 15.7% caused complete arrest of blood flow. Bora et al. (1980) found the maximal elongation of normal and operated nerves to be approximately 20%. Despite the ability to elongate, intraneural blood flow is altered when nerves are elongated more than 8% of their resting length, and blood flow ceases at 15% elongation. (Lundborg & Rydevik 1973). Clearly, nerves may sustain permanent damage from stretching.

Nerve compression of 20–30 mm Hg has been found to reduce venular blood flow in the epineurium. At pressures of 30–50 mm Hg, axonal transport may be inhibited and blood flow impaired (Rydevik et al. 1981). Complete cessation of intraneural circulation has been observed with compression of 50–70 mm Hg or 60–70% mean arterial pressure (Ogata & Naito 1986). Different postures influence compressive factors. For example, pronation of the forearm induces pressures greater than a neutral forearm position. Therefore, typists with suspected carpal tunnel syndrome are advised to use "split keyboards," which encourages a neutral forearm position that reduces pressure within the carpal canal (Markison 1990).

Effect on Axoplasmic Transport. Axoplasmic transport is affected by anoxia and ischemia because of its dependence on microvascular circulation. Alterations in transport may lead to morphologic and biochemical changes in the cell body. For instance, compression may alert the cell body through retrograde axonal transport to produce new Schwann cells (Lundborg & Dahlin 1992). Changes in axonal flow or in the cell body also may make other parts of the nerve more susceptible to trauma (Dahlin & Lundborg 1990). Nerves may experience double or multiple crush injuries, indicating that more than one region of the nerve may be impaired (Upton & McComas 1973; Osterman 1988; Rydevik et al. 1990; Mackinnon 1992). Individuals with chronic compressive neuropathy may present with diffuse symptoms due to the presence of multiple segments of nerve damage (Anderson & Tichenor 1994).

Neural Reorganization Secondary to Compression

Given alterations in sensory input experienced in peripheral nerve compressions, related regions of the CNS will reorganize (Merzenich & Jenkins 1993). Through invasive animal studies, researchers have found that massive cortical reorganization occurs following sensory deafferentation. Current hypotheses regarding mechanisms for reorganization in the somatosensory cortex can be divided into four categories:

1. There may be migration of cells that serve other functions, into the deafferented region of the cortex (Allard et al. 1991; Ramachandran et al. 1992; Mogilner et al. 1993). For example, the face may become more sensitive to light touch if the index finger has lost its sensibility.
2. Inhibitory controls in the affected region may be removed (Rothe et al. 1990; Turnbull & Rasmusson 1990, 1991; Calford & Tweedale 1991; Garraghty et al. 1991; Rasmusson et al. 1992; Zarzecki et al. 1993).
3. Existing subthreshold excitatory inputs and connections may be strengthened on the basis of experience postcompression (Jenkins et al. 1990; Merzenich & Sameshima 1993; Pascual-Leone & Torres 1993).
4. There may be subcortical reorganization, as in the basal ganglia, which project input to the cortex. (Merzenich et al. 1978; Garraghty et al. 1991; Pons et al. 1991; Rasmusson et al. 1992).

Because of the massive central reorganization after injury, it is not surprising that individuals may have difficulty in regaining full sensibility and motor control even with removal of compressive forces and regrowth of the axon.

Motor control is affected by the lack of sensory input, as documented in patients with large-fiber neuropathy (Sainburg et al. 1993; Gordon et al. 1995). Lack of sensory input requires the use of adaptive strategies to maximize motor function. Until further research is done, it is important to recognize that nerve compressions do induce CNS re-

organization, which has an effect on function and may impede full recovery.

Classification of Nerve Injuries

Traditional Classification. Classification of nerve injuries enhances accurate communication between professionals. Seddon (1943) classified nerve injuries into three groups: neuropraxia, axonotmesis, and neurotmesis. Sunderland (1978) further separated nerve lesions into five categories. Both classifications are summarized in Figure 5.7. *Neuropraxia* (Sunderland I) is considered a conduction block induced by compression or stretching. *Axonotmesis* (Sunderland II) refers to an advanced nerve compression or traction injury. It suggests a loss of axonal continuity, with wallerian degeneration and intact endoneurial tubes. Neurotmesis (Sunderland III–V) indicates loss of axonal continuity, with select loss of remaining elements of the nerve trunk. It refers also to cases of total nerve severance. Although this classification system is used widely, it is too extreme to describe sufficiently the subtle deficits found in mild compressive neuropathies.

Classification of Mild Compressions. A more useful classification may be that proposed by Butler (1991), which is based on mild nerve compressions (Table 5.2). The four general categories, which may occur in sequence, are (1) the potential lesion, (2) physiologic pain, (3) the inflamed and irritated nerve, and (4) fibrosis of various areas. The *potential lesion* can be exemplified by edema in the carpal tunnel or blood around a nerve that induces *physiologic pain.* This pain may involve either the connective or neural tissue. Edema in the epineurial layer is the first sign of nerve injury. The potential lesion caused by edema may reduce blood flow. Irritation of the epineurium may develop secondary to mild compression or friction. A break in the perineurium may lead to persistent irritation or nerve pressure. If an irritation persists, intraneural or extraneural fibrosis may develop. Extraneural fibrosis may alter the ability of the nerve to glide against its surrounding tissues.

Acute Versus Chronic Conditions. Nerve compressions often are regarded as acute or chronic,

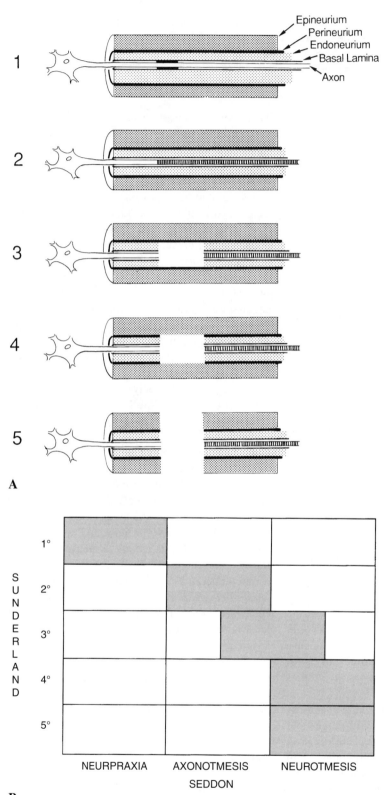

Figure 5.7. A. Classification of nerve injuries by Seddon and Sunderland. 1. First-degree injury: local conduction blockade with minimal structural disruption. Prognosis: complete recovery within days to months. 2. Second-degree injury: complete axonal disruption with wallerian degeneration; basal lamina remains intact. Prognosis: complete recovery in months. 3. Third-degree injury: axonal and endoneurial disruption with interruption of the basal lamina. Prognosis: intrafascicular axonal admixture with regeneration yields mild to moderate reduction in function. 4. Fourth-degree injury: axonal, endoneurial, and perineurial disruption. Prognosis: moderate to severe functional loss due to interfascicular axonal admixture; microsurgical manipulation can improve prognosis. 5. Fifth-degree injury: complete structural disruption. Prognosis: No return without microsurgical manipulation. **B.** Comparison between Sunderland's and Seddon's classifications. First-degree injuries correspond to neurapraxic injuries. Second-degree injuries are comparable to axonotmetric injuries. Third-degree injuries may be either axonotmetric or neurotmetric, and fourth- and fifth-degree injuries are neurotmetric. (Reprinted with permission from JK Terzis & KL Smith [1990]. *The Peripheral Nerve: Structure, Function, and Reconstruction* [p. 40]. New York: Raven Press.)

Table 5.2. Pathophysiology of Mild Nerve Compressions

Potential Lesion	→ Physiologic Pain	Inflamed and → Irritated Nerve	→ Fibrosis
Edema in carpal tunnel	Irritation of connective or neural tissue	Epineurial irritation; breach of perineurium with persistent irritation or nerve pressure	Intraneural or extraneural, which limits nerve gliding
Blood around a nerve	Reduced blood flow		

Source: Modified from DS Butler (1991). *Mobilisation of the Nervous System*. New York: Churchill Livingstone.

with an intermediate subacute stage. The main difference between the two lies in the onset and progression of signs and symptoms.

As with tendinitis, injured nerves undergo an initial inflammatory response that will alter tissue integrity if the compressive forces or entrapping conditions are not alleviated. Secondary to entrapment, nerves undergo focal slowing and display histologic signs of demyelinization and remyelinization (Nakano 1991).

Long-standing peripheral nerve compression or entrapment may result in wallerian degeneration. The components of wallerian degeneration involve disintegration of the axon, shrinkage of the endoneurial tubes, breakdown of the myelin sheath, and disintegration of the end organs. In cases of nerve compression, degeneration may occur within select fascicles only and may not effect the entire nerve. The cell body reaction may be minimal, yet there may be alterations in CNS representation.

Major Upper-Limb Nerves with Potential Compression and Entrapment Sites

Cervicobrachial Region.   The thoracic outlet (inlet) is a three-dimensional, triangular region that forms the superior opening of the thorax (Howell 1991). Included in the medial wall of this triangle are the anterior scalene anteriorly, the middle scalene posteriorly, and the first rib inferiorly. The anterior-lateral wall extends from the second cervical vertebra to the clavicle and pectoralis minor. Finally, the posterior-lateral wall extends from the occiput to the attachments of the trapezius muscle (Pratt 1991).

The subclavian artery and the brachial plexus, made up of spinal rami of C5, C6, C7, C8, and T1, travel together within the thoracic outlet, as seen in

Figure 5.8 (Dawson et al. 1990; Pratt 1991). After exiting the spinal cord, the spinal rami quickly combine into the upper, middle, and lower nerve trunks that, along with the subclavian artery, pass between the anterior and middle scalene musculature. All three trunks separate into posterior and anterior divisions before crossing over the first rib and beneath the clavicle in the region, termed the *costoclavicular interval*. As they travel beneath the pectoralis minor, the divisions combine to form the posterior, lateral, and medial cords. This region is termed the *axillary interval*. Within the axilla region, the cords eventually divide into terminal peripheral nerves.

The potential sites of compression or entrapment of the neurovascular structures that pass within this region include the interscalene triangle, the costoclavicular interval, and the axillary interval, as pictured in Figure 5.9 (Sanders & Haug 1991; Walsh 1994). Along with the listed sites, the presence of such anatomic anomalies as a cervical rib or a prefixed plexus (large C4 contribution) may exacerbate symptoms further.

Radial Nerve.   The radial nerve is a continuation of the posterior cord of the brachial plexus (Pratt 1991; Matloub & Yousif 1992). As depicted in Figure 5.10, it courses through the axilla, then moves medial to lateral on the posterior humerus in the spiral groove, where it innervates the triceps. The nerve then travels anteriorly at the elbow, where it innervates the brachioradialis, extensor carpi radialis longus (ECRL), and extensor carpi radialis brevis (ECRB). Distal to the elbow, it rests on the head of the radius, where it divides into a superficial and a deep branch. The deep branch (posterior interosseous nerve) travels beneath the edge of the ECRB. After it innervates and pierces the supinator muscle, it innervates the extensor carpi ulnaris, the extensor digi-

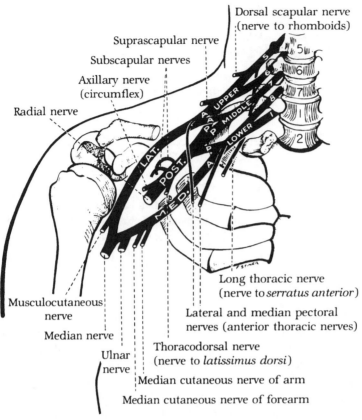

Dorsal scapular nerve
(nerve to rhomboids)

Suprascapular nerve

Subscapular nerves

Axillary nerve
(circumflex)

Radial nerve

Musculocutaneous
nerve

Median nerve

Ulnar
nerve

Long thoracic nerve
(nerve to *serratus anterior*)

Lateral and median pectoral
nerves (anterior thoracic nerves)

Thoracodorsal nerve
(nerve to *latissimus dorsi*)

Median cutaneous nerve of arm

Median cutaneous nerve of forearm

Figure 5.8. Brachial plexus. (Reprinted with permission from DM Dawson, M Hallett, and LH Millender [1990]. *Entrapment Neuropathies* [2nd ed, p. 233]. Boston: Little, Brown.)

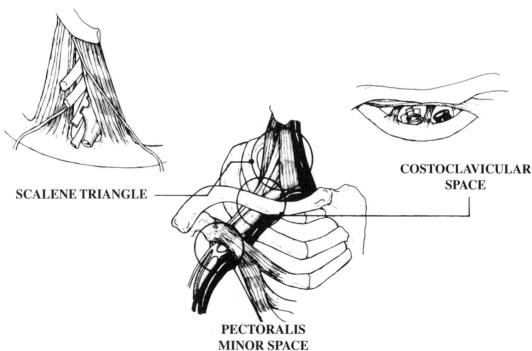

SCALENE TRIANGLE

PECTORALIS
MINOR SPACE

COSTOCLAVICULAR
SPACE

Figure 5.9. Three major spaces for entrapment in thoracic outlet (inlet) region. (Reprinted with permission from RJ Sanders & CE Haug [1991]. *Thoracic Outlet Syndrome: A Common Sequela of Neck Injuries* [p. 34]. Philadelphia: Lippincott.)

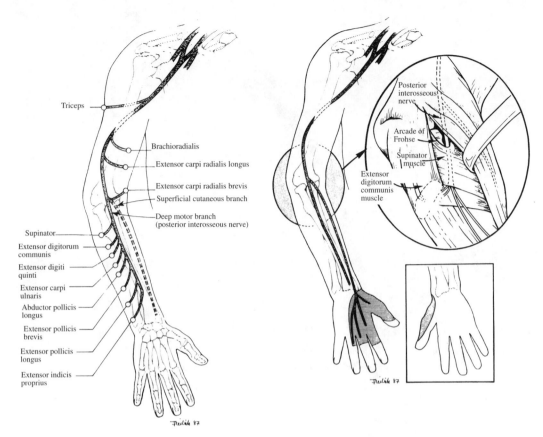

Figure 5.10. Radial nerve innervation patterns and vulnerable anatomic sites. (Reprinted with permission from G Lundborg [1988]. *Nerve Injury and Repair* [p. 135]. New York: Churchill Livingstone.)

torum communis, the extensor digiti minimi, the abductor pollicis longus (APL), the extensor pollicis longus, and extensor pollicis brevis and the extensor indicis. The superficial branch travels underneath the brachioradialis and emerges distally between the attachment of the brachioradialis and the ECRB, near the anatomic snuff-box. This sensory branch serves the cutaneous portion of the radial three and one-half digits, excluding the nail beds.

The potential sites of radial nerve entrapment include the axilla region between the heads of the triceps, the radial tunnel (region of supinator) between the tendons of the ECRL and BR in the forearm, and the region near the anatomic snuff-box. The posterior interosseous branch may also become entrapped or compressed after it branches off from the radial nerve. The supinator muscle region and the anatomic snuff-box region are the most vulnerable areas (see Figure 5.10).

Median Nerve. The median nerve receives branches off the lateral and medial cords of the brachial plexus, with spinal nerve contributions from C5, C6, C7, C8, and T1 (Pratt 1991; Matloub & Yousif 1992). The median nerve courses through the axilla and progresses medial to the humerus in the upper arm. Distally, it travels between the brachialis and the biceps until it passes beneath the ligament of Struthers. After this landmark, it begins to innervate the forearm muscles (Figure 5.11). In the cubital fossa, the nerve rests medial to the biceps tendon, then traverses under the bicipital aponeurosis. After passing through the two heads of the pronator teres, the median nerve plunges beneath the edge of the flexor digitorum superficialis (FDS). After traveling beneath the FDS in the forearm, the median nerve emerges 5 cm proximal to the carpal tunnel. It courses through the tunnel to serve the cutaneous portion of the radial three and

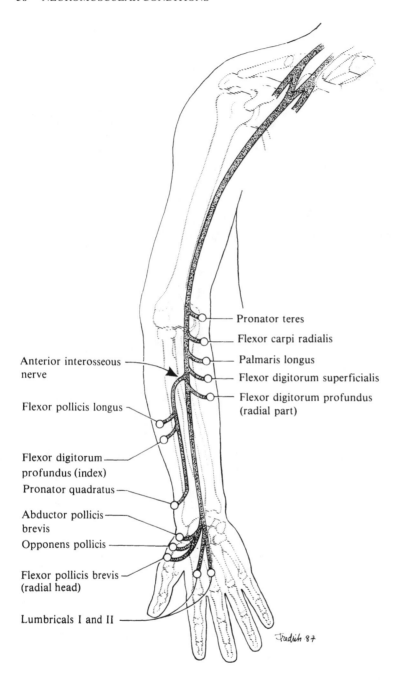

Figure 5.11. Median nerve innervation patterns. (Reprinted with permission from G Lundborg [1988]. *Nerve Injury and Repair* [p. 113]. New York: Churchill Livingstone.)

Anterior interosseous nerve

Flexor pollicis longus

Flexor digitorum profundus (index)

Pronator quadratus

Abductor pollicis brevis

Opponens pollicis

Flexor pollicis brevis (radial head)

Lumbricals I and II

Pronator teres

Flexor carpi radialis

Palmaris longus

Flexor digitorum superficialis

Flexor digitorum profundus (radial part)

one-half digits, lumbricals I and II, and the thenar muscle group: opponens pollicis, abductor pollicis brevis, and superficial portion of the flexor pollicis brevis. The palmar cutaneous branch, which serves the skin of the thenar eminence, does not course through the carpal tunnel (Figure 5.12). The anterior interosseous branches off from the median nerve approximately 5 cm distal to the medial epicondyle and innervates the flexor pollicis longus (FPL), the flexor digitorum profundus (FDP) to the index and long fingers, and the pronator teres.

Potential sites of entrapment (see Figure 5.12) are beneath the ligament of Struthers, the proximal forearm (location of pronator syndrome), and the

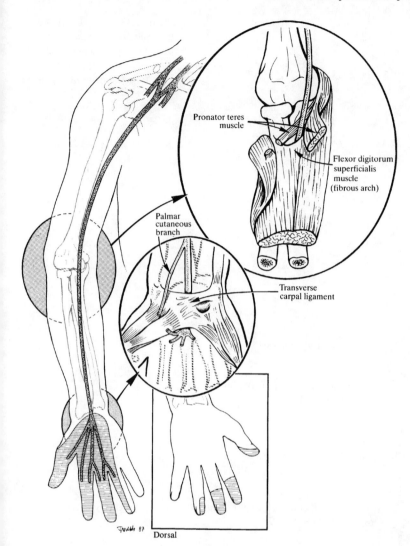

Figure 5.12. Median nerve cutaneous innervation and critical anatomic areas. (Reprinted with permission from G Lundborg [1988]. *Nerve Injury and Repair* [p. 114]. New York: Churchill Livingstone.)

Pronator teres muscle

Flexor digitorum superficialis muscle (fibrous arch)

Palmar cutaneous branch

Transverse carpal ligament

Dorsal

carpal tunnel. The anterior interosseous nerve may become compressed as it branches off from the median nerve.

Ulnar Nerve.   The ulnar nerve is a continuation of the medial cord of the brachial plexus, with C8 and T1 spinal contributions (Pratt 1991; Matloub & Yousif 1992). The ulnar nerve courses through the axilla medially to the triceps before moving posteriorly behind the medial epicondyle through the cubital tunnel. In the forearm, it traverses between the heads of the flexor carpi ulnaris and travels distally deep to this muscle. The muscles served in the forearm include flexor carpi ulnaris and the FDP to the ring finger and small fingers (Figure 5.13). Approximately 2 cm proximal to the wrist, it sends off a dorsal cutaneous branch to serve the dorsal one and one-half digits (Figure 5.14). The volar branch then continues its course through Guyon's tunnel. The ulnar nerve eventually innervates the ulnar side of the fifth digit and the ulnar half of the fourth digit. In the hand, the ulnar nerve serves the following muscles: flexor digiti minimi, adductor digiti minimi, opponens digiti minimi, dorsal and palmar interossei, lumbricals III and IV, the deep portion of the flexor pollicis brevis, and the adductor pollicis. Potential sites of entrapment

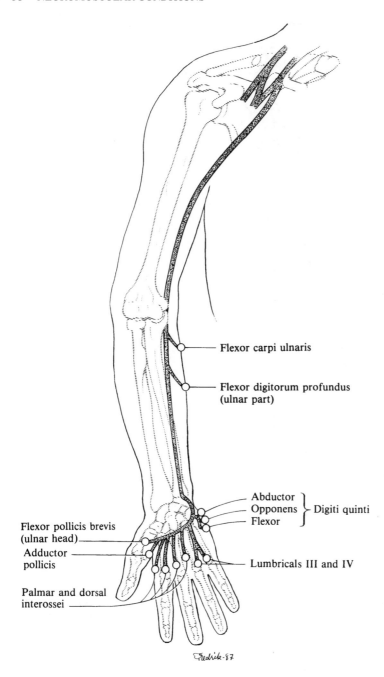

Figure 5.13. Ulnar nerve innervation patterns. (Reprinted with permission from G Lundborg [1988]. *Nerve Injury and Repair* [p. 129]. New York: Churchill Livingstone.)

Flexor carpi ulnaris

Flexor digitorum profundus (ulnar part)

Abductor ⎱
Opponens ⎰ Digiti quinti
Flexor ⎰

Flexor pollicis brevis (ulnar head)

Adductor pollicis

Lumbricals III and IV

Palmar and dorsal interossei

or compression of the ulnar nerve include the cubital tunnel region and the region of Guyon's tunnel (see Figure 5.14).

Anastomosis.   The median nerve may form connections with the ulnar nerve in the forearm. The most well-known is the Martin-Gruber anastomosis, a motor connection between the two in the proximal forearm (Matloub & Yousif 1992). It is also possible that the anterior interosseous connects with the ulnar nerve more distally. Other less common anastomoses may be responsible for entrap-

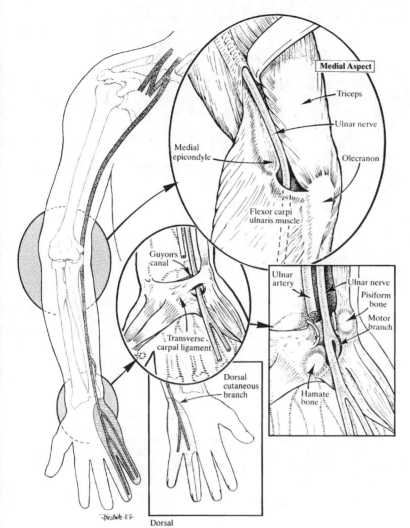

Figure 5.14. Ulnar nerve cutaneous innervation and critical anatomic area. (Reprinted with permission from G Lundborg [1988]. *Nerve Injury and Repair* [p. 130]. New York: Churchill Livingstone.)

ment syndromes, causing symptoms that do not follow a logical pattern. Diagnosis of these unusual anastomoses is difficult. If symptoms are severe enough and impeding function, surgical intervention may be warranted.

Differentiating Between Tendinitis and Nerve Entrapments

Peripheral nerve compressions or entrapments can be mistaken for tendinitis or tendinosis. Verification of the existence of neural or contractile tissue involve-

ment requires a thorough evaluation. Findings from sensibility and resistance tests provide the most useful information. Test results for tendinitis and compression/entrapment are summarized in Table 5.3.

History and Subjective Assessment

An accurate history is key to addressing most injuries. Specific information regarding pre-existing conditions and interventions as well as work, self-care, and leisure histories may be obtained through an interview or a health history form (Kasch 1995).

Table 5.3. Differentiating Tendinitis from Peripheral Nerve Compression or Entrapment

Finding	Tendinitis	Nerve Compression or Entrapment
Pain at rest	Possibly	Yes
Pain with resistive manual muscle test	Yes	Possibly
Weakness on manual muscle test	Possibly	Yes
Symptoms reproduced with provocative maneuvers	Yes	Yes
Abnormal sensibility tests	No	Yes
Abnormal electromyography/nerve conduction velocity	No	Yes

Sources: Modified from G Lundborg & LB Dahlin (1992). The pathophysiology of nerve compression. *Hand Clin*, 8,215–227; and RP Nirschl (1992). Elbow tendinosis/tennis elbow. *Clin Sports Med*, 11,851–870.

Table 5.4. Levels of Cumulative Trauma Based on Activity Tolerance and Associated Pain

Level one
    Constant pain (dull aching) and pain or paresthesia that disturbs sleep
    Intermittent pain or paraesthesia at rest that does not disturb sleep
    Pain or paresthesia caused by light activities of daily living
Level two
    Pain or paresthesia caused by heavy activities of daily living
    Pain or paresthesia with exercise or activity that alters performance of the activity
    Pain or paresthesia with exercise or activity that does not alter performance of the activity
Level three
    Pain or paresthesia after activity that persists beyond 48 hours yet resolves with rest
    Mild pain or paresthesia after exercise or activity that resolves within 24 hours

Notes: Under each level are descriptors of activity tolerance, in decreasing order of severity. Level one represents the most restrictive level of activity. Reported symptoms may be compared against this list in order to plan for treatment by level.
Sources: Modified from M Lindsay (1993). Radial tunnel versus lateral epicondylitis. *Newsletter of the Section on Hand Rehabilitation of the American Physical Therapy Association*, 10(39),1; and RP Nirschl (1992). Elbow tendinosis/tennis elbow. *Clin Sports Med*, 11,851–870.

Activity Tolerance

An important aspect of the interview is to obtain information about how the disorder has progressed. Tasks or activities that exacerbate signs and symptoms should be highlighted. Specifically, one should ask for the location, duration, and description of symptoms. Nirschl (1992) outlined phases of tendon pathology on the basis of pain induced by specific activities. These phases have been incorporated into levels of recovery associated with tendinitis or nerve compressions (Table 5.4). For example, an individual may complain of pain in the lateral forearm after carrying a bag of groceries, an activity categorized under level 2 as a heavy activity of daily living. Lateral forearm pain may imply compression of the radial nerve or tendinitis of the common extensor tendon. As treatment continues, this task could be used to evaluate tolerance to loads, either through task simulation or verbal report. An accurate history enables one to begin isolating tendinous conditions from those of neurogenic origin and to determine whether the disorder's onset was insidious or traumatic.

Pain Assessment

Measurement of pain provides a means of documenting subjective complaints, identifying the source(s), and establishing a baseline for treatment. A rating scale, such as the visual analog scale (VAS) is a simple means of documenting either the intensity or affective quality of pain (Gracely 1979; Scott & Huskisson 1979; Newton 1990). Although there are variations, typically an unmarked 10-cm line is drawn vertically or horizontally on a sheet of paper, which is placed in front of an individual. Descriptive words are placed at either end of the line, and the individual is asked to place a mark on the line that indicates which word best describes the patient's condition, and to what degree. For example, if one wishes to measure pain intensity, the description at one end of the line might read "No pain," and the opposite description read "Intense pain." Following completion, the line may be measured and placed in the individual's chart for later comparison. Although the VAS is viewed as a sensitive indicator of pain, the reader is advised that cultural influences and expectations also play a role in pain and are difficult to measure.

The McGill pain questionnaire (MPQ) attempts to measure multiple aspects of pain in four parts (Melzack 1975). In part one, descriptive words are divided into 3 categories and 20 subcategories. The three main categories include sensory, evaluative, and affective pain components. In each subcategory, there are six similar words that rank pain in descending order according to intensity. The individual is asked to circle one word from each applicable category and to leave blank any category that does not apply. Quantitative scoring involves the number of words chosen and a pain rating index. Part two of the MPQ is the pain diagram. On a front and back diagram of the upper quadrant, the individual marks the exact location and type of pain through designated symbols. The therapist reviews the diagram with the individual after completion. In part three, the subject verbally describes the duration of pain and the activities that influence it. Part four asks the individual to rate pain on a five-point scale according to its intensity, to determine the present pain index. The scale is marked with descriptive terms: *mild, discomforting, distressing, horrible,* and *excruciating.* If all four parts of the MPQ are given, the test provides a more sensitive measure of pain than does the VAS alone.

Related History

It is important to obtain information regarding previous treatment and formal testing. For example, in cases of nerve compression or tendinitis, the physician may have injected the region with anti-inflammatory medication. Although this may serve to reduce inflammation and

pain, three repeated injections may influence healing of the injured tissue. Electromyography (EMG) and nerve conduction studies (NCSs) are formal tests frequently used by physicians in combination with other clinical tests to confirm or refute nerve impairment. Although EMG and NCS results may guide early treatment, electrodiagnostic testing is not valuable the first 2 weeks after nerve injury, and specificity cannot be assumed. Redmond and Rivner (1977) reported that one-third of normal subjects tested demonstrated a false-positive result on at least one electrodiagnostic factor. Thus, electrodiagnostic test results must be evaluated against signs and symptoms and objective clinical findings.

Electromyography

Invasive EMG uses a needle electrode placed in muscle to record electrical potentials produced by innervated and denervated muscle fibers (Brumback et al. 1992). The needle of the EMG will record activity from adjacent muscle fibers on insertion, during relaxation, and during minimal or strong contractions (Figure 5.15). Abnormal EMG findings include fibrillations and positive sharp waves, fasciculations, polyphasic motor units, and poor recruitment. Fibrillations are small-amplitude, short-duration, biphasic or triphasic potentials with a discharge rate 13–15 times per second. Fibrillations are seen in cases of nerve disease and other conditions that may increase excitability of the nerve cell membrane. Positive sharp waves are similar to fibrillations, except that typically there is an initial positive deflection. Fasciculations are the visible twitching of muscle bundles as a result of spontaneous initiation of an action potential in a nerve axon branch. This activity eliminates the normal anterograde propagation. Instead, the propagation occurs in both directions: anterograde (toward the nerve terminal) and retrograde (toward the spinal cord). The size and duration of the motor unit as well as the number of phases may change in cases of nerve or muscle disease.

Nerve Conduction Studies

NCSs record the conduction velocity of nerve fiber action potentials by myelinated fibers (Figure 5.16). As a rule, conduction velocity is six times the diameter of a myelinated fiber (in micrometers per sec-

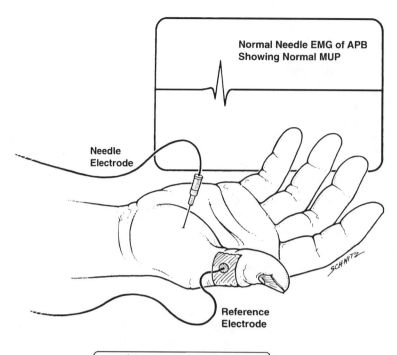

Figure 5.15. Electromyogram (EMG). (APB = abductor pollicis brevis; MUP = motor unit potentials.) (Reprinted with permission from JW Hilburn [1996]. General principles and use of electrodiagnostic studies in carpal and cubital tunnel syndromes: with special attention to pitfalls and interpretation. *Hand Clin,* 12,210.)

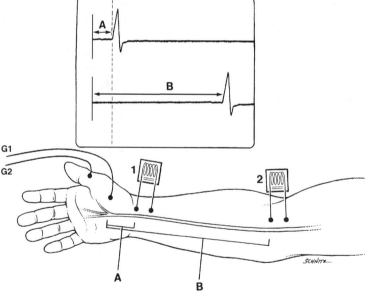

Figure 5.16. Median nerve conduction study. (A = distal motor latency; B = proximal motor latency; G1 = active point; G2 = reference point; 1 = distal stimulation site; 2 = proximal stimulation cite.) (Reprinted with permission from JW Hilburn [1996]. General principles and use of electrodiagnostic studies in carpal and cubital tunnel syndromes: with special attention to pitfalls and interpretation. *Hand Clin,* 12,212.)

ond), and myelinated fiber diameter varies between 1 and 20 μm (Brumback et al. 1992). Thus, the largest myelinated fiber can conduct up to 120 μm per second. Nerve conduction velocity for an individual with suspected nerve compression is often evaluated against the uninvolved extremity because there is a large age variance among normative data.

Objective Clinical Assessments

In addition to a good history and activity tolerance screen, a physical assessment should be obtained. This portion of the evaluation may begin with visual inspection and progress to ROM and strength testing. In some instances, it may be necessary to conduct an

Table 5.5. Upper-Quadrant Screen

Observation and inspection
    Body build: endomorph, ectomorph, or mesomorph
    Weight:_____ Height:_____ (unusual features)
    Assistive devices or orthotics
    General mobility and static limb posture (on entrance into clinic or during interview)
    Alterations in skin (e.g., scars, edema)
    Reported functional use
    Static posture (lateral, posterior, and anterior)
        Scapular position (elevated, abducted, etc.)
        Head position (forward head posture, tilted)
        Pelvic position (anterior or posterior pelvic tilt, lateral tilts, or rotations)
        Position of arm and shoulder
        Asymmetries
Function tests
    Cervical spine (rule out pathology related to cervical spine): degree and quality of motion, pain location and severity
        recorded
        Active cervical motion followed by overpressure (e.g., forward bend, backbend, rotations, and lateral flexion)
        Axial compression and distraction (performed manually)
    Neurologic evaluation via a quick manual muscle test to check for weakness: therapist positioned behind patient and
        giving resistance bilaterally
        Motor:
            C2: axial flexion
            C3–4: shoulder shrug
            C5: shoulder abduction at 90 degrees
            C6: elbow flexion
            C7: elbow extension
            C8: wrist extension
            T1: finger abduction
        Sensory:
            Dizziness: yes or no
            Tinnitus: yes or no
            Light touch (may use monofilaments): tested via dermatome mapping and recorded
                C4: top of shoulder
                C5: deltoid area
                C6: lateral arm to thumb
                C7: middle finger
                C8: ulnar aspect of hand
                T1: medial upper arm
        Reflex (hammer):
            C5–C6: biceps tendon
            C7: triceps tendon
        Provocative thoracic outlet tests (see text)

Source: Reprinted from C Moran & SR Saunders (1991). Evaluation of the shoulder: a sequential approach. In RA Donnatelli (Ed). *Physical Therapy of the Shoulder* (2nd ed, pp. 19–62). New York: Churchill Livingstone.

upper-quadrant screen, as outlined in Table 5.5. To discriminate between a neurogenic disorder and tendinitis, sensibility and adverse neural tension tests may be done. Findings may be supported further with palpation and observation of prehension patterns during select tasks. Each portion of the assessment provides important clues about the tissue involved and the activities that provoke signs and symptoms.

Visual Inspection

Before the initiation of any physical tests, it is wise to survey the reported region of involvement. With long-standing tendinitis or nerve compression, there may be observable signs of muscle atrophy in comparing the involved to the uninvolved side. Visual inspection of the involved extremity may

Table 5.6. Interpretation of Resistive Tests

Response to Resistance	Interpretation
Painless	Muscle-tendon unit may be normal
Painful on repetition of resistance	Questionable neurovascular disorder
Strong and painful	Minor lesion of muscle-tendon unit
Weak and painful	Partial rupture of tendon (if passive joint range is normal)
Weak and painless	Complete rupture of muscle-tendon unit or nerve involvement

Source: Modified from J Cyriax (1982). *Textbook of Orthopaedic Medicine, Vol 1: Diagnosis of Soft-Tissue Lesions* (8th ed). London: Bailliere Tindall.

also reveal sites of biomechanical deformity, edema, skin discoloration, or burns. These warning signals should be supported with further testing.

Range of Motion Tests

Extensibility of the muscle-tendon unit is assessed through active and passive ROM tests. Because tendons are contractile tissue, pain will be elicited with passive stretching on injury. To assess muscle-tendon units that cross two or more joints, it is necessary to induce a stretch across all the joints they cross before measuring the most involved joint. For example, the finger flexors cross the wrist and digits. To assess them at maximum length, the fingers and wrist must be extended simultaneously. In this position, wrist extension can be measured to document changes in tissue extensibility with treatment.

Strength Assessment

In the clinic, the tools used to assess strength are manual muscle tests, grip-pinch dynamometers, and isokinetic dynamometers. With the exception of the isokinetic dynamometer, these tests are designed primarily to elicit an isometric contraction. Active contraction of the muscle-tendon unit against resistance may elicit pain or weakness (Cyriax 1982). Response to resistance done in the midrange may be interpreted according to a scale used by Cyriax (Table 5.6). Weakness or poor endurance is often discovered in cases of nerve compression. For example, the subject may not be able to complete a three-cycle segment of testing on the involved side or may not be able to hold a grip on the dynamome-

ter for at least 1 minute during a sustained grip test (Harris 1994). As pain subsides and the injured tissue is allowed to recover or as the nerve compression is lifted, strength measures should improve.

In cases of mild tendinitis or nerve compressions, task simulation may be used to test functional limitations adequately. Task analysis may reveal the method of treatment required to promote full healing of the involved tissue. For example, in acute tendinitis, pain during select tests may be induced secondary to small microtears and subsequent inflammation. In chronic conditions, tissue shortening may be noted, with an inability to sustain loads without significant pain or weakness. The strength and biomechanics of distant areas of the kinetic chain, such as the proximal shoulder girdle, given distal involvement, might be altered and affect performance (Kibler et al. 1992).

Adverse Neural Tension Assessment

Assessment of adverse neural tension is important, especially if a neurogenic disorder is suspected (Elvey et al. 1986; Butler 1991). Adverse neural tensions are those abnormal physiologic and mechanical responses produced by nervous system structures when their extensibility and range is tested (Butler & Guth 1993). Elvey and Butler advise putting tension into the nervous system through selective passive placement techniques, to reproduce the signs and symptoms that the individual is experiencing frequently. Figure 5.17 is an example of a sequential upper-limb tension test 1 for the median nerve. It requires passive depression of the scapula in steps 1 and 2, followed by wrist extension and shoulder external rotation in steps 3 and 4. At this point, the tension is now directed at the elbow. When elbow

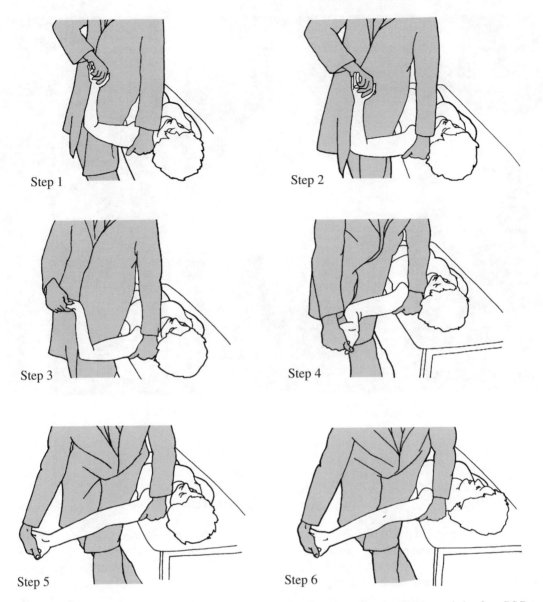

Figure 5.17. Sequential upper-limb tension test (ULTT) 1 for the median nerve. (Reprinted with permission from DS Butler [1991]. *Mobilisation of the Nervous System* [p. 149]. New York: Churchill Livingstone.)

extension begins to create a pins-and-needles sensation or other neurogenic sign, the clinician should stop the stretch and measure the elbow extension. The range available provides an objective assessment of tension tolerance. Treatment via nerve gliding would begin at the point of maximum tension, followed by a hold for 1 second, then an ease in the tension by flexion of the elbow for 1 second. This process continues for 20 seconds. The subject should be asked to report any neurogenic signs during the tension tests or the treatment phase. After an initial assessment, ongoing evaluation should coincide with treatment, especially as compressive forces are alleviated and nerve function begins to increase.

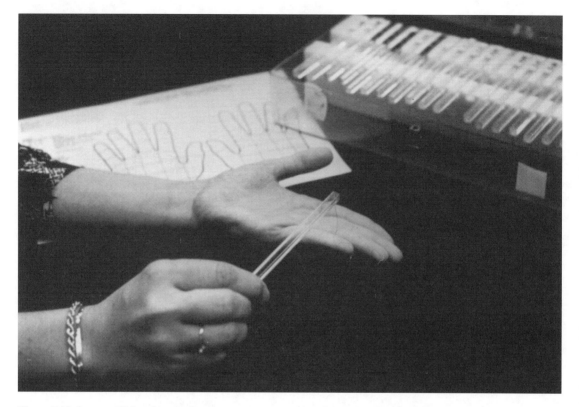

Figure 5.18. Semmes-Weinstein monofilaments used to measure sensibility threshold for light touch.

Sensibility Tests

Sensibility is the conscious appreciation and interpretation of a stimulus that produces sensation. Both academic and functional sensibility tests may be used to identify the extent of nerve damage and to document return. *Academic sensibility* involves interpretation of passive tactile stimuli. It may be assessed via threshold tests, innervation density tests, provocative tests, and tests of sympathetic function. *Functional sensibility* refers to the use of tactile information for active exploration in daily activities and work (Bowden 1954; Seddon 1954; Zachary 1954). Often it is measured by using specific functional or dexterity tests. Following nerve injury, it is possible to achieve recovery of academic sensibility with minimal recovery of functional sensibility (Moberg 1962). The reader is referred to Stone (1992) for a summary of test administration and scoring of common sensibility tests discussed later.

Threshold Tests

Threshold tests are performed to determine the minimal tactile stimulus perceived by an individual with occluded vision (Callahan 1990). Threshold testing is used to demonstrate a gradual or progressive change following nerve compression (Szabo & Gelberman 1987). Classic threshold tests include those used to measure pain, temperature, touch-pressure, and vibratory sensibility. The most reliable and repeatable clinical tool used is the Semmes-Weinstein monofilaments test, which is a test of light touch (Bell-Krotoski 1990). The Semmes-Weinstein monofilaments (Figure 5.18) bend when they reach a peak force and maintain a constant force until recovery. The test is the only hand-held test in which the application force is controlled (Bell-Krotoski et al. 1993). The monofilaments require frequent calibration to ensure accurate length and diameter. The Weinstein enhanced sensory test (WEST) has been introduced as an alternative test of light touch (Weinstein 1993). It is a pocket-sized version of the full 20–nylon filament set. In the WEST, the surface area of the contacting tip is textured to prevent slippage and is hemispheric in shape rather than smooth and flat, like the monofilaments. On bending of the new WEST filaments, the same surface area of the tip remains in contact with the skin. To make the results easier to interpret, the forces (in milligrams) used to bend the monofilaments are printed on the device itself (Weinstein 1993, p. 18). This assessment is not as widely used as the Semmes-Weinstein monofilaments test; as yet, studies of reliability and validity have not been completed.

Innervation Density Tests

Tests of innervation density are based on a select region of nerve innervation and its cortical representation. The most widely used density tests assess static two-point discrimination (Weber 1835) and moving two-point discrimination (Dellon 1978). Weber's test originally required that two compass points be moved inward until the subject could no longer detect two points; this was modified to touching the individual with either one point or two. Although the two-point discrimination test has frequently been referred to as a strong measure of tactile gnosis, it is considered to have only fair reliability and validity because of the variation in force application of the hand-held test device. Moving two-point discrimination varies in both rate and force of application, further compromising its reliability and validity. Despite the caution, Dellon et al. (1987) demonstrated improved reliability in testing two-point discrimination by using the "Disk-Criminator" with a specific protocol. The reader should be cognizant of the concerns addressed when interpreting the results of two-point discrimination tests.

Provocative Tests

Provocative tests are screening tools that invoke a signal or sign of sensation or lack of sensation on the basis of response to a specific movement. Common provocative tests are those of nerve percussion, nerve compression, and stress testing. Nerve percussion was introduced by Tinel (1915) and involves tapping over the nerve (at either a superficial

location or the location to which the nerve end has regenerated). A positive result induces tingling or paresthesias in the distal nerve distribution. Tinel's sign has become a popular method of detecting the presence of axons and serves as an indication of regeneration. Compression tests are used to provoke signs of nerve involvement by placing the involved region in compromising positions (Callahan 1990). One example is Phalen's wrist flexion test (1966), which "squeezes" the median nerve between the flexor tendons, the radius, and the transverse carpal ligament. The subject is requested to hold the forearms vertically, leaning on the elbows and allowing both hands to drop into complete flexion. The subject is asked to hold this position for 1 minute (Phalen 1966, p. 214). Phalen's test may induce feelings of numbness and paresthesia if the median nerve already is somewhat compressed.

Because some nerve compressions and cases of tendinitis are caused by repetitive motion over a period, it may be necessary to replicate the cause of symptoms through stress tests. A stress test combines sensibility testing with activities that may induce symptoms of nerve compression (Callahan 1990). If stress testing is performed, prebaseline and postbaseline measurements are taken. For example, to induce the symptoms associated with radial tunnel or pronator syndrome, repetitive forearm rotation for a sustained period may have to be used. Baseline measurements may include sensibility testing, pain assessment, or volume measurements. Results from the baseline measurements may or may not implicate structures affected by repetitive activity that may be addressed through treatment or activity modification.

Sympathetic Signs of Nerve Injury

Sympathetic signs of nerve injury may be highlighted by select objective tests. Three categories of sympathetic testing include vasomotor tests of skin color or temperature; sudomotor or sweat tests; tests for pilomotor (or gooseflesh response); and tests for trophic changes, such as alterations in skin texture, soft-tissue atrophy, nail changes, hair growth, and rate of healing. Two tests, the sweat test and the wrinkle test, are used commonly. The Ninhydrin sweat test of sudomotor (sweat) function was introduced by Guttman in 1940 and modified by Moberg in 1954 (Moran & Callahan

1983). The O'Riain wrinkle test (1973) was based on O'Riain's observation that the skin of denervated tissue did not wrinkle when immersed in water. Of the two tests, the Ninhydrin sweat test has been used most frequently in pediatric cases and in cases of malingering to verify nerve injury.

Functional (Dexterity) Tests

Functional sensibility (or tactile gnosis) was first described by Broman in 1945 (Moran & Callahan 1983). It is defined as the quality of cutaneous sensibility needed for a precision sensory grip or "seeing" with the fingers (Moberg 1960, p. 357). There are varied tests used to determine manual or finger dexterity (Dellon & Kallman 1983; Apfel & Carranza 1992). These tests differ as to required tool use and grasp patterns; thus, a combination of tests may help to correlate individual prehensile skill and the status of the nerve. Common tests include the Purdue pegboard test, the Crawford small parts test, the Moberg pick-up test, the nine-hole peg test, and the Minnesota rate of manipulation test. Specific functional tests include the Jebsen-Taylor hand function test, the modified Moberg picking-up test, the Sollerman grip and function test, and the Apfel 19-item pick-up test. The reader is referred to Apfel and Carranza (1992) for information about administration and scoring. Rider and Linden (1988) compared standardized administration of the Jebsen-Taylor Test of Hand Function (JTHF) (Jebsen et al. 1969) to nonstandardized methods. Because plastic checkers and 1.25-in. paper clips often are used in place of wooden checkers or 1-in. paper clips, the authors investigated the effects of these substitutions. They found a significant difference in test scores using plastic rather than wooden checkers. Although all groups displayed faster pick-up of 1.25-in. paper clips, the results were not significant. Until the JTHF is restandardized with the substitute items, therapists are cautioned against comparing scores to the prescribed norms. For accurate verification of one's functional status, more comprehensive tests with up-to-date functional tasks may have to be designed.

Dellon (1993) has proposed a grading scale of peripheral nerve function. Scores on a 0–10 scale would be calculated on the basis of findings from the clinical assessment. A score of 0 would be equated with findings in the normal range. A score of 10 would be given for severe atrophy and severely limited sensibility test findings. Although this scale has yet to be validated, it may enhance communication among professionals regarding findings from multiple sources of assessment.

Palpation

Because palpation is the least reliable method of determining the nature of the disorder and may introduce bias, it should be the last item performed in a physical examination (Cyriax 1982; Rodineau 1991). Palpation of the involved region may induce pain or reveal alterations in tissue integrity (including atrophy). Tenderness over select sites may reveal the source of pain or indicate an area of referred pain. Trigger points and sites of specific tendon or nerve irritation may be localized. For example, in cases of tennis elbow, the lateral epicondyle may be particularly sensitive to touch pressure.

Adaptive Changes in Nearby Tissue

Adaptive changes in regions away from the local site of pain may influence the effectiveness of rehabilitation if not evaluated and addressed. Such alterations may include muscle strength, tissue flexibility, and biomechanics of nearby regions. For instance, shoulder weakness and inflexibility in the individual with lateral epicondylitis may delay healing because the shoulder musculature may not contribute fully during upper-limb resistive tasks. Therefore, excess stress may be imparted to the vulnerable common extensor tendon, the bony attachment of which lies very close to the myotendinous junction.

Therapeutic Intervention

Therapeutic intervention for CTDs requires careful consideration of tissue involvement and its condition. Because recovery from injury may follow a course resembling the stages of wound healing, it is reviewed here for reference. The stages are reviewed, along with treatment corresponding to these stages. Separate sections will address select intervention strategies for tendinitis and nerve compressions and entrapments.

Stages of Wound Healing

The three phases of wound healing—inflammation, proliferation, and remodeling—overlap. For example, there may be some inflammatory cells present in a healing wound as it begins to proliferate new fibroblasts (Fyfe & Stanish 1992). Acute injuries follow a relatively sequential process of wound healing in the absence of further stress. However, chronic injuries typically do not follow this course, and healing is often halted at one phase or another. It is possible that conservative treatment may promote sequential wound repair. If unsuccessful, surgical intervention may be needed to remove degenerative or compressive tissue and to induce tissue repair.

Inflammatory Phase (Acute)

The postinjury inflammatory phase lasts approximately 5–7 days (Peacock 1965). The cardinal signs of inflammation (redness, pain, heat, swelling) are induced by an enzymatically driven sequence, led by the production of arachidonic acid, phospholipids, and other metabolites (Rubin & Faber 1988). In this phase, the vascular disruption initiates platelet activation and a clotting mechanism. A fibrin clot is formed when fibronectin or adhesive molecules cross-link with collagen. During this phase, any tissue damaged in the initial trauma is removed from the region. In addition, endothelial sites and fibroblasts are recruited and stimulated to divide (Martens et al. 1982).

Proliferation (Subacute)

The subacute phase, which lasts from 3 days to 6–8 weeks, has been termed *fibroplasia*. This phase begins with the production of collagen by the third day. The relative hypoxia within the wound and the increase in lactate levels are the critical operating forces (Hunt & Hussain 1992). During this stage, vascularity is increased, and by day 12, there is a significant reduction in inflammatory cells. The teknocyte is the reparative cell, determined to be the source of collagen production, protein mediators, and matrix proteoglycans. The mobile macrophage directs the sequence of events leading to wound repair (Martens et al. 1982; Rubin & Faber 1988). It is able to release

growth factors, chemoattractants, and proteolytic enzymes when needed, to activate fibroblasts or tendon repair. If the provocative activity causing the injury is modified or avoided during this phase, the tissue should mature and recondition.

Remodeling

This stage of healing continues throughout life. However, 17–28 days after injury, the collagen content is weaker than normal (Peacock 1965). During this period, cellularity and synthetic activity are decreased. There is an increase in extracellular matrix organization and normalization of the biochemical profile (Laurent 1987). Longitudinal tension induced through select activity aids remodeling. If the tissue is allowed to progress through this phase, collagen matures, and linear realignment of fibers is noted by 2 months.

Intervention for Tendinitis and Related Conditions

Management of tendinitis and related conditions is often difficult because injury often occurs in regions frequently used to accomplish daily activities. Therefore, it may be difficult to advance an individual through the phases of wound healing in a predictable manner.

Treatment of tendinitis or tendinosis may follow a conservative nonsurgical course. The overall goal of nonsurgical treatment is to promote revascularization and collagen repair, allowing the formation of a strong yet mobile scar that can withstand the loads induced in functional activity and recreation (Cyriax 1982). Treatment level is based on clinical findings. As a general guide, tendinitis or tendinosis can be treated in three levels that follow the phases of wound healing. General goals and methods for conservative treatment are listed in Table 5.7. Restriction of the provocative activity is primary. Key restrictions for most types of upper-limb tendinitis are listed in Table 5.8.

If signs and symptoms persist or are severe enough, surgical intervention may be warranted. The primary goal of surgical treatment is to remove degenerated tissue and to promote a renewed cycle of wound repair so as to alter the cell matrix of the tendon (Leadbetter 1991). Goals following surgical treat-

Table 5.7. Management of Tendinitis and Tendinosis

Goal	Method
Level one	
Protect and rest affected regions	Restrict provocative activities
	Splint affected areas
	Provide ergonomic equipment
	Encourage frequent breaks
Reduce pain and inflammation	Rest and support affected areas
	Ice
	Transcutaneous electrical nerve stimulation
	Phonophoresis or pulsed ultrasound
	Iontophoresis
Level two	
Increase mobility and length of the involved tissue	Superficial heat modalities
	Continuous low-level ultrasound
	Massage
	Myofascial release techniques
	Active range of motion with stretching
Increase knowledge of cause and prevention of tendinitis	Perform task analysis
	Educate
Level three	
Increase tolerance to controlled stress	Graded strengthening
Enhance motor control in work-related and sports tasks and activities of daily living	Practice
Promote return to premorbid function	Task simulation

Note: At all levels, it is important to monitor pain associated with activity.
Sources: Modified from M Lindsay (1993). Radial tunnel versus lateral epicondylitis. *Newsletter of the Section on Hand Rehabilitation of the American Physical Therapy Association*, 10(39),1; and M Kasch (March 1993). Nerve compressions. Presented at the Rehabilitation of the Hand annual meeting, sponsored by the Hand Center of Thomas Jefferson University, Philadelphia, PA.

ment resemble those for nonsurgical treatment, with the additional goal of postoperative scar management.

Intervention for Nerve Compressions and Entrapments

Most of the research regarding regeneration has been done on nerve lacerations and repairs. In terms of compressions, inferences often are made because there is much variation in terms of recovery. Recovery can begin when the compressive forces or entrapping structures have been removed. Decompression may involve removal of causative factors, such as edema or fibrosis. If the nerve compression is not relieved with removal of the presumed cause or provocative activity, surgical decompression may be necessary. Once decompressed, the nerve may follow the course of wound repair. However, it is vital that regeneration of the damaged axon occur.

Anatomic Considerations in Nerve Regeneration

Ideally, regeneration results in a reversal of changes that may have occurred during the period of compression. The type and location of the peripheral nerve compression determines the outcome of the reinnervation. Proximal lesions have a better chance of full return than do distal lesions, because of their proximity to the cell body. Recovery of sensation will be determined by the number and types of axons that establish functional connections with cutaneous receptors. In addition, changes in the encoding properties of regenerated fibers and the response of the somatosensory cortex to deprivation of input also will affect return (Braune & Schady 1993). Motor function will be determined by the number and type of reconnections to the end organs serving the muscles. In compressions, there is a strong possibility that some endoneurial tubes were left intact. With the tube intact, the axon has a better

Table 5.8. Key Restrictions in Upper-Limb Tendinitis

Disorder	Restriction
Rotator cuff tendinitis	Overhead activities
Bicipital tendinitis	Resisted elbow flexion and shoulder flexion with elbow extended
Lateral epicondylitis	Resisted gripping, wrist extension, and excessive elbow motion
Medial epicondylitis	Resisted wrist flexion, pronation, and excessive elbow motion
Intersection syndrome	Thumb and wrist flexion
Flexor paratendinitis (tenosynovitis)	Resisted gripping
de Quervain's disease	Resisted pinching
Trigger thumb or finger	Resisted thumb or finger flexion

chance of regrowing toward the correct target tissue (Brandenburg & Mann 1989).

Regeneration following nerve lacerations and repair typically is preceded by a 2- to 3-week latency period. Following this latency period, the nerve should regrow at a rate of 1–3 mm per day. Insidious onset of nerve compression alters this typical concept of nerve regeneration. Instead of the entire nerve, it may be only one axon or fascicle that has suffered damage. Intraneural fibrosis will effect the ability of the axon to regrow. After a period of compression, the regenerating nerve may also undergo a latency period before regeneration secondary to the effects of fibrosis (Braune & Schady 1993). As research continues, one explanation may prove more valid than the others.

Factors Affecting Regeneration

Successful nerve regeneration requires that specific conditions be in place:

1. The central neuron must survive.
2. The environment must be able to support axonal sprouting and growth.
3. The regenerated axon must make appropriate distal contact with receptors.
4. The CNS must integrate the signals from the PNS appropriately.

Axon regeneration is encouraged through contact guidance and neurotropism. In studies of nerve lacerations, factors within the distal nerve stump seem to be associated with regrowth of the proximal segments. Humoral, cellular, and molecular factors may serve to guide the regenerating axon.

In addition, cell bodies of regenerating nerves send out chemical messengers that make their way down the axon by traveling within the axoplasm (see Figure 5.4), directed by the distal segment (Lundborg et al. 1986; Mackinnon et al. 1986). Because some component of the connective tissue surrounding the axon is often intact in compression injuries, it is hypothesized that regeneration guided through neurotropism is achieved with greater success.

Enhancement of the environment surrounding the axon is currently being researched. Investigations regarding local drug application to nerve sites damaged by crush injuries or lacerations have begun. In animal studies, Kanje et al. (1988) injected a regenerating sciatic nerve encased in a silicone tube. The authors found the rate of regeneration to be on the order of 3.5 mm per day, which followed an initial delay of 1.6 days. They further supported the notion that proliferation and protein synthesis of cells around the affected axon were required for regeneration. Fortunately, in compression there is often some continuity of connective tissue structures that allows for the regeneration without the need for such intervention. However, future research may prove the benefit of drug injection to be the enhancement of the environment surrounding the nerve.

Given the conditions outlined earlier, a damaged nerve will eventually grow back into its former location. Unfortunately, nerve regeneration is often delayed and unpredictable. The complications to regeneration include shrinkage of the endoneurial tubes; mismatching of motor, sensory, and sympathetic nervous system fibers; degeneration of end receptors; the presence of scarring at the injury site; and ineffective central reorganization.

Table 5.9. Management of Nerve Compression or Entrapment

Goal	Method
Level one	
Protect and rest affected regions	Restrict provocative activities
	Splint affected areas
	Provide ergonomic equipment
	Encourage frequent breaks
Reduce pain and inflammation	Rest and support affected areas
	Ice
	Transcutaneous electrical nerve stimulation
	Phonophoresis or pulsed ultrasound
	Iontophoresis
Reduce pressure	Viscoelastic inserts, ergonomic tools
Level two	
Increase circulation	Active range-of-motion exercises
	Thermal modalities (monitor decreased sensation)
	Avoid caffeine and nicotine
	Aerobic exercises
Promote soft-tissue mobility	Massage
	Myofascial release techniques
	Stretching, range of motion
Enhance nerve gliding	Nerve-gliding techniques (passive and active)
	Myofascial release techniques
Level three	
Enhance motor control and function	Task simulation
	Work-site evaluation

Note: At all levels, it is important to monitor edema, sensitivity, motor recovery, and strength.
Sources: Modified from M Lindsay (1993). Radial tunnel versus lateral epicondylitis. *Newsletter of the Section on Hand Rehabilitation of the American Physical Therapy Association*, 10(39),1; and M Kasch (March 1993). Nerve compressions. Presented at the Rehabilitation of the Hand annual meeting, sponsored by the Hand Center of Thomas Jefferson University, Philadelphia, PA.

Promoting Regeneration

Clinicians are always looking for methods to improve function conservatively, given peripheral nerve compressions and entrapments. General goals and methods for conservative treatment by levels are listed in Table 5.9. Splints are used to reduce the effects of muscle imbalances. Extensive sensory programs follow individuals from absent through protective sensation before return of light touch. Once the finger exhibits protective sensation (as detected by a 4.3-gauge filament from the Semmes-Weinstein monofilament test), a sensory re-education program is initiated. Although touch pressure thresholds cannot be improved by means of re-education or functional use, sensory re-education can enhance central reorganization (Bell-Krotoski et al. 1993; Pascual-Leone & Torres 1993). Enhancement of central

reorganization may involve an increase in receptive field representation for the involved nerve or an increase in the number of central regions recruited during select tasks.

Besides sensory re-education, what can be done to promote quicker and more accurate regeneration of peripheral nerves? Walker et al. (1994) found axonal regeneration in the sciatic nerve could be accelerated via pulsed electromagnetic fields (PEMF), as evaluated through functional outcomes. The functional measures they used included toe abduction, duration of the stance phase during gait, and a sciatic function index based on footprint analyses (see Walker et al. 1994 for details). Throughout the 43-day recovery period, gains were made in both toe abduction and duration of stance. However, the sciatic function index proved insignificant. How PEMF enhances nerve regeneration is unknown and currently is under investigation by the authors. Pending adequate efficacy studies, PEMF may become available for use within clinical populations.

Treatment by Levels

Although many have divided treatment into acute versus chronic phases, this chapter uses the concept of treatment levels described by Lindsay (1994). Designation by levels allows guidance through sequential treatment while monitoring pain and activity tolerance. Although there is a distinct difference between treatment of tendinous and neurogenic disorders, there are enough similarities to warrant discussion of the available treatment strategies in a combined fashion.

Level 1: Inflammatory Phase

The primary goals of conservative treatment at this level are to reduce pain and inflammation and to prevent further injury, whether neurogenic or tendinous. It is also important to protect and monitor the acute condition.

Activity Modification.   During this phase, it is best to avoid activities or tasks that provoke or exacerbate signs and symptoms. This avoidance may be accomplished via supportive splinting or activity modification. Static splinting may be indicated to protect the region from repetitive trauma or compressive forces and to reduce inflammation or edema. The afflicted individual should thoroughly understand all tasks that may interfere with tendon or nerve healing. Because of the negative effects of immobilization, ROM maintenance of uninvolved regions and nerve mobilization away from the injured site should be encouraged. According to Butler (1991), nerve mobilization at this level requires taking up slack in the neural system away from the site of pain and mobilizing the neural system for brief intervals (e.g., 1-second pressure on, 1-second pressure off, for a total of 20 seconds).

Modalities.   Pain and inflammation may be reduced via steroidal or nonsteroidal anti-inflammatory drugs (NSAIDs), phonophoresis, cryotherapy techniques, pulsed ultrasound, transcutaneous electrical nerve stimulation (TENS) and rest. Exact clin-ical applications of the modalities vary, depending on the individual case.

Anti-Inflammatory Medication.   Local injections are one method used to reduce inflammation in cases of tendinitis and inflammation surrounding a nerve. In select cases, a mixture of anesthetic and water-soluble corticosteroid is used. To avoid negative side effects, the number of injections is frequently limited to three, with a 6-week interval between injections (Warhold et al. 1993). For cases of tenosynovitis, corticosteroids work by interacting with the synovial fluid; thus, they should be injected only into the tendon sheath. It has been postulated that postinjection ultrasound might enhance the benefits of the injected corticosteroid (Newman et al. 1958; W Nagler, personal communication, 1995).

To avoid the effects of needle injection, ultrasound may be used to drive anti-inflammatory medication through the skin to the involved tendon or nerve region, a process termed *phonophoresis* (Ziskin & Michlovitz 1986; Kahn 1991). Theoretically, the molecular transmission across the skin occurs because of changes in tissue permeability with ultrasound heating and because the radiation pressure of the ultrasound beam forces the medication away from the transducer. Although hydrocortisone and dexamethasone are commonly used, lidocaine and zinc oxide are also suitable molecules for phonophoresis. The strength of medication that should be used is controversial. In the case of hydrocortisone, some advocate that at least 10% be used, yet others report no difference in penetration between 5 and 10% hydrocortisone (Davick et al. 1988). Despite the use of a coupling agent, the amount of medication that penetrates the tissue via ultrasound is minimal because of the entrapment of air at a microscopic level, which serves as a blocking mechanism. To enhance the effects of transmission, some have advocated massaging the medication into the site first, then applying the ultrasound, using a coupling gel (Warren et al. 1976; Edwards 1991; Kahn 1991). Because the benefits of phonophoresis remain questionable, further research is warranted.

Iontophoresis (or ion transfer) involves the use of direct current to drive in medication (Kahn 1994). The process uses the physics principle: *like charges repel*. The desired anti-inflammatory medication is repelled from beneath an electrode with an identical

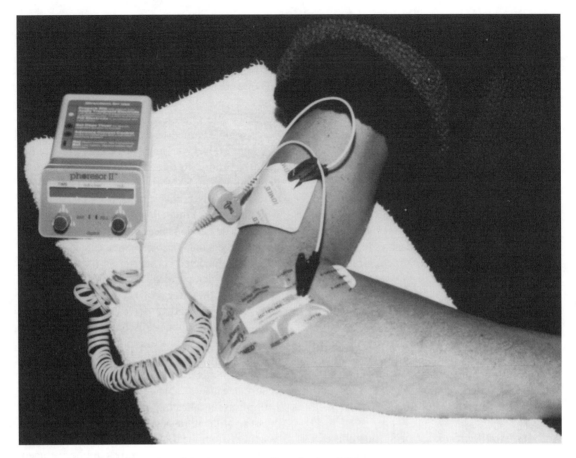

Figure 5.19. Example of iontophoresis in the treatment of lateral epicondylitis.

charge into the skin subdermally. Although the medication penetrates to a depth of less than 1 mm, deeper absorption occurs through transmembrane transport and capillary circulation. Therapeutic compounds are formed as the ions recombine with ions and radicals in the bloodstream. The ionic charge of the medication and the pathology determine whether the positive (anode) or negative (cathode) electrode should be used. For example, hydrocortisone contains positive ions, thus the positive electrode is used; dexamethasone contains negative ions, thus the negative electrode is used. The anode (+) produces a weak hydrochloric acid, is sclerotic or tends to harden tissue, and serves as an analgesic on the basis of the local release of oxygen. The cathode (−) releases hydrogen and is sclerotic, tending to soften tissue. The cathode is considered ideal for use as the active electrode, yet can lead to chemical burns due to the formation of sodium hydroxide at the elec-

trode site. Other complications from iontophoresis include heat burns from excess tissue resistance; sensitivities; and allergic reactions. Units designed exclusively for use with iontophoresis have made the modality easier and safer to use, thus more popular during the acute condition. An example of the setup of iontophoresis to treat lateral epicondylitis is pictured in Figure 5.19.

Other Modalities.   Cryotherapy, or the use of cold agents, can be used effectively to reduce pain and decrease inflammation (Michlovitz 1986). In addition, cold alters the synaptic activity and conduction velocity of peripheral nerves. Popular clinical methods of cryotherapy include cold packs, ice massage, and vapocoolant sprays. The location and size of the body part to be treated determines the best method. If commercial cold packs are used, a moist towel interface between the cold pack and the skin will eliminate much of the air interface and will facilitate energy transfer. Typically, ice massage is done over small areas, such as tendons, using water frozen in a paper cup. Ice massage will induce four separate sensations: intense cold, burning, aching, and analgesia. Vapocoolant sprays are often used to inactivate trigger points and to increase passive ROM of the muscle-tendon unit. The *stretch-and-spray technique* first places the muscle on stretch, then the muscle is sprayed two to three times from its proximal to distal attachment and over the region of referred pain, in parallel unidirectional sweeps. The spray is angled at approximately 30 degrees, 18 in. from the skin, and is moved at a rate of 10 cm per second (Travell & Simons 1983). Precautions against cryotherapy include cold insensitivity (e.g., Raynaud's phenomenon). Local hypersensitivity is indicated by wheals (small regions with erythematous raised borders and blanched centers). Cold treatment should be used cautiously in hypertensive individuals and in the early stage of wound healing, because of its effect on blood flow.

A pulsed mode of ultrasound at 20 or 50% without medication can be used to treat tendinitis successfully on the basis of its nonthermal effects (Ziskin & Michlovitz 1986). Within the pulsed mode, it is advisable to extend the application period to allow for maximal penetration of the sound waves.

TENS can also be used to reduce pain. Two theories attempt to explain the positive effect of TENS: the gate theory by Melzack and Wall (1965) and the endorphin concept (Sjolund & Eriksson 1979; Adler 1982). The gate theory proposes that pressure or touch input from large A beta fibers can modulate the specific or diffuse pain signals sent by small A delta or C fibers. Melzack and Wall (1965) postulated that T cells or second-order neurons within the spinal cord serve as transmission junctions for nerve fibers carrying the sensation of pain to the thalamus. Further, both large- and small-diameter sensory neurons are primary afferents that impinge on the substantia gelatinosa and the T cell. The substantia gelatinosa interneurons act to modulate or gate the sensory message sent to the brain via presynaptic inhibition on the large- and small-diameter fibers before they reach the T cell. A reduction in substantia gelatinosa activity, as influenced by a high percentage of small-fiber "pain" input, results in a decrease in presynaptic control. This allows the gate

to be open and the sensory input to the T cell to go unaltered. With the gate open, pain sensations can reach the thalamus. If the substantia gelatinosa is activated through large-fiber input (touch, pressure), there is greater presynaptic control on the first-order neurons, and the gate is in a closed position. This results in a decrease in T-cell sensory input and a reduction in pain sensation. TENS works by increasing the input to A beta fibers, which closes the gate through its action on the substantia gelatinosa. This theory has required modifications due to advances in neuroscience; however, it provides a general framework for the use of TENS in treatment of acute and chronic pain. Endorphins, morphine-like molecules produced by the body, serve as endogenous analgesics to pain. Levels of endorphins increase in the blood when afferent brain signals indicate pain. Low-frequency TENS of 1–4 Hz have been found to increase endorphin production. For those with chronic tendinitis and pain due to nerve compressions and entrapments, low-rate TENS would provide the most pain relief (Wolf 1984).

Level 2: Proliferative Phase

During the proliferative phase, the primary goals are to increase mobility and length of the involved tissue while preventing recurrence of the injury and resultant inflammation.

Superficial or deep heating may increase blood flow before massage, stretching, or myofascial release techniques to prepare the tissue for exercise. Due to its vasodilation effect, heat is best used after the threat of inflammation has subsided sufficiently. Superficial heat penetrates to depths of 1 cm. Methods include hot packs, paraffin wax, or "fluidotherapy." Deeper heating may be obtained with continuous ultrasound, which can penetrate tissues 3–5 cm in depth (Ziskin & Michlovitz 1986). In addition to increasing blood flow, low-intensity ultrasound may induce tissue growth in involved structures (Dyson et al. 1968). It has been postulated that acoustic streaming, a nonthermal effect of ultrasound, may alter ion fluxes across tissue membranes, thereby facilitating repair.

In cases of tendinitis, deep-friction (cross-fiber) massage theoretically breaks up adhesions that typically form during healing of small tendon tears (Cyriax 1982). Soft-tissue massage and isometrics increase blood flow in the region of the myotendinous junction and tendon, wherein blood flow typically is much less than that of the muscle belly. Forcing blood into the undernourished myotendinous-tendon regions may be achieved by massaging from the muscle belly toward the tendon. This technique would be followed by a stretch, to the involved muscle-tendon unit.

Myofascial release is another method of intervention that addresses restrictions within the loose connective tissue associated with the muscle-tendon unit and peripheral nerves. Several techniques may be used, including unwinding and cross-stretch. In cases of peripheral nerve compression, it may be advantageous to first perform adverse neural tension tests, then to perform myofascial release techniques to address the interfacing tissues associated with the nerve.

Researchers have found that isometric warm-ups with follow-up stretching give the muscle greater toleration of force before failure (Safran et al. 1988). If isometrics or nonresisted eccentric-concentric loading induces pain, it may be best to follow the treatment with ice. An ideal sequence of treatment may be massage followed by stretching or myofascial release, initiation of isometrics, or nonresisted eccentric-concentric loading and ending with ice. When the individual does not have pain with simple stretching or moderate loading, it may be safe to reintroduce the activity or task that typically caused the most pain.

During level 2, active exercise should be included in the program to restore range of motion and to strengthen uninvolved muscles. Active and passive nerve mobilization at the site of compression may be performed as long as it does not provoke symptoms. As stated, myofascial release techniques may also be used to enhance nerve gliding via its reported effect on the loose connective tissue. In select cases, it may be necessary to continue protection of the involved site and to avoid the provocative activity.

Level 3: Recovery Stage

During level 3 treatment, the primary goals are to increase tolerance to controlled stress of involved regions and to enhance motor control within work, sports, and activities of daily life. In addition, it is important to educate the individual as to the cause of injury and methods of prevention.

Healing tendon and myotendinous regions requires a controlled loading stimulus to form an organized scar. Weak tissue with a poorly organized scar may be at risk for reinjury if repetitive forceful activity is resumed prematurely. Strengthening the involved areas may begin best with isometrics, as in level 2, and progress through eccentric work and general progressive resistive exercise. Controlled loading should be introduced and progressed. In addition, strengthening of proximal regions may reduce distal signs and symptoms significantly. Curwin and Stanish (1984) outlined in detail the components of an eccentric exercise program for tendinitis. Their program highlighted key features: length, load, and speed of contraction. In sequence, the program involves stretch, eccentric exercise, stretch, and ice. Although each region has unique features and individuals have various levels of activity, an ongoing problem-solving approach is best to assess and treat these disorders. Research into effective treatment methodology is somewhat controversial. Almekinders and Almekinders (1994) found that neither activity modification nor NSAIDs with stretching and strengthening was associated with a positive result on the basis of a questionnaire. Because the best method of treatment has yet to be determined, individual cases of tendinitis should be treated separately. The methods that promote full healing and conditioning of the injured tendon unit may not be the same for all people.

During the phase of recovery from nerve injury, regeneration should be monitored in terms of motor, sensory, and sympathetic function. In some cases, relearning of movement and prehension patterns must be addressed. Sensory re-education may be indicated to promote desensitization and to enhance protective and discriminative sensibility through cortical reorganization. It may be necessary to incorporate postural concepts and ergonomics as they pertain to causative factors. Aerobic exercise and proper breathing strategies may further enhance the recovery of function.

Finally, preparation for regular occupations, including work and recreation, are indicated. Enhancing motor control and the timing of muscle recruitment may be the key to promoting carryover of any rehabilitation procedures. In preparing an individual to return to work or sports activity, simulation of the related tasks is vital. In addition, it may be necessary to evaluate the size and weight of tools

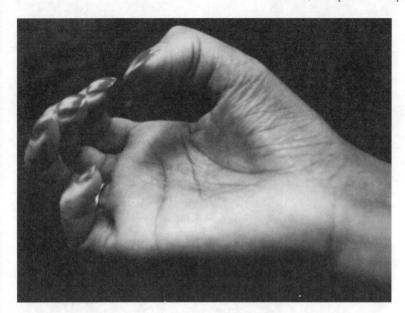

Figure 5.20. Result of long-standing cervical rib compression of the brachial plexus. Note flattened thenar eminence, adducted thumb, and claw position of the fingers as this woman attempts to make a fist.

or sports implements used and to redesign the work and recreation space, because the set-up itself may be perpetuating injury. These issues are addressed in later chapters.

Interventions for Common Upper-Limb Cumulative Trauma Disorders

Cervicobrachial Region

Thoracic Outlet Syndrome. Typically, signs and symptoms of thoracic outlet syndrome (TOS) fall under a larger category termed *neurovascular entrapment syndromes of the upper quadrant* (Edgelow 1995). This author emphasizes that TOS is actually a problem of reversible or irreversible stenosis or rigid narrowing from acquired or congenital conditions. Figure 5.9 highlights common regions of stenosis. Despite Edgelow's clear distinction of TOS as a problem of stenosis, others continue to separate TOS into either a compressive or an entrapment disorder.

Compressions usually implicate postural deficits that may perpetuate signs and symptoms induced from repetitive strain disorders. In compressions, pain is often nocturnal or activity-related. Because of its location, the lower plexus (including nerve fibers from C8 to T1) is at a greater risk of com-

pression. However, it is possible that any region of the plexus may be implicated (Kelly 1979; Szabo 1989). Entrapments often have some association with cervical-shoulder trauma or an anatomic abnormality. It is possible that they are also related to long-standing repetitive stress (Walsh 1994). Figure 5.20 exemplifies the severe damage that may ensue from long-standing nerve entrapment, in this case from a cervical rib. Pain associated with entrapments can be divided into nerve trunk pain and dysesthetic pain. Nerve trunk pain occurs secondary to increased activity in the nociceptive endings of the nerve nervorum (sheath). Dysesthetic pain occurs by virtue of impulses from damaged or regenerating afferent fibers (Asbury & Fields 1984). Further subjective and objective findings of TOS are outlined in Table 5.10.

Findings from cervical x-rays and other diagnostic tests should be obtained before a physical examination is conducted. Confirmation of TOS should include assessment of static and active posture, shoulder–cervical spine active ROM, grip and pinch strength, sensibility, provocative testing, and endurance testing. For example, the individual pictured from the side in Figure 5.21 presented with neurogenic signs and subtle postural deficits, such as a dowager's hump, rounded shoulders, abducted scapulas, and slight forward

Table 5.10. Cervicobrachial Syndromes: Subjective and Objective Findings

Thoracic outlet syndrome

    Pain, paresthesias, and numbness in an ulnar nerve distribution

    Occasional transitory ischemia and edema

    Burning pain over select dermatomal regions

    Progressive sensory and motor loss in distal sites

    Possible positive findings with provocative maneuvers

Cervical radiculopathy

    Neck pain and referred pain of a dermatomal nature rather than a diffuse one

    Symptoms of cervical disc protrusion *reproduced* with neck bending to the opposite side

    Spinal stenosis symptoms *relieved* with neck bending to the opposite side

    Often, muscle group weakness (rhomboids, trapezius) and abnormal tendon reflexes

    Symptoms from cervical disc and stenosis relieved with cervical traction and exacerbated with compression

    Provocative thoracic outlet syndrome tests negative

    Possible coexistent cervical nerve compression and distal site of compression

Sources: Thoracic outlet syndrome information modified from RM Szabo (1989). *Nerve Compression Syndromes: Diagnosis and Treatment*. Thorofare, NJ: Slack, Inc.; and MT Walsh (April–June 1994). Therapist management of thoracic outlet syndrome. *J Hand Ther,* 7(2),131–144. Cervical radiculopathy information modified from R Cailliet (1991). *Shoulder Pain* (3rd ed). Philadelphia: Davis; and ARM Upton & AJ McComas (1973). The double crush in nerve entrapment syndromes. *Lancet,* 2,359–362.

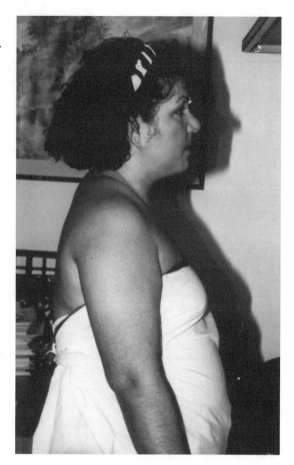

Figure 5.21. Side-view posture of woman with suspected thoracic outlet syndrome. Note her rounded shoulders, dowager's hump, and forward head posture.

head posture. These postural deficits may be related to TOS signs and symptoms.

Provocative tests should be used cautiously because they can produce a high incidence of false-positive results. Adson's maneuver (1951) tests for nerve compression within the scalene triangle. It requires a 30-second palpation of the radial artery while the individual takes a deep breath, elevates the chin, and rotates the head first in the direction of pain, then in the opposite direction. A positive test involves a reduction in palpable pulse rate or exacerbation of symptoms during extremes of movement. This test supposedly induces upper-trunk symptoms versus those of the lower trunk. Wright's maneuver requires neck rotation to the opposite side and passive abduction above 90 degrees while changes in the radial pulse and neurogenic symptoms are monitored (Wright 1945; Walsh 1994). This maneuver tests for nerve compression beneath the pectoralis minor muscle at less than 90 degrees humeral abduction and compression between the clavicle and first rib at more than 90 degrees. The costoclavicular compression test attempts to rule out compression between the first rib and the clavicle. With the arms at the side, an individual actively retracts and depresses the scapula while the radial pulse and symptoms are monitored. Harris (1994) recommended that endurance be tested through timed grasping of a 10-lb gripper (normal: 5 minutes) and the Roos elevated stress test. The Roos test (1966) (or the 3-minute elevated-arm stress test) is the most reliable provocative test for evaluating for TOS. In the "surrender" position (arms abducted and externally rotated to 90 degrees with the forearms pronated), the subject is asked to open and close the hands once every 2 seconds and to describe symptoms during the 3-minute test. This position accentuates the abnormal compressions affecting the brachial plexus and vessels. It narrows the costoclavicular space and tenses the neck and shoulder muscles. In most positive tests, the individual cannot complete 3 minutes without reproduction of symptoms. With positive TOS, there are complaints of heaviness or fatigue in the involved extremity. Feelings of pins and needles or numbness may follow, along with a progressive ache.

Within level 1, treatment may involve restriction of aggravating activities, such as humeral hyperabduction, static neck flexion, and repetitive overhead shoulder flexion. It is recommended that pressure on the plexus be minimized through elbow propping, avoidance of carrying or lifting, and the use of a backpack or pull cart rather than a shoulder bag. Muscular and nerve inflammation as well as edema may be addressed via NSAIDs, ice, or TENS. Edgelow (1995) stressed the importance of relaxing the scalene muscle(s) (or other related musculature) if inflamed or enlarged. Although nerve gliding away from the involved region may be introduced at this level, myofascial release may relieve compression and thus promote relief of symptoms. By level 2, the inflammatory phase has typically subsided and heat and stretch techniques, along with myofascial release strategies, may be used to enhance circulation and tissue extensibility. Postural deficits such as rounded shoulders and forward head posture can be addressed through correctional exercises. This activity may involve the lengthening of shortened tissues and the strengthening of weakened muscles. For example, the pectoralis major may be lengthened and the middle and lower trapezius may be strengthened. Nerve gliding in the involved region may be done as pictured in Figure 5.22. By level 3, modality treatment should be discontinued. General conditioning through aerobic exercise may be used. Given the high incidence of work-related TOS, posture and ergonomics related to occupational tasks should be emphasized. Work-site evaluations and subsequent modifications may be required to ensure adequate carryover of the treatment program.

Cervical Disc and Foraminal Stenosis.   At the cervical level, nerve roots may be irritated secondary to entrapment within the foramen, cervical disc herniation, cervical spondylosis, or post-traumatic sub-luxation (Cailliet 1991). Cervical root involvement may mimic signs of brachial plexopathy or distal peripheral nerve compressions.

It is possible to differentiate cervical disc–foraminal stenosis from more distal disorders through an upper-quadrant screen (see Table 5.5). Suspected findings may include neck pain and referred pain of a dermatomal rather than diffuse nature. Dermatomal symptoms of numbness, tingling, and pain may be reproduced by bending the neck to the opposite side in cases of cervical disc protrusion. Alternatively, bending the neck to the opposite side may relieve spinal stenosis symptoms. In addition, abnormal neurologic signs may be reflected as muscle group tenderness or weakness or abnormal tendon reflexes (Cailliet 1991). For example, there may be tenderness through the rhomboids or the trapezius. In both types of disorders, symptoms are relieved with cervical traction and exacerbated with compression. Provocative TOS tests will be negative. Although it is important to differentiate between the presence of cervical and distal nerve involvement, it also is possible to have a proximal (cervical) nerve compression coexist with a distal site of compression (Osterman 1988).

Treatment may progress through all three levels. Treatment at level 1 typically involves providing relief from symptoms. This may involve the use of thermal agent modalities or the use of cervical traction, if indicated. Some clinicians prefer to treat via joint mobilization from day one (Maitland 1991). At level 1, it is important to address posture and avoidance of provocative positions. Once the individual begins to feel relief, he or she may be ready for simple cervical ROM exercises and postural correctional exercises. Myofascial release strategies and soft-tissue mobilization techniques may be preceded by heat modalities or TENS to prepare the tissue and reduce pain. This level of treatment may continue for some time until the individual is ready for level 3. Once the pain no longer limits activity or if it resolves within 24 hours, afflicted individuals are ready to tolerate upper-body conditioning if needed and work-simulation activities. Level 3 treatment for those with cervical radiculopathy will vary widely.

Shoulder Region

Typical injuries that occur within the shoulder region, secondary to overuse, include rotator cuff tendinitis

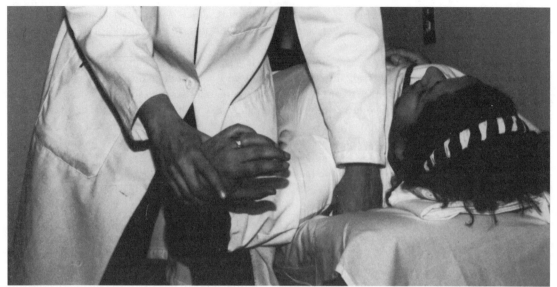

A

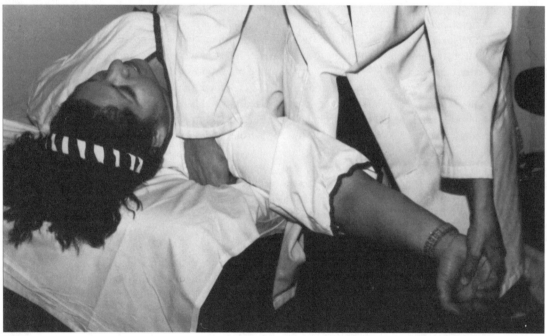

B

Figure 5.22. Upper-limb tension test, median nerve bias. **A.** Initial position. Note therapist's fisted hand and her arm depressing the shoulder while she begins to passively externally rotate the patient's shoulder and extend the wrist. **B.** Final position. Note elbow extension. The therapist's hand remained in neutral secondary to the patient's low tolerance to lateral side bending.

and bicipital tendinitis (Table 5.11). Associated conditions include trigger points and bursitis. Risk factors associated with shoulder overuse include awkward or static postures, direct load bearing, overhead work, heavy work, repetitive movements, and lack of rest (Sommerich et al. 1993).

Rotator Cuff Tendinitis.   Tendinitis of the rotator cuff has been linked to impingement of structures within the suprahumeral (subacromial) space. This tight space lies between the head of the humerus and the coracoacromial arch. The arch is formed by the coracoid process, the acromion, and the coracoacromial ligament. Superiorly to inferiorly, this space contains the subacromial (subdeltoid) bursa, the supraspinous muscle and tendon, the superior part of the shoulder joint capsule, the tendon of the long head of the biceps brachii, and, possibly, the anterior portion of the infraspinous tendon (Neer & Welsh 1982; Pratt 1991). Narrowing of the subacromial space may occur secondary to posterior joint capsule tightness, congenital malformation of the acromion into a downward arc, spur development beneath the acromion, or humeral head elevation relative to the glenoid fossa. If the muscular depressors of the humeral head are weaker than the elevators, the humeral head may tend to ride in an elevated position within the glenoid fossa, predisposing the suprahumeral space to compression. The depressors of the humeral head are the long head of the biceps muscle, the infraspinous, the latissimus dorsi, and the teres minor and major muscles. The elevators are the deltoid and the supraspinous muscles.

Neer and Welsh (1982) have devised a classification system for impingement, as outlined in Table 5.12. Impingement of subacromial structures typically occurs in those individuals who engage in overhead activities, such as are required in baseball pitching, swimming, tennis, and painting. In the presence of impingement, nutrition to the distal end of the tendon may be restricted. Given this restriction of blood supply, an injured supraspinous tendon may heal slowly. In elderly individuals, degeneration of the tendon may have occurred secondary to repeated bouts of tendon microtrauma that resulted in a defect in the tendon rather than a true tear (Schmelzeisen 1990).

Rotator cuff impingement may be associated with tendinitis or tears to the cuff's related tendons.

Table 5.11. Shoulder Disorders in Tendinitis: Subjective and Objective Findings

Rotator cuff tendinitis (tendinosis)
Supraspinous
   A painful arc of abduction
   Pain with resisted abduction and internal rotation
      combined
   Pain with full passive elevation
   Pain on palpation to tendon (lateral to acromion or
      anterior humeral head given position of humeral
      extension)
   Positive impingement test (passive flexion with internal
      rotation)
Infraspinous
   Pain with resisted external rotation
   Pain on tendon palpation (lateral humeral head given
      position of horizontal adduction)
Bicipital tendinitis (tendinosis)
   Pain with isotonic shoulder flexion, which increases
      with resistance
   Pain with resisted elbow flexion and forearm supination
   Painless passive movement
   Possible tenderness to touch over proximal biceps
      tendon

Source: Modified from J Cyriax (1982). *Textbook of Orthopaedic Medicine, Vol 1: Diagnosis of Soft-Tissue Lesions* (8th ed). London: Bailliere Tindall.

Typically, the supraspinous tendon is implicated, although the infraspinous tendon may be involved. The signs and symptoms of supraspinous tendon impingement include a painful arc of abduction, pain with combined resistance to abduction and internal rotation, pain with full passive elevation, and pain on palpation. The impingement test reported by Hawkins and Kennedy (1980) notes that symptoms can be reproduced from a position of 90 degrees of humeral flexion with forceful passive internal rotation, which causes the humeral head to drive the rotator cuff underneath the coracoacromial ligament. The supraspinous tendon may be palpated in its superior position on the humeral head lateral to the acromion process or from a position of shoulder extension. If involved, the supraspinous tendon may be tender to palpation. Complete rupture of the supraspinous tendon is indicated by an inability to maintain humeral abduction after passive placement of the arm in this position (drop-arm test). If one suspects involvement of the supraspinous tendon but there is not a painful arc or pain with passive eleva-

Table 5.12. Classification of Subacromial Impingement

Stage	Anatomic Changes	Primary Complaint	Signs and Symptoms
Stage 1	Edema and hemorrhage	Anterior shoulder ache Occasional radiation to posterior capsule and pain following activity	Painful arc 70–120 degrees abduction Positive impingement sign
Stage II	Subacromial (subdeltoid) bursa involved	Pain during and after activity	Weakness
	Fibrosis and thickening of rotator cuff		Painful abduction arc Positive impingement sign
Stage III	Permanent thickness of rotator cuff	Pain during and after activity	Persistent weakness
	Spurring of acromion		Painful abduction arc
	Calcification of rotator cuff and biceps tendon		Positive impingement sign
	1-cm tears in rotator cuff		
Stage IV	Muscle atrophy	Pain during and after light activities of daily living	Severe weakness
	Rotator cuff tears >1 cm		Minimal active range of motion against gravity
	Bicep tears, partial or full		May develop adhesive capsulitis

Source: Modified from CS Neer & RP Walsh (1982). The shoulder in sports. *Orth Clin North Am,* 8,439.

tion, the myotendinous junction may be implicated (Cyriax 1982).

Treatment for supraspinous tendinitis (partial tear) may be approached in levels, as outlined previously. At level 1, overhead activities are restricted, and inflammation may be reduced by use of NSAIDs or other inflammation-reducing modalities such as iontophoresis, phonophoresis, or pulsed ultrasound. At level 2, cross-fiber massage or massage from the supraspinous muscle belly toward the tendon will enhance blood flow. To enhance mobility of the muscle-tendon unit, stretching into shoulder adduction after massage is recommended. Isometrics may be initiated at this treatment level. Postural correctional exercises are initiated as indicated. Isotonic resistive loading of the rotator cuff is begun at the third treatment level. Eccentric activities generally are not used for supraspinous tendinitis. Instead, training of scapular depressors and retractors is used to strengthen and balance the scapular and glenohumeral muscles around the shoulder region. Once the tendon shows signs of tolerance to resistance, conditioning of the supraspinous muscle itself can be undertaken. Because supraspinous tendinitis is often induced by overhead work, job or task simulation should be incorporated into the treatment program. Ergonomic

redesign of work tasks may be necessary to avoid recurrence.

Infraspinous tendinitis is associated with pain on resisted external rotation. The posteriorly located infraspinous tendon can be palpated over the humeral head if the humerus is horizontally adducted. This tendon may be tender to palpation if involved. Treatment may be followed as above, with the replacement of external rotation for abduction, at levels 2 and 3.

Bicipital Tendinitis. Bicipital tendinitis involves the long head of the biceps tendon in the proximal anterior humeral region. The long head of the biceps might become inflamed as it is recruited during resisted shoulder flexion and elbow flexion.

Signs and symptoms include pain elicited on resisted elbow flexion and forearm supination as well as on isotonic shoulder flexion (Figure 5.23). Passive movement is typically painless (Cyriax 1982). The region over the proximal biceps tendon may be tender to touch.

During the first level of treatment for bicipital tendinitis, the provocative activity must be avoided. However, because of the large number of movements for which the long head of the biceps is recruited, it may be difficult to determine which

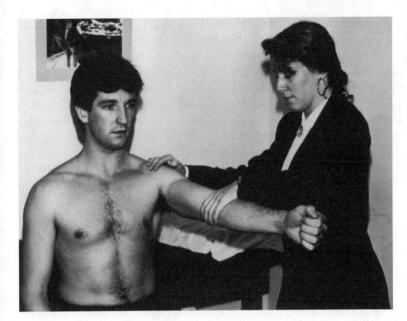

Figure 5.23. Test for bicipital tendinitis. Manual resistance during isotonic shoulder flexion. Positive test reproduces pain in the region of the biceps tendon or referred areas.

activity is implicated. To reduce inflammation, methods such as NSAIDs, phonophoresis, iontophoresis, pulsed ultrasound, and ice may be used. An injection of corticosteroid also may be given. At treatment level 2, cross-friction massage over the tendon may assist in reducing adhesions, and massage from the muscle belly proximally toward the tendon can help to increase blood flow. It is best to stretch the biceps tendon immediately after these therapeutic interventions to take advantage of the increased blood flow. The stretch may be accomplished by extending the elbow and shoulder in forearm pronation. During treatment level 3, conditioning may ensue once symptoms have subsided. Treatment should include eccentric training because eccentric activities often are the cause of bicipital tendinitis. Reconditioning for work or recreational tasks should be incorporated into level 3 activities.

Myofascial Trigger Points.   To inactivate the trigger points, treatment should be directed at the muscle itself. The stretch-and-spray technique involves stretch of the muscle followed by the application of a vapocoolant spray (Travell & Simons 1983). Ischemic compression or firm digital pressure to the trigger point causes ischemia with hypoxia and may be followed by a reactive hyperemia. Other modalities such as TENS, laser, or acupuncture may prove very effective at activating trigger points. Acupunc-

ture involves injection of a dry needle, saline, or local anesthetic. As stated earlier, some centers advocate using pulsed ultrasound for 3 consecutive days following injection of trigger points (W Nagler, personal communication, 1995). Ultrasound applied at low intensities over a sustained period may inactivate the trigger point through thermal and nonthermal effects.

After trigger point inactivation, the muscle and its fascia should be addressed. Moist heat may be used, followed by myofascial release strategies. As one progresses into treatment levels 2 and 3, reconditioning of the involved muscle as well as retraining should be undertaken to enhance muscle balancing during activities of daily living and work activities.

Subacromial Bursitis.   Goals for treatment of subacromial bursitis include reducing pain and inflammation, preventing further injury, increasing active and passive range of motion, increasing strength, enhancing motor control, and returning the patient to functional activities. The methods for reaching these goals are similar to those prescribed for tendinitis secondary to impingement.

The primary method of treatment for acute or chronic bursitis is protection from further injury through avoidance of provocative activities or, in the case of olecranon bursitis, use of a padded elbow sleeve. Anti-inflammatory agents or cortisone injections (or both) may be prescribed by a physician. Some physicians opt to drain the bursa. Pulsed ultrasound, iontophoresis, or phonophoresis can be used during the acute inflammatory period. Some individuals with chronic bursitis develop calcium deposits, which also may be resolved with ultrasound (Cyriax 1982). Once the initial pain and inflammation subside, the individual may tolerate simple active ROM exercises against gravity, progressing to general conditioning as needed. The reader is referred to the previous section on rotator cuff tendinitis for conditioning strategies applicable to bursitis in the glenohumeral joint region because of its association with impingement.

Elbow-Forearm Region

The elbow region is vulnerable to injury because of its intermediate position within the upper limb. Most upper-limb movements involve elbow structures, and so the region is susceptible to many forms of tendinous and neurogenic cumulative trauma including cubital tunnel syndrome, lateral epicondylitis, radial tunnel syndrome, medial epicondylitis, pronator syndrome, and anterior interosseous syndrome.

The two typical forms of tendinitis occurring within the elbow-forearm region are lateral epicondylitis (tennis elbow) and medial epicondylitis (golfer's elbow). These two repetitive injuries stem from different provocative activities and implicate separate anatomic regions. The frequency with which medial epicondylitis occurs is approximately 10–20% that of lateral epicondylitis (Powell & Burke 1991).

Common nerve compressions in this region involve three distinct peripheral nerves: radial, median, and ulnar. Because of the close proximity of structures and the similarity of causative activities, some conditions may have both a tendinous and a neurogenic component, both of which must be evaluated and treated. It may be necessary to treat the neurogenic signs first and then to treat the tendon injury (Lindsay 1993).

Cubital Tunnel Syndrome. The cubital tunnel lies between the medial epicondyle of the humerus and the olecranon process of the ulna. The floor of the tunnel consists of the medial collateral ligament of the elbow (Pratt 1991). The two heads of the flexor carpi ulnaris make up the sides, and the triangular arcuate ligament composes the roof. In full elbow extension, the triangular arcuate ligament is slack whereas, at 90 degrees of elbow flexion, this ligament is taut and the medial collateral ligament bulges, raising the tunnel floor, while the medial triceps pushes the ulnar nerve anteromedially. Because of their superficial position beneath the arcuate ligament, the motor fibers to the intrinsic hand muscles and the cutaneous sensory fibers to the hand are vulnerable to external compression (Szabo 1989). Although the cubital tunnel region is frequently implicated, there are an additional four potential sites of ulnar nerve compression around the elbow, as pictured in Figure 5.24.

Signs and symptoms of ulnar nerve compression in this region (listed in Table 5.13) include a numbness or tingling in the ulnar nerve distribution of the volar and dorsal small finger and half of the ring finger as well as the ulnar side of the palm. There may be weakness in the muscles innervated by the ulnar nerve below the elbow, limiting ulnar deviation and flexion of the wrist; distal interphalangeal joint (DIP) flexion of the fourth and fifth digits; finger abduction; finger-thumb adduction; metacarpophalangeal joint (MP) flexion of the thumb, ring, and small fingers; and small-finger abduction and opposition. In general, gross grasp and prehensile functions such as lateral pinch and handwriting may be affected. Sensibility in the ulnar distribution will be diminished. On physical examination, a positive Tinel's sign will be found, and symptoms will be reproduced with the sustained elbow flexion test (wrists extended), which increases pressure within the cubital tunnel. The test position of elbow flexion is held for 1 minute while the subject reports any symptoms (Szabo 1989).

Treatment during level 1 involves reducing the nerve compression and avoiding provocative activities. Typically, to reduce the compression and rest the region, a long arm splint is fabricated (Figure 5.25). Some authors advocate a position of 45 degrees of flexion when splinting because this puts minimal pressure on the ulnar nerve within the cubital tunnel. The 90-degree position may also be recommended. NSAIDs or other modalities can be used to reduce pain, inflammation, and edema. In addition, associated regions of involvement may require attention at level 1. For example, the distal

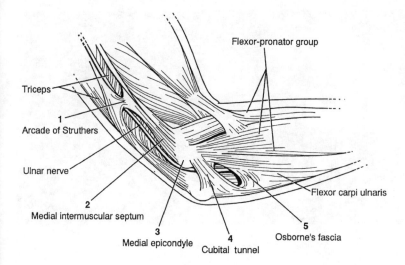

Figure 5.24. Five potential sites of nerve compression around the elbow. (Reprinted with permission from AL Osterman & CA Davis [1996]. Subcutaneous transposition of the ulnar nerve for treatment of cubital tunnel syndrome. *Hand Clin,* 12,422.)

Table 5.13. Ulnar Nerve Compressions: Subjective and Objective Findings

Cubital tunnel syndrome
- Sharp or aching pain in medial-proximal forearm, with possible proximal or distal radiation exacerbated by elbow flexion and extension
- Sensibility diminished through dorsal and volar regions of the hand in the ulnar one and a half digits
- Numbness and tingling in an ulnar nerve distribution
- Weakness in intrinsics of hand, possibly causing:
  - Altered grip and pinch strength
  - Slight atrophy of hypothenar eminence
  - Hyperextension of fourth and fifth metacarpophalangeal joints
- Weakness of flexor carpi ulnaris and flexor digitorum profundus to small and ring fingers
- Altered nerve conduction
- Tinel's sign in cubital tunnel
- Froment's sign (excess flexion of thumb interphalangeal joint secondary to weak adductor pollicis noted on lateral pinch)
- Wartenberg's sign (excess small-finger abduction secondary to overpull of the extensor digiti minimi and weak dorsal interossei muscles)
- Jeneau's sign

Guyon's tunnel syndrome
- Diminished sensibility of volar cutaneous distribution of fifth digit and half of the fourth digit (dorsal cutaneous branch spared as it originates 5 cm proximal to Guyon's tunnel)
- Strong flexor digitorum profundus to fourth and fifth digits and flexor carpi ulnaris
- Weakness in intrinsics of hand, possibly causing:
  - Altered grip and pinch strength
  - Atrophy of hypothenar eminence
  - Hyperextension of fourth and fifth metacarpophalangeal joints (less prominent than cubital tunnel)
- Tinel's sign near Guyon's tunnel
- Froment's sign (excess flexion of thumb interphalangeal joint secondary to weak adductor pollicis during lateral pinch)
- Wartenberg's sign (excess small-finger abduction secondary to overpull of the extensor digiti minimi and weak dorsal interossei muscles)

Source: Modified from GM Rayan (1992). Proximal ulnar nerve compression. Cubital tunnel syndrome. *Hand Clin,* 8,325–336.

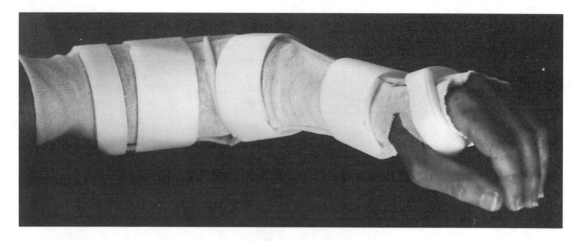

Figure 5.25. Long arm splint. Often used in cases of cubital tunnel or severe cases of lateral epicondylitis.

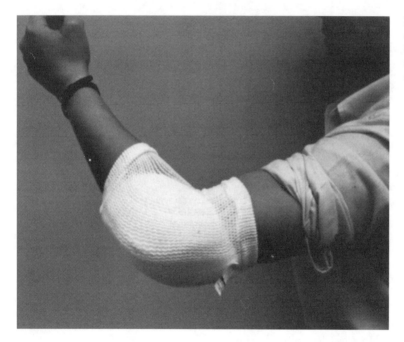

Figure 5.26. "Heelbo," which cushions the elbow in cases of cubital tunnel and olecranon bursitis or provides neutral warmth in cases of lateral or medial epicondylitis.

medial triceps may be tender and show signs of edema or enlargement. Nerve mobilization away from the site of injury may be used.

Once the inflammation has subsided and the significant signs of paresthesia have diminished, heat treatments and massage may be used at level 2. The patient may be able to tolerate a "heelbo" or soft splint (Figure 5.26), which prevents direct elbow pressure yet allows greater mobility than a plastic splint. Nerve mobilization and myofascial release techniques may be used near the site of injury and throughout the site of the involved region.

Once the patient's activity tolerance begins to increase, he or she may begin aerobic and muscular reconditioning (level 3). The primary precaution is avoidance of excessive or repetitive elbow flexion and extension. As stated previously, the final rehabilitative phase should include task simulation and work-site evaluation, as needed, to avoid recurrence of signs and symptoms. If conservative treatment is unsuccessful, the individual may require surgical decompression. One common form of decompression is an ulnar nerve transposition, which typically involves relocating the ulnar nerve to a more protected anterior position. Treatment after surgical intervention resembles the treatment by levels as just outlined.

Olecranon Bursitis.   Olecranon bursitis has been described by Cyriax (1982). If the bursa has not been drained, the primary goal at level 1 is to protect the bursa from further insult. This may be accomplished by use of a long arm splint with a cutout for the enlarged elbow or by use of a heelbo if a small enough size is available. If the excess fluid is not absorbed by the system, the bursa may need to be drained or surgically treated. As the pain subsides, level 2 strategies of ROM exercises and gentle forearm and upper-arm conditioning exercises may be done. Level 3 treatment may not be indicated.

Lateral Epicondylitis.   The lateral epicondyle serves as the attachment site for the common extensor tendon and includes the extensor carpi radialis longus and brevis, extensor digitorum, and extensor digiti minimi (Pratt 1991). Microrupture and subsequent fibrosis of the ECRB and the common extensor tendon of the lateral epicondyle are considered primary pathologic causes of tennis elbow, as first noted by Cyriax in 1936 and later confirmed by Nirschl and Pettrone (1979) through histologic evidence of pathologic alteration of the ECRB muscle tissue. The anterior extensor digitorum and the ECRL typically are affected less than the ECRB. The work of Nirschl and Pettrone (1979) supported the belief that tennis elbow was a degenerative process; these researchers labeled the condition *angiofibroblastic tendinosis.*

Lateral epicondylitis is often found in less accomplished tennis players who exhibit poor backhand mechanics, in which eccentric forces cause a lesion to the wrist extensors. However, lateral epicondylitis is not isolated to tennis players; activities unrelated to sports, including repetitive assembly work and typing, have also been implicated as causes (Powell & Burke 1991).

Among the key signs and symptoms of lateral epicondylitis are pain and weakness experienced with excessive gripping and resisted wrist extension, point tenderness on the lateral epicondyle, and

Table 5.14. Elbow Tendon Disorders: Subjective and Objective Findings

Lateral epicondylitis
  Pain and weakness experienced with excessive gripping and resisted wrist extension
  Point tenderness over lateral epicondyle
  Pain with stretching of wrist extensors, given elbow extension and finger flexion (may have extrinsic shortening)
  Must rule out impingement of the radial nerve in the region of the radial tunnel due to its close proximity to the extensor carpi radialis brevis
Medial epicondylitis
  Pain with resisted wrist flexion and finger flexion and, possibly, resisted pronation
  Pain with passive elbow, wrist, and finger extension
  On supination with the elbow extended, possible replication of symptoms secondary to stretch of the pronator teres
  Point tenderness over medial epicondyle

Sources: Modified from M Lindsay (1993). Radial tunnel versus lateral epicondylitis. *Newsletter of the Section on Hand Rehabilitation of the American Physical Therapy Association,* 10(39),1; and SG Powell & AL Burke (1991). Surgical and therapeutic management of tennis elbow. An update. *J Hand Ther,* 4,64–68.

pain with stretching of the wrist extensors (Table 5.14). The long-finger extension test is positive (Powell & Burke 1991). Symptoms will be reproduced with wrist extension and radial deviation and with elbow extension and finger flexion. Pain also may occur with resisted supination and wrist extension. The signs and symptoms of lateral epicondylitis might have a neurogenic basis: Because of the lateral epicondyle's close proximity to the radial nerve, impingement of the radial nerve in the proximal forearm must be ruled out, as must cervical nerve involvement.

Treatment at level 1 may include rest within a wrist support or counterforce brace with a clasp or cuff placed over the origin of the ECRB (common extensor tendon). Counterforce bracing serves to reduce pain and control tendon overload. It also constrains the involved muscle groups and maintains muscle balance. Groppel and Nirschl (1986) reported that counterforce bracing of the elbow decreased angular acceleration of the elbow and reduced EMG activity in the wrist extensors (Figure 5.27). In conditions that are resistant to low-level immobilization, a long arm splint may be

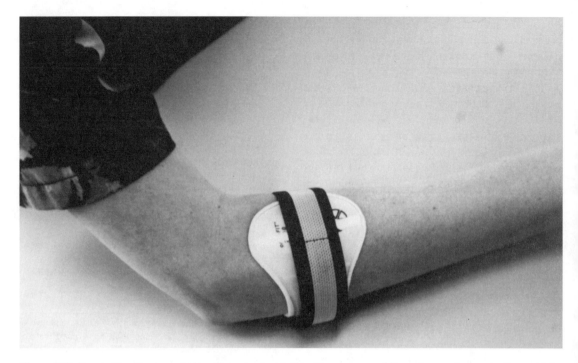

Figure 5.27. Counterforce brace used to treat lateral epicondylitis. Clasp acts as an alternative attachment site from which the muscle can pull, thus allowing for tendon healing.

used. Anti-inflammatories, ice, phonophoresis, and iontophoresis (see Figure 5.19) may be used to reduce inflammation.

At level 2, extensibility of the tissue should be emphasized. Cross-friction massage may help to restore mobility between tissue interfaces. With the patient's elbow flexed and the forearm supinated, the therapist uses his or her index or long finger or thumb to massage perpendicular to the ECRB tendon for 6–12 minutes (Cyriax 1982). Because the common extensor tendon has a limited blood supply and lacks a synovial sheath, massage from the muscle belly (ECRB) toward the lateral epicondyle may be the most effective. Stretching of the common extensor tendon is best achieved with "alphabet exercises": With the shoulder flexed to approximately 90 degrees and the elbow extended, the individual draws the capital letters of the alphabet with his or her index finger, moving the wrist into flexion and extension, while the MP and IP are maintained in extension.

At level 3, conditioning of the extensor region follows the concept of isometric to eccentric loading (Fyfe & Stanish 1992). Wrist extension with the elbow flexed as well as extended should be emphasized. Because strong gripping is a common cause of pain, sustained grip activities should be included in the conditioning program. It may be necessary to use a flexible wrist support during select tasks (Figure 5.28) to allow use of the extensor muscle group in a modified wrist range of motion. Finally, the program should be completed with job or recreational simulation and follow-up work-site analysis, as needed.

Radial Tunnel Syndrome. The radial tunnel region extends from the elbow to the insertion of the posterior interosseous nerve into the supinator. It involves compression of the deep motor or posterior interosseous branch of the radial nerve, induced primarily through repetitive forearm rotation (Peimer & Wheeler 1989; Pratt 1991). One activity that may induce this disorder is repetitive supination and pronation, performed routinely by checkout clerks who scan items.

Signs and symptoms include pain in the proximal-dorsal forearm that increases with rotational activities or at night (Table 5.15). On physical examination, symptoms will be reproduced with resisted supination

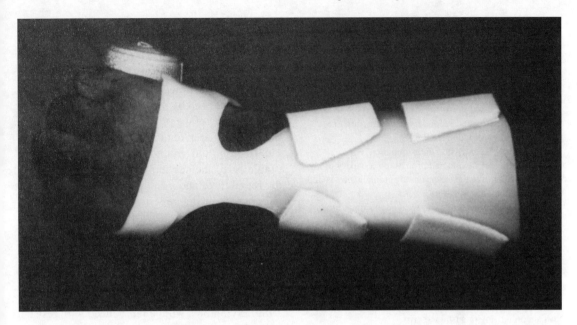

Figure 5.28. Semimobile wrist splint allows use of wrist extensors in functional tasks in a protected range of motion. Note that 1-in. bar at wrist allows for movement.

and resisted middle-finger extension with the wrist flexed or extended (ECRB). Pressure on the supinator or between the brachioradialis and ECRB may reproduce symptoms in the dorsal radial nerve distribution (Peimer & Wheeler 1989).

Radial tunnel syndrome may be differentiated from lateral epicondylitis by physical examination. In cases of lateral epicondylitis, resistance specific to the ECRL and ECRB may invoke pain. Palpation of the lateral epicondyle will be painful and, at rest, the pain will be localized to the epicondyle region. In cases of radial tunnel syndrome, the signs and symptoms are listed above.

At level 1, the treatment strategies for radial tunnel syndrome include restriction of forearm supination and extension, possible provision of a dorsal or volar wrist cock-up splint to restrict extension of the wrist and to provide external support, NSAIDs, and modalities to reduce inflammation (i.e., ice, phonophoresis, iontophoresis). Pulsed ultrasound may be initiated. Myofascial release strategies also might be effective. Nerve gliding should be performed away from the site of pain.

Once the individual progresses to level 2, local radial nerve–gliding technique may be used while myofascial release strategies are continued. Massage may be done according to the patient's tolerance, followed by active stretching of the proximal-dorsal forearm musculature.

At level 3, reconditioning of the weakened extensors and supinator may be undertaken. If tolerated, job simulation and a work-site evaluation can be conducted.

Medial Epicondylitis. The medial epicondyle serves as the attachment site of the pronator teres, flexor carpi radialis, flexor carpi ulnaris, FDS, and palmaris longus muscles (Pratt 1991). Medial epicondylitis is frequently caused by overuse of the wrist flexors or pronator teres muscle-tendon units that attach to the medial epicondyle. Powerful forehand strokes and golfing and typing are examples of activities that can contribute to this disorder. This form of tendinitis may be induced by acute forceful injury more often than is lateral epicondylitis. Nerve compression of the ulnar nerve and, occasionally, of the median nerve will need to be ruled out because of the similarities in symptomatology.

On physical examination, pain is often reproduced with resisted wrist flexion, resisted finger flexion and, possibly, resisted pronation (see Table 5.14). Passive stretching into elbow, wrist, and fin-

Table 5.15. Radial Nerve Compressions: Subjective and Objective Findings

Radial tunnel syndrome
    Pain at rest over the mobile extensor muscle mass, which increases with activity
    Pain with resisted third-finger extension if elbow and wrist are extended secondary to contraction of extensor carpi radialis brevis
    Pain with wrist extension and supination
    Pain with wrist flexion and pronation secondary to stretching over the extensor carpi radialis brevis and supinator
    Functional loss secondary to weakened supination, thumb abduction, and wrist, finger, and thumb extension
    Restriction in proximal-dorsal forearm, given adverse neural tension testing of the radial nerve
    No sensory deficits
Superficial radial nerve compression
    Pain over the dorsal radial aspect of the hand
    Pain on writing or sustained grip
    Sensory loss over the distribution of the radial nerve
    Positive Tinel's sign over the nerve near the snuff-box
    Positive Finkelstein's test
    No pain with thumb extension and no tenderness over the first dorsal compartment

ger extension also may induce pain secondary to an extreme muscle stretch. Supination with the elbow extended may replicate symptoms secondary to stretching of the pronator teres; therefore, it is important to rule out pronator syndrome.

Treatment follows that listed for lateral epicondylitis, with a few exceptions. Counterforce bracing typically is unsuccessful in medial epicondylitis. In some conditions, a soft elbow support may provide the necessary cushioning and neutral warmth during levels 1 and 2 and might help to enhance blood flow for healing of involved tissues once the inflammatory phase resolves. At level 2, heat and massage from the flexor-pronator muscle group toward the medial epicondyle may be an effective preparation for myofascial release strategies and gentle stretching. Reconditioning of the tissue in this region through treatment levels 2 and 3 should be carried out cautiously. It is advisable to avoid full-range stretching into elbow extension unless pain is minimal. In addition, strengthening should be done in a slow, graded fashion to avoid reinjury. Because of the vulnerability of the affected site, medial epi-

condylitis may take a long time to heal fully but, once reconditioning is successful, retraining for job and recreational tasks may be undertaken.

Pronator Syndrome. The median nerve can become compressed by the lacertus fibrosus between the two heads of the pronator teres and underneath the proximal arch to the FDS (Johnson & Spinner 1989). Signs and symptoms of pronator syndrome (Table 5.16) include numbness or paresthesias in the radial three and a half digits, weakness in grip and pinch during repetitive writing or related tasks, and pain in the volar forearm that increases with activity. On physical examination, likely findings include firmness with tenderness to palpation over the enlarged pronator teres, a positive Tinel's sign over the distal margin of the pronator teres, and a negative Phalen's test (Johnson & Spinner 1989). Symptoms will be reproduced with resisted pronation (and will increase with movement from flexion to extension, implicating the pronator teres), isolated flexion of the long and ring proximal interphalangeal (PIP) joints (indicating entrapment at the FDS), active elbow flexion with supination (indicating entrapment by the lacertus fibrosus), and resisted elbow flexion past 120 degrees (indicating entrapment by the ligament of Struthers). Rarely is a conduction defect found on electrodiagnostic testing.

Treatment at level 1 includes strategies to reduce inflammation such as NSAIDs and other modalities (e.g., ice, phonophoresis, iontophoresis, pulsed ultrasound). TENS may assist in pain reduction. Avoidance of provocative activities may require task modification and supportive splinting. At this treatment level, nerve mobilization should be performed away from the injury site. However, myofascial release techniques may be done within the affected region.

By level 2, continuous ultrasound may be substituted for pulsed ultrasound to induce a heating effect. Massage may be used to enhance muscle blood flow before stretching in a direction of supination and elbow flexion. (Elbow flexion may remain tender for an extended period.) Isometrics may be initiated.

By level 3, the patient should be ready to advance from isometrics to isotonic resistive exercises. Reconditioning for work or recreational tasks that require forearm rotation should be undertaken.

Table 5.16. Median Nerve Compressions: Subjective and Objective Findings

Pronator syndrome
    Numbness or paresthesias in the radial three and a half digits
    Weakness in grip and pinch during repetitive writing or related task
    Firmness and tenderness to palpation over enlarged pronator teres
    Positive Tinel's sign over distal margin of the pronator teres
    Negative Phalen's test
    Symptoms reproduced with the following resisted movements:
        Pronation (increases with movement from flexion to extension, implicating pronator teres)
        Isolated flexion of long and ring proximal interphalangeal joints (flexor digitorum superficialis), indicating
            entrapment at the flexor digitorum superficialis
        Elbow flexion with supination, indicating entrapment by the lacertus fibrosus of the biceps brachii
    Rarely, conduction defect on electrodiagnostic testing
Anterior interosseous syndrome
    Weakness: possible denervation seen on electromyographic studies of flexor pollicis longus, index and long flexor
        digitorum profundus, and pronator quadratus
    Abnormal pinch patterns with decreased dexterity
    Elbow pain with resisted pronation (elbow flexed to isolate the pronator quadratus)
    No cutaneous deficits
    Negative nerve conduction studies
Carpal tunnel syndrome
    Intermittent paresthesias or pain
    Numbness, particularly nocturnal burning pain
    Inability to sustain grip on objects, with thenar atrophy, weak abductor pollicis brevis, and strong flexor pollicis longus
        and flexor digitorum profundus
    Positive Tinel's sign and Phalen's test
    Abnormal sensibility in median nerve distribution, with diminished sudomotor activity (normal sensibility in proximal
        palm)
    Abnormal electromyographic and nerve conduction studies in median nerve distribution

Surgical decompression may need to be performed if conservative treatment is ineffective.

Anterior Interosseous Syndrome.   The anterior interosseous nerve branches off the median nerve approximately 5 cm distal to the medial epicondyle. It innervates the FPL, the pronator quadratus, and the FDP to the index and long finger. Although such compressions are uncommon, this nerve may be compressed by the deep head of the pronator teres, the origin of the FDS, the origin of the flexor carpi radialis, and accessory muscles from the FDS to the FDP, including Gantzer's muscle (FPL) (Spinner 1970). Other causes of the anterior interosseous syndrome include trauma and vascular insufficiency. The onset of this entrapment syndrome is often insidious.

In approximately one-third of reported cases, there is an insidious onset of proximal forearm pain followed by several hours of weakness or paralysis to the affected muscles. In the other two-thirds; individuals often recall a bout of strenuous or repetitive forearm activity, prolonged forearm pressure, or trauma. Some individuals report having difficulty only with handwriting. On further examination, thumb interphalangeal (IP) flexion is weak or absent (Chidgey & Szabo 1989). Index DIP flexion may or may not be affected. The characteristic pinch deformity involves collapse of the thumb IP joint and index DIP joint into extension. There may be a positive Tinel's sign over the proximal forearm with distal radiation toward the pronator quadratus. Proximal forearm pain may be reproduced by the Mills' test, which involves wrist and finger flexion with the forearm hyperpronated or extension of the elbow from a flexed position (see Table 5.16). The differential diagnosis includes partial lesion of the median nerve or lateral cord.

Treatment at level 1 primarily involves avoidance of provocative activities, particularly forearm rota-

Table 5.17. Wrist Tendon Disorders: Subjective and Objective Findings

Flexor tenosynovitis
  Pain with sustained grip activities
  Pain with resisted finger flexion
  Tenderness over the flexor tendons in the palm
  Possible edema in the region of the palm or carpal tunnel (may be a precursor to carpal tunnel syndrome)
Intersection syndrome
  Pain, tenderness, swelling, and crepitus over the radial-dorsal aspect of the distal forearm 4–8 cm proximal to Lister's tubercle
  Possible symptoms with resisted thumb extension and Finkelstein's test
  Differentiated from de Quervain's as the palpable point of tenderness is more proximal
  Provocative tests: resisted wrist radial deviation and resisted wrist extension with rotation

Sources: Flexor tenosynovitis information modified from DS Butler (1991). *Mobilisation of the Nervous System.* New York: Churchill Livingstone. Intersection syndrome information modified from AB Grundberg & DS Reagan (1985). Pathologic anatomy of the forearm: intersection syndrome. *J Hand Surg [Am],* 10,299–305.

tion. The use of TENS and other modalities may be required to reduce inflammation, edema, and pain. Myofascial release techniques may be tolerated.

When the initial symptoms have subsided, treatment level 2 may be initiated. This involves heat application, such as a hot pack or continuous ultrasound, followed by anterior forearm massage.

Progression to level 3 involves reconditioning of palmar pinch and forearm pronation. During this level of treatment, one must be alert for recurrence of signs and symptoms. The individual who tolerates reconditioning well should be ready to perform job simulation tasks, such as handwriting. If conservative treatment fails or EMG and NCSs indicate an unresolvable entrapment, surgical intervention may be warranted.

Wrist and Hand Regions

Common injuries of the wrist and hand region include flexor peritendinitis (tenosynovitis) that may precede carpal tunnel syndrome, carpal tunnel syndrome, Guyon's tunnel syndrome, intersection syndrome, de Quervain's disease, and trigger finger or thumb.

Flexor Tenosynovitis.   Flexor peritendinitis (tenosynovitis) is an inflammation of the flexor tendon synovial sheaths from repetitive use or frequent high force when engaged in such prehensile activities as typing and playing musical instruments. Inflammation may lead to edema and fibrotic changes in the tissue itself. Because the flexor tendons ride in the carpal tunnel, edema may reduce the available room in the canal (Butler 1991). With pressure in this region, the median nerve can become compressed because it is soft and lies close to the volar transverse carpal ligament (Pratt 1991).

The site of pain varies along the length of the tendons and may be present at rest or may increase with resistive/sustained grip activities. There often is point tenderness along the volar palm in a select region of the flexor tendons. Table 5.17 lists most symptoms.

At level 1, rest is best accomplished with avoidance of provocative activities and splinting. Tendon-gliding exercises, exemplified by hook fisting, may prevent formation of adhesions. Strategies such as phonophoresis or iontophoresis may be used to reduce inflammation. As the individual progresses, stretching and reconditioning strategies, as advocated at treatment levels 2 and 3, may be used.

Carpal Tunnel Syndrome.   The floor of the carpal tunnel is formed by an arch of carpal bones. It is covered in the volar aspect by the transverse carpal ligament that attaches in the ulnar aspect to the pisiform bone and hook of the hamate bone and radially to the scaphoid tubercle and trapezium (Pratt 1991). The median nerve traverses the carpal tunnel along with the eight long finger flexor tendons and the FPL. The palmar cutaneous branch to the thenar region does not traverse the carpal canal; rather it courses above it.

Causes of carpal tunnel syndrome include inflammatory and metabolic disorders, repetitive trauma, tumors, and developmental disorders. To confirm carpal tunnel syndrome, the differential diagnosis includes testing for diabetic neuropathy, cervical root impingement, pronator syndrome, and anterior interosseous syndrome.

Signs and symptoms of carpal tunnel syndrome (see Table 5.16) include numbness or nocturnal burning pain through the radial-volar side of the hand; pain and paresthesias in the median nerve distribution of the hand that occasionally radiate proximally; and reports of dropping objects or an inability to sustain grip of objects. On physical examination, there may be thenar atrophy with weakness of the abductor pollicis brevis, diminished sensibility within the median nerve distribution of the hand, a positive Phalen's test, a positive Tinel's sign, and diminished sudomotor activity. The FPL and FDP will be strong. Sensibility will be normal in the proximal palm. Diagnostic confirmation may be accomplished using EMG or NCSs.

Initial conservative treatment includes dorsal or volar cock-up splinting to hold the wrist in neutral to 10 degrees of extension. Methods to reduce inflammation may include the use of NSAIDs or corticosteroid injections and avoidance of pinching, gripping, or repetitive wrist motions. Some have advocated the use of phonophoresis or iontophoresis instead of injections. Symptoms might be reduced and gliding of the nerve promoted through myofascial release or nerve-gliding techniques. Tendon-gliding exercises for the long finger flexors should be done. If symptoms begin to resolve, therapy may progress through levels 2 and 3, including ROM exercises and reconditioning with theraputty and resistive grip tasks. If the signs and symptoms progress, however, surgical decompression may be indicated through either direct or endoscopic technique. In either case, workplace modifications and proper hand use should be addressed to avoid further problems with the disease.

Guyon's Tunnel Syndrome.   Guyon's tunnel is located between the hook of the hamate and the pisiform bone. The transverse carpal ligament makes up the floor and the pisohamate ligament makes up the roof of this tunnel. In addition to the volar sensory ulnar nerve and the deep motor branch, Guyon's tunnel contains the ulnar artery and vein (Pratt 1991). Activities that can induce nerve compression include long-distance cycling, use of the palm as a hammer, and pressure from the head of a screwdriver or pliers.

Signs and symptoms include paresthesias and diminished sensibility in the ulnar nerve distribution on the volar side only (see Table 5.13), and weak finger abduction and adduction, weak fourth and fifth MP flexion, weak small-finger opposition, and

thumb adduction. Froment's sign, which is exaggerated thumb IP flexion with attempted thumb adduction, may be present. Grip strength and lateral pinch strength will be significantly reduced.

Treatment at level 1 includes avoidance of provocative activities, splinting of the wrist in neutral, and the application of inflammation-reducing methods such as NSAIDs, cortisone injections, or other modalities. Progression to level 2 may involve ulnar nerve–gliding techniques and easy prehensile tasks. As tolerance increases, level 3 resistive tasks (e.g., theraputty and sustained grip tasks) should be incorporated into treatment. Job simulation may be undertaken according to the patient's tolerance. If conservative treatment is not successful, surgical decompression might be attempted. Treatment after decompression is similar to the presurgical conservative treatment plan.

Dorsal Radial Sensory Nerve Compression and Entrapment.   The dorsal radial sensory nerve (DRSN) passes between the dense fascia of the forearm and the tendons of the brachioradialis and ECRL muscles before it becomes superficial at the anatomic snuff-box. In this superficial position, it is vulnerable to radial-side injury, compressive forces, and neuritis. More proximally, forearm pronation may squeeze the DRSN between the tendons of the brachioradialis and ECRL. The resultant tethering of the distal segment of the nerve can lead to entrapment, known as *Wartenberg's syndrome* (Ehrlich 1986).

Signs and symptoms of entrapment include pain over the dorsal and radial aspect of the hand that is exacerbated by writing or sustained grip tasks (see Table 5.15). If the DRSN is irritated, as in neuritis, tingling or burning pain may be distributed over the dorsal and radial aspect of the thumb. On examination, sensitivity over the distribution of the radial nerve may be diminished, and there may be a positive Tinel's sign near the attachment of the brachioradialis. Finkelstein's test will be positive. This test involves a stretch into forearm hyperpronation with ulnar deviation and thumb flexion, which may provoke symptoms significantly. It is important to differentiate nerve involvement from de Quervain's disease. The absence of pain with thumb extension and the absence of tenderness over the first dorsal compartment are indicative of nerve entrapment.

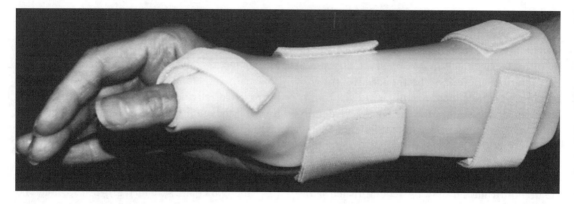

Figure 5.29. Thumb spica splint used in cases of de Quervain's disease, intersection syndrome, and dorsal radial sensory nerve irritation and compression.

Table 5.18. Hand Tendon Disorders: Subjective and Objective Findings

de Quervain's Disease
    Pain with resisted thumb abduction or extension
    Positive Finkelstein's test (thumb flexion with wrist ulnar deviation), pain induced
    Pain when performing specific tasks such as writing
    Possible palpable pain near tendons of first dorsal compartment (near snuff-box)
    Might be confused with irritation of dorsal radial sensory nerve; latter must be ruled out
Trigger finger (thumb)
    Either locking in flexion or "catch" and "snap" to release on attempted extension
    Possible palpable nodule at volar base of metacarpophalangeal joint
    Possible weakness and pain when performing sustained grip or pinch tasks

Sources: de Quervain's disease information modified from M Anderson & CJ Tichenor (1994). A patient with de Quervain's tenosynovitis: a case report using an Australian approach to manual therapy. *Phys Ther*, 74,314–326; and R Cailliet (1975). *Hand Pain and Impairment* (2nd ed). Philadelphia: Davis. Trigger finger information modified from R Cailliet (1975). *Hand Pain and Impairment* (2nd ed). Philadelphia: Davis; J Cyriax (1982). *Textbook of Orthopaedic Medicine, Vol 1: Diagnosis of Soft-Tissue Lesions* (8th ed). London: Bailliere Tindall; and RB Evans, JM Hunter, & WE Burkhalter (1988). Conservative management of the trigger finger: a new approach. *J Hand Ther*, 1(2),59–74.

Treatment at level 1 for superficial radial nerve compression includes rest and avoidance of the provocative activity; a thumb spica splint should be worn (Figure 5.29). NSAIDs or other modalities may be used to reduce inflammation.

Ice and TENS work well if the radial nerve is irritated or compressed. However, other modalities may also be useful, including iontophoresis or phonophoresis. As symptoms subside, the patient may be able to engage in gentle reconditioning through treatment levels 2 and 3. Wearing of the thumb spica at night through levels 2 and 3 is advisable to promote full recovery. If conservative treatment is not effective, surgical decompression may be necessary.

de Quervain's Disease.   de Quervain's disease affects the extensor pollicis brevis and APL within the first dorsal compartment of the wrist. It is caused by an abrasion of the tendons and their sheath as they angle around the radial styloid process during simultaneous pinch and wrist motions. Movements that create stress on the first dorsal compartment include thumb abduction and extension, wrist radial and ulnar deviation, and forearm pronation and supination. Muckart (1964) found that a firm gross grasp with radial wrist deviation creates the greatest stress on the structures of the first dorsal compartment. This position causes the taut APL tendon to apply a tensile force to the fibrous extensor retinaculum. The extensor retinaculum thickens to resist the strain, resulting in more pain and pressure.

Signs and symptoms of de Quervain's disease (Table 5.18) include localized tenderness and swelling in the region of the radial styloid and radial wrist pain radiating proximally into the forearm and distally into the thumb (Cailliet 1975; Anderson & Tichenor 1994). Finkelstein's test stretches the tendons in the first dorsal compartment; the test requires that the thumb be held in flexion by the fingers during wrist ulnar deviation, which increases symptoms if positive. Resisted thumb abduction or extension may also reproduce symptoms. Active thumb abduction may be decreased at the carpometacarpal (CMC) joint. Palpable thickening of the extensor sheath and the tendons distal to the first dorsal compartment may occur secondary to reduced vascularity and edema. Crepitus is rare. It is important to rule out DRSN irritation, extensor pollicis longus tenosynovitis, and CMC arthritis.

Treatment at level 1 consists primarily of rest in a thumb spica (see Figure 5.29). This may be coupled with anti-inflammatory treatment via phonophoresis, iontophoresis, or physician-administered cortisone injection. In addition, massage may be done along the length of the tendon (longitudinally). As the inflammation subsides, levels 2 and 3 may be initiated through active motion and conditioning with light resistance (theraputty). Because de Quervain's disease is exacerbated easily, therapists are cautioned against quick progression through the treatment program and encouraged to educate clients about the disease process.

Intersection Syndrome. Intersection syndrome is caused by an abrasion of the tendons within the second dorsal wrist compartment as the muscle bellies of the APL and extensor pollicis brevis cross over it during thumb and wrist flexion or repetitive wrist flexion and extension (Grundberg & Reagan 1985). Specifically, the second compartment contains the ECRL and ECRB.

The signs and symptoms (see Table 5.17) include pain, tenderness, swelling, and crepitus over the radial-dorsal aspect of the distal forearm 4–8 cm proximal to Lister's tubercle, which is where the first compartment crosses over the second (Grundberg & Reagan 1985). Provocative tests include resisted wrist radial deviation and resisted wrist extension with rotation. Intersection syndrome is frequently misdiagnosed as de Quervain's disease because resistive thumb extension and Finkelstein's test may reproduce symptoms in either condition. However, the two are differentiated by the more proximal location of the palpable point of tenderness in intersection syndrome (as described previously).

Treatment during level 1 may include rest in a thumb spica and avoidance of the provocative activity. In addition, anti-inflammatory medications, injections, ice, iontophoresis, or phonophoresis may be used. The affected area often is very tender in the acute stages, making massage intolerable. At level 2, tendon gliding may be done as tolerated. Flexibility and strength reconditioning may be undertaken as symptoms subside, per level 3. If conservative treatment is not effective, some surgeons perform a synovectomy to the APL muscle (Wulle 1993).

Trigger Finger (Thumb). Triggering or snapping of a flexor tendon occurs primarily in the thumb or long or ring finger. It is caused by a nodule that forms on the tendon. This nodule often is located near the volar MP joint and prevents smooth gliding under the A1 pulley located at the head of the metacarpal. The region of involvement, between the A1 and A2 pulleys, has been termed the *hypovascular watershed area* because of its limited vascular supply (Littler 1977; Evans et al. 1988). Occasionally, a trigger may form near the thumb IP joint, preventing smooth gliding during IP flexion and extension.

Signs and symptoms may range from a stiffness in the affected digit to a painful snap on fist making or re-extension; occasional locking may prevent either flexion or extension (see Table 5.18). Complications include intrinsic tightness with limited IP motion (Cailliet 1975; Cyriax 1982; Evans et al. 1988).

Conservative treatment of this disorder, at level 1, typically includes injection with local steroid, NSAIDs, splinting, and tendon gliding. In addition, phonophoresis or iontophoresis may be used to reduce inflammation. It often is advisable to avoid the use of resistive devices or sustained grip tasks because those are usually the activities that cause the trigger to form (Cailliet 1975; Cyriax 1982; Evans et al. 1988). For example, a trigger may be induced through use of a cane with a small handle diameter. Altering the cane to incorporate a wider handle may help to resolve the problem.

Once the trigger has resolved, it is best to guide the individual gradually into normal activities at level 2. Some do not advocate the use of resistive devices such as theraputty (level 3) because the tendon may be degenerated and thus susceptible to further injury as well as to rupture. If conservative treatment fails, surgical resection of the A1 pulley is performed.

Table 5.19. Trigger Finger Protocol

1. Provocative activities requiring repetitive grasping or acute flexion are avoided.
2. A hand-based static splint is used to immobilize the involved metacarpophalangeal joints at 0 degrees, allowing full interphalangeal flexion. Within this splint, the individual is instructed to make a "hook fist" and to repeat this maneuver 20 times every 2 hours. The splint is to be worn during waking hours for at least 3 weeks (up to 6). (Theoretically, this splint encourages maximal differential tendon gliding of the superficialis and profundus tendons and promotes circulation of the synovial fluid within the tendon sheath.) Flexion contractures at the proximal interphalangeal joints are managed with finger-based volar static extension splints worn at night.
3. Every 2 hours, the splint is removed for place-and-hold full-fist exercises and massage. Longitudinal massage of the digit is performed to soften the pulley area and increase circulation.
4. After 3 weeks, the finger is checked for triggering. If triggering persists, the protocol may be continued for another 6 weeks.

Source: Modified from RB Evans, JM Hunter, & WE Burkhalter (1988). Conservative management of the trigger finger: a new approach. *J Hand Ther,* 1(2),59–74.

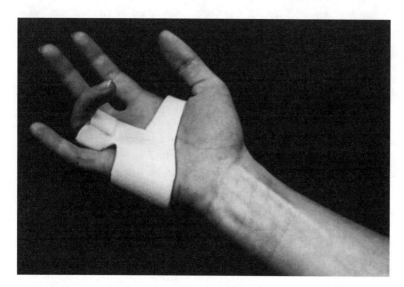

Figure 5.30. Single-finger block splint used to promote tendon gliding within the trigger finger protocol.

Evans et al. (1988) advocate conservative management of trigger finger that alters the mechanical pressures of the proximal pulley systems and encourages differential tendon gliding. The authors conducted a prospective study of 54 digits with triggering in 38 (nonrheumatoid) individuals managed with a 3- to 6-week treatment protocol. In 52% of the reported cases, there was an excellent result or resolution of the trigger at an average follow-up of 8.8 months. Further study has not yet been reported for trigger thumb. The treatment protocol followed in the study is now widely used clinically (Table 5.19). In this protocol, the individual makes use of an MP block splint that prevents MP flexion but allows PIP and DIP flexion (Figure 5.30). This protocol may be considered to be a progression through levels 1 and 2 only. Resistive activities such as theraputty are not advocated.

Treatment of a trigger at the thumb IP joint may involve rest in a small IP block splint (Figure 5.31), which prevents IP motion and redirects the tendon to the MP joint. Treatment also may involve progression through pulsed to continuous ultrasound over a longer time period. Longitudinal massage along the thumb may follow ultrasound and precede ROM. Active ROM exercises through a minimal range can be initiated. Unfortunately, this type of trigger often recurs because the provocative activity is difficult to avoid.

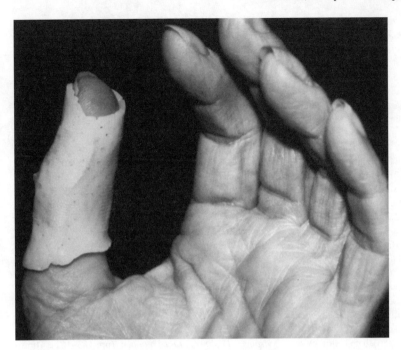

Figure 5.31. Block splint for treating distal interphalangeal joint trigger.

Future Trends

Tendinitis and nerve compression/entrapments are being diagnosed and referred for treatment more frequently then ever before. As the public becomes better educated about the types of activities that may lead to cumulative trauma, the incidence may begin to drop. It also is possible that if acute injuries are treated early, the problems associated with chronic conditions may be avoided.

Currently, the key components to a speedy recovery are early diagnosis, avoidance of provocative activities, and reconditioning. Because of the nature of the injuries, it is often difficult to predict success in treating these cases. With greater ability to differentiate clearly between a tendinous and a neurogenic disorder, treatment may be better directed and more effective from the outset.

As the medical community begins to explore further the healing process associated with tendinitis and nerve compression disorders, greater variations in treatment are expected. The research on reorganization of the somatosensory cortex following functional use and peripheral nerve injury is exciting and has tremendous implications for recovery from nerve compressions and entrapments. Clinicians who use sensory re-education strategies have already taken advantage of the plasticity within the nervous system to promote recovery. Knowledge of the extreme significance of functional use to reorganization should motivate therapists working with nerve-injured patients to ensure that their clinic and home treatment programs are rich in sensorimotor exploration and manipulation. As researchers continue their investigations of pulsed electromagnetic fields and other methods, there may soon be available treatment modalities that truly promote quicker growth of axons, resulting in greater gains toward functional recovery.

References

Adler MW (1982). Endorphins, enkephalins and neurotransmitters. *Med Times,* 110,32.

Adson AW (1951). Cervical ribs: symptoms, differential diagnosis and indications for section of the insertion of the scalenus anticus muscle. *J Int Coll Surgeons,* 16,546–559.

Allard T, Clark SA, Jenkins WM, & Merzenich MM (1991). Reorganization of somatosensory area 3b representations in adult owl monkeys after digital syndactyly. *J Neurophysiol,* 66,1048–1058.

Almekinders LC & Almekinders SV (1994). Outcome in the treatment of chronic overuse sports injuries: a retrospective study. *J Orthop Sports Phys Ther,* 19(3),157–161.

Anderson M & Tichenor CJ (1994). A patient with de Quervain's tenosynovitis: a case report using an Australian approach to manual therapy. *Phys Ther,* 74,314–326.

Apfel ER & Carranza J (1992). Dexterity. In JS Cassanova (Ed). *Clinical Assessment Recommendations* (2nd ed, pp. 85–94). Chicago: American Society of Hand Therapists.

Asbury A & Fields H (1984). Pain due to peripheral nerve damage—a hypothesis. *Neurology,* 34,1587–1590.

Backman C, Boquist L, Friden J, Lorentzon R, & Toolanen G (1990). Chronic achilles paratenonitis with tendinosis: an experimental model in the rabbit. *J Orthop Res,* 8,541–547.

Backman C, Friden J, & Widmark A (1991). Blood flow in chronic achilles tendinosis. Radioactive microsphere study in rabbits. *Acta Orthop Scand,* 62,386–387.

Baker PF, Ladds M, & Rubinson KA (1977). Measurement of the flow properties of isolated axoplasm in a defined chemical environment. *J Physiol (Lond),* 269,10–11.

Bell-Krotoski JA (1990). Sensibility testing: state of the art. In JM Hunter, LH Schneider, EM Mackin, & AD Callahan (Eds). *Rehabilitation of the Hand* (3rd ed, pp. 575–584). St. Louis: Mosby.

Bell-Krotoski J, Weinstein S, & Weinstein C (1993). Testing sensibility, including touch-pressure, two-point discrimination, point localization and vibration. *J Hand Ther,* 6(2),114–123.

Benjamin M, Evans EJ, & Copp L (1986). The histology of tendon attachments to bone in man. *J Anat,* 149,89–100.

Birk DE & Zycband E (1994). Assembly of the tendon extracellular matrix during development. *J Anat,* 184,457–463.

Bisby MA & Keen P (1986). Regeneration of primary afferent neurons containing substance P–like immunoreactivity. *Brain Res,* 365,85–95.

Bora FW, Richardson W, & Black J (1980). The biomechanical responses to tension in a peripheral nerve. *J Hand Surg [Am],* 5,21–25.

Borynsenko M & Beringer T (1989). *Functional Histology* (3rd ed, pp. 105–112). Boston: Little, Brown.

Bowden REM (1954). Factors influencing functional recovery. In HJ Seddon (Ed). *Peripheral Nerve Injuries* (pp. 298–353). London: Her Majesty's Stationery Office.

Brandenburg GA & Mann MD (1989). Sensory nerve crush and regeneration and the receptive fields and response properties of neurons in the primary somatosensory cerebral cortex of cats. *Exp Neurol,* 103,256–266.

Braune S & Schady W (1993). Changes in sensation after nerve injury or amputation: the role of central factors. *J Neurol Neurosurg Psychiatry,* 56,393–399.

Brumback RA, Bobele GB, & Rayan GM (1992). Electrodiagnosis of compressive nerve lesions. *Hand Clin,* 8,241–254.

Butler DS (1991). *Mobilisation of the Nervous System.* New York: Churchill Livingstone.

Butler DS & Guth BP (May 1–2, 1993). Mobilization of the Nervous System. Course sponsored by Summit Physical Therapy, PC. Syracuse, NY.

Cailliet R (1975). *Hand Pain and Impairment* (2nd ed). Philadelphia: Davis.

Cailliet R (1991). *Shoulder Pain* (3rd ed). Philadelphia: Davis.

Calford MB & Tweedale R (1991). Immediate expansion of receptive fields of neurons in area 3b of macaque monkeys after digit denervation. *Somatosens Mot Res,* 8,249–260.

Callahan AD (1990). Sensibility testing: clinical methods. In JM Hunter, LH Schneider, EJ Mackin, & AD Callahan (Eds). *Rehabilitation of the Hand* (3rd ed, pp. 594–610). St. Louis: Mosby.

Carlstedt CA (1987). Mechanical and chemical factors in tendon healing. Effects of indomethacin and surgery in the rabbit. *Acta Orthop Scand Suppl,* 224,1–75.

Carlstedt CA, Madsen K, & Wredmark T (1986a). The influence of indomethacin on collagen synthesis during tendon healing in the rabbit. *Prostaglandins,* 32,353.

Carlstedt CA, Madsen K, & Wredmark T (1986b). The influence of indomethacin on collagen synthesis during tendon healing. A biomechanical and biochemical study. *Arch Orthop Trauma Surg,* 105,332.

Carlstedt CA & Nordin M (1989). Biomechanics of tendons and ligaments. In M Nordin & VH Frankel (Eds). *Basic Biomechanics of the Musculoskeletal System* (2nd ed, pp. 59–74). Philadelphia: Lea & Febiger.

Chidgey LK & Szabo RM (1989). Anterior interosseous nerve palsy. In RM Szabo (Ed). *Nerve Compression Syndromes: Diagnosis and Treatment* (pp. 153–162). Thorofare, NJ: Slack, Inc.

Clancy WG (1990). Tendon trauma and overuse injuries. In WB Leadbetter, JA Buckwalter, & SL Gordon (Eds). *Sports-Induced Inflammation: Clinical and Basic Science Concepts* (p. 609). Park Ridge, IL: Academy of Orthopedic Surgeons.

Curwin S & Stanish WD (1984). *Tendinitis: Its Etiology and Treatment.* Lexington, MA: Collamore Press/DC Heath.

Cyriax J (1982). *Textbook of Orthopaedic Medicine, Vol 1: Diagnosis of Soft-Tissue Lesions* (8th ed). London: Bailliere Tindall.

Cyriax JH (1936). The pathology and treatment of tennis elbow. *J Bone Joint Surg Am,* 18,921–940.

Dahlin LB & Lundborg G (1990). The neurone and its response to peripheral nerve compression. *J Hand Surg [Br],* 15,5–10.

Davick JP, Martin RK, & Albright JP (1988). Distribution and deposition of tritiated cortisol using phonophoresis. *Phys Ther,* 68,1672–1675.

Dawson DM, Hallett M, & Millender LH (1990). *Entrapment Neuropathies* (2nd ed.). Boston: Little, Brown.

Dellon AL (1978). The moving two point discrimination test: clinical evaluation of the quickly adapting fiber/receptor system. *J Hand Surg [Am],* 3,474–481.

Dellon AL (1993). A numerical grading scale for peripheral nerve function. *J Hand Ther,* 6(2),152–160.

Dellon AL & Kallman CH (1983). Evaluation of functional sensation in the hand. *J Hand Surg [Am],* 8,865–870.

Dellon AL, MacKinnon SE, & Crosby PM (1987). Reliability of two point discrimination measurements. *J Hand Surg [Am],* 12,693–696.

Droz B, Rambourg A, & Koenig HL (1975). The smooth endoplasmic reticulum: structure and role in the renewal of axonal membrane and synaptic vesicles by fast axonal transport. *Brain Res,* 93,1–13.

Dyck PJ, Lais AC, Giannini C, & Engelstand JK. (1990). Structural alterations of nerve during cuff compression. *Proc Natl Acad Sci U S A*, 87,9828–9832.

Dyson M, Pond JB, Joseph J, & Warwick R (1968). The stimulation of tissue regeneration by means of ultrasound. *Clin Sci*, 35,273–285.

Edgelow PI (February 1995). Thoracic outlet syndrome: thoughts on cause and correction. Presented at the American Physical Therapy Association's Combined Section Meeting, Reno, NV.

Edwards NT (August 1991). Phonophoresis . . . let me count the ways. *Phys Ther Forum*, 4–7.

Ehrlich W (1986). Cheiralgia parasthetica (entrapment of the radial sensory nerve). *J Hand Surg [Am]*, 11,196.

Elliott DH (1967). The biomechanical properties of tendon in relation to muscular strength. *Ann Phys Med*, 9,1.

Elvey RL, Quintner JL, & Thomas AN (1986). A clinical study of RSI. *Aust Fam Physician*, 15,1314–1322.

Evans RB, Hunter JM, & Burkhalter WE (1988). Conservative management of the trigger finger: a new approach. *J Hand Ther*, 1(2),59–74.

Fyfe I & Stanish WD (1992). The use of eccentric training and stretching in the treatment and prevention of tendon injuries. *Clin Sports Med*, 11,601–624.

Garraghty PE, Lachica EA, & Kaas JH (1991). Injury-induced reorganization of somatosensory cortex is accompanied by reductions in GABA staining. *Somatosens Mot Res*, 8,347–354.

Garrett W & Tidball J (1988). Myotendinous junction: structure, function, and failure. In SL-Y Woo & JA Buckwalter (Eds). *Injury and Repair of the Musculoskeletal Soft Tissues* (pp. 171–212). Park Ridge, IL: American Academy of Orthopedic Surgeons.

Garrett WE Jr, Nikolaou PK, Ribbeck BM, Glisson RR, & Seaber AV (1988). The effect of muscle architecture on the biomechanical failure properties of skeletal muscle under passive tension. *Am J Sports Med*, 16(1),7–12.

Gelberman RH (1991). *Operative Nerve Repair and Reconstruction*, Vols 1 & 2. Philadelphia: Lippincott.

Gerber G, Gerber G, & Altman KI (1960). Studies on the metabolism of tissue proteins: I. Turnover of collagen labeled with proline-U-C14 in young rats. *J Biolog Chem*, 235,2653–2656.

Gordon AM, Huxley AF, & Julian FJ (1966). Tension development in highly stretched vertebrate muscle fibers. *J Physiol*, 184,143–169.

Gordon J, Ghilardi MF, & Ghez C (1995). Impairments of reaching movements in patients without proprioception: I. Spatial errors. *J Neurophysiol*, 73,347–360.

Gracely RH (1979). Psychophysical assessment of human pain. In JJ Bonica (Ed). *Advances in Pain Research and Therapy*, Vol 3 (pp. 805–824). New York: Raven Press.

Grafstein B & Forman DS (1980). Intracellular transport in neurons. *Physiol Rev*, 60,1167.

Groppel JL & Nirschl RP (1986). A mechanical and electromyographical analysis of the effects of various joint counter force braces on the tennis player. *Am J Sports Med*, 14(3),195–200.

Grundberg AB & Reagan DS (1985). Pathologic anatomy of the forearm: intersection syndrome. *J Hand Surg [Am]*, 10,299–305.

Haak RA, Kleinhaus FW, & Ochs S (1976). The viscosity of mammalian nerve axoplasm measured by electron spin resonance. *J Physiol*, 263,115–137.

Harris L (Aug 13, 1994). Treating thoracic outlet syndrome. Lecture given at the conference, Current Topics in Hand Rehabilitation, sponsored by the Section on Hand Rehabilitation of the American Physical Therapy Association. New Orleans, LA.

Hawkins R & Kennedy J (1980). Impingement syndrome in athletes. *Am J Sports Med*, 8,151–157.

Howell JW (1991). Evaluation and management of thoracic outlet syndrome. In R Donatelli (Ed). *Physical Therapy of the Shoulder* (2nd ed, pp. 151–190). New York: Churchill Livingstone.

Hunt TK & Hussain Z (1992). Wound micro environment. In IK Cohen, RF Diegelmann, & WJ Lindblad (Eds). *Wound Healing* (p 274). Philadelphia: Saunders.

Jebsen RH, Taylor N, Trieschmann RB, Trotter MJ, & Howard LA (1969). An objective and standardized test of hand function. *Arch Phys Med Rehabil*, 50,311–319.

Jenkins WM, Merzanich MM, & Raconzone G (1990). Neocortical representational dynamics in adult primates. *Neuropsychologia*, 28,573–584.

Johnson RK & Spinner M (1989). Median nerve compression in the forearm: the pronator tunnel syndrome. In RM Szabo (Ed). *Nerve Compression Syndromes: Diagnosis and Treatment* (pp. 137–151). Thorofare, NJ: Slack, Inc.

Jozsa L, Reffy A, Kannus P, Demel S, & Elek E (1990). Pathological alterations in human tendons. *Arch Orthop Trauma Surg*, 110,15–21.

Kahn J (August 1991). Response to NT Edwards' "Phonophoresis . . . let me count the ways." *Phys Ther Forum*, 7.

Kahn J (1994). *Principles and Practice of Electrotherapy* (3rd ed). New York: Churchill Livingstone.

Kanje M, Lundborg G, & Edstrom A (1988). A new method for studies of the effects of locally applied drugs on peripheral nerve regeneration in vivo. *Brain Res*, 439,116–121.

Kasch M (1995). Therapist's evaluation and treatment of upper extremity cumulative trauma disorders. In J Hunter, J Schneider, E Mackin, & A Callahan (Eds). *Rehabilitation of the Hand* (4th ed, pp. 1725–1737). St. Louis: Mosby.

Kastelic J & Baer E (1980). Deformation in tendon collagen. *Symp Soc Exp Biol*, 34,397–435.

Kastelic J, Galeski A, & Baer E (1978). The multicomposite structure of tendons. *Connect Tissue Res*, 6,11–23.

Kelly T (1979). Thoracic outlet syndrome: current concepts of treatment. *Ann Surg*, 190,657–662.

Kennedy JC & Baxter-Willis R (1976). The effects of local steroid injections on tendons: a biochemical and microscopic correlative study. *Am J Sports Med*, 4,11–18.

Kibler WB, Chandler TJ, & Pace BK (1992). Principles of rehabilitation after chronic tendon injuries. *Clin Sports Med*, 11,661–670.

Laurent TC (1987). Structure, function and turnover of the extracellular matrix. *Adv Microcirc*, 13,15–34.

Leadbetter W (1991). Physiology of tissue repair. In *Athletic Training and Sports Medicine*. Park Ridge, IL: American Academy of Orthopedic Surgeons.

Leadbetter WB (1992). Cell-matrix response in tendon injury. *Clin Sports Med*, 11,533–578.

Lindsay M (November 1993). Radial tunnel versus lateral epicondylitis. *Newsletter of the Section on Hand Rehabilitation of the American Physical Therapy Association*, 10(39),1.

Lindsay M (June 1994). Evaluation and management of elbow disorders. Presented at the American Society of Hand Therapists' Upper Extremity Expo, Atlanta, GA.

Littler JW (1977). Stenosing digital tendovaginitis. In JM Converse & JW Littler (Eds). *Reconstructive Plastic Surgery, Vol 6: The Hand and Upper Extremity* (pp. 3440–3443). New York: Saunders.

Lundborg G (1979). The intrinsic vascularization of human peripheral nerves: structural and functional aspects. *J Hand Surg*, 4(1),34.

Lundborg G & Dahlin LB (1992). The pathophysiology of nerve compression. *Hand Clin*, 8,215–227.

Lundborg G, Dahlin LB, Danielsen N, & Nachemason AK (1986). Tissue specificity in nerve regeneration. *Scand J Plast Reconstr Surg*, 20,279–283.

Lundborg G & Rank F (1978). Experimental intrinsic healing of flexor tendons based on synovial fluid nutrition. *J Hand Surg [Am]*, 3,21–31.

Lundborg G & Rydevik B (1973). Effects of stretching the tibial nerve of the rabbit: a preliminary study of the intraneural circulation and the barrier function of the perineurium. *J Bone Joint Surg Br*, 55,390–401.

Mackinnon SE (1992). Double and multiple entrapment neuropathies. *Hand Clin*, 8,369–390.

Mackinnon SE, Dellon AL, Lundborg G, Hudson AR, & Hunter DA (1986). A study of neurotropism in a primate model. *J Hand Surg [Am]*, 6,888–894.

Maitland GD (1991). *Peripheral Mobilization* (3rd ed). Boston: Butterworth-Heinemann.

Markison RE (1990). Treatment of musical hands: redesign of the interface. *Hand Clin*, 6,525–544.

Markison RE (1992). Tendinitis and related inflammatory conditions seen in musicians. *J Hand Ther*, 5(2),80–83.

Martens M, Wouters P, Burssens A, & Mulier JC. (1982). Patellar tendinitis: pathology and results of treatment. *Acta Orthop Scand*, 53,445–450.

Matloub HS & Yousif NJ (1992). Peripheral nerve anatomy and innervation pattern. *Hand Clin*, 8,201–214.

Melzack R (1975). The McGill Pain Questionnaire: major properties and scoring methods. *Pain*, 1,277.

Melzack R & Wall PD (1965). Pain mechanisms: a new theory. *Science*, 150,971.

Merzenich MM & Jenkins WM (1993). Reorganization of cortical representation of the hand following alterations of skin inputs induced by nerve injury, skin island transfers and experience. *J Hand Ther*, 6(2),89–104.

Merzenich MM, Kaas JH, Sur M, & Lin C-S (1978). Double representation of the body surface within cytoarchitectonic areas 3b and 1 in "S1" in the owl monkey (*Aotus trivirgatus*). *J Comp Neurol*, 181,41–74.

Merzenich MM & Sameshima K (1993). Cortical plasticity and memory. *Curr Biol* 3,187–196.

Michlovitz SL (1986). Cryotherapy: the use of cold as a therapeutic agent. In SL Michlovitz (Ed), *Thermal Agents in Rehabilitation* (pp. 73–98). Philadelphia: Davis.

Millesi H, Zoch G, & Rath TH (1990). The gliding apparatus of peripheral nerve and its clinical significance. *Ann Hand Surg*, 9(2),87–97.

Moberg E (1960). Evaluation of sensibility in the hand. *Surg Clin North Am*, 40,357–361.

Moberg E (1962). Criticism and study of methods for examining sensibility of the hand. *Neurology*, 12,8–9.

Mogilner A, Grossman JA, Ribary U, Joliot M, Volkmann J, Rapaport D, Beasley RW, & Llinas RR (1993). Somatosensory cortical plasticity in adult humans revealed by magnetoencephalography. *Proc Natl Acad Sci U S A*, 90,3593–3597.

Moran CA (1994). Using myofascial techniques to treat musicians. *J Hand Ther*, 5(2),97–101.

Moran CA & Callahan AD (1983). Sensibility measurement and management. In CA Moran (Ed). *Hand Rehabilitation* (pp. 45–68). New York: Churchill Livingstone.

Muckart RD (1964). Stenosing tendovaginitis of abductor pollicis longus and extensor pollicis brevis at the radial styloid (de Quervain's disease). *Clin Orthop*, 33,201–208.

Nakano KK (1991). Peripheral nerve entrapments, repetitive strain disorder, occupation-related syndromes, bursitis and tendonitis. *Curr Opin Rheumatol*, 3,226–239.

Neer CS & Welsh RP (1982). The shoulder in sports. *Orthop Clin North Am*, 8,439.

Newman MK, Kill M, & Frampton G (1958). Effects of ultrasound alone and combined with hydrocortisone injections by needle or hydrospray. *Am J Phys Med*, 37,206.

Newton RA (1990). Contempory views on pain and the role played by thermal agents in managing pain symptoms. In SL Michlovitz (Ed). *Thermal Agents in Rehabilitation* (pp. 19–48). Philadelphia: Davis.

Nirschl RP (1992). Elbow tendinosis/tennis elbow. *Clin Sports Med*, 11,851–870.

Nirschl RP & Pettrone FA (1979). Tennis elbow: the surgical treatment of lateral epicondylitis. *J Bone Joint Surg Am*, 61,832–839.

Noonan TJ & Garrett WE Jr (1992). Injuries at the myotendinous junction. *Clin Sports Med*, 11,783–806.

Noyes FR, Torvi P, Hyde WB, & DeLucas JL (1974). Biomechanics of ligament failure. II. An analysis of immobilization, exercise, and reconditioning effects in primates. *J Bone Joint Surg Am*, 56,1406–1418.

O'Brien M (1992). Functional anatomy and physiology of tendons. *Clin Sports Med*, 11,505–520.

Ogata K & Naito M (1986). Blood flow of peripheral nerve effects of dissection, stretching and compression. *J Hand Surg [Br]*, 11(1),10–14.

Ohkawa S (1982). Effects of orthodontic forces and anti-inflammatory drugs on the mechanical strength of the periodontium in the rat mandibular first molar. *Am J Orthodont*, 81,498.

Olsson Y & Kristennson K (1971). Permeability of blood vessels and connective tissue sheaths in the peripheral nervous system to exogenous proteins. *Acta Neuropathol*, 5,61–69.

O'Riain S (1973). New and simple test of nerve function in the hand. *BMJ*, 3,615–616.

Osterman AL (1988). The double crush syndrome. *Orthop Clin North Am*, 19,147–155.

Otten U (1984). Nerve growth factor and the peptidergic sensory neurons. *Trends Pharmacol*, 7,307–310.

Pascual-Leone A & Torres F (1993). Plasticity of the sensorimotor cortex representation of the reading finger in Braille readers. *Brain,* 116,39–52.

Peacock EE (1965). Biological principles in the healing of long tendons. *Surg Clin North Am,* 45,461.

Peimer CA & Wheeler DR (1989). Radial tunnel syndrome (posterior interosseous nerve compression). In RM Szabo (Ed). *Nerve Compression Syndromes: Diagnosis and Treatment.* (pp. 177–192). Thorofare, NJ: Slack, Inc.

Phalen GS (1966). The carpal tunnel syndrome: seventeen years' experience in diagnosis and treatment of six hundred fifty four hands. *J Bone Joint Surg Am*, 48,211–228.

Pons TP, Garraghty PE, Ommaya AK, Kaas JH, Taub E, & Mishkin M (1991). Massive cortical reorganization after sensory deafferentation in adult macaques. *Science*, 252,1857–1860.

Powell SG & Burke AL (1991). Surgical and therapeutic management of tennis elbow. An update. *J Hand Ther,* 4,64–68.

Pratt NE (1991). *Clinical Musculoskeletal Anatomy.* Philadelphia: Lippincott.

Puddu G, Ippolito E, & Postacchini P (1976). A classification of achilles tendon disease. *Am J Sports Med*, 4,145–150.

Ramachandran VS, Rogers-Ramachandran D, & Stewart M (1992). Perceptual correlates of massive cortical reorganization. *Science*, 258,1159–1160.

Rasmusson DD, Webster HH, & Dykes RW (1992). Neuronal response properties within subregions of raccoon somatosensory cortex 1 week after digit amputation. *Somatosens Mot Res*, 9,279–289.

Rath T & Millesi H (1990). The gliding tissue of the median nerve in the carpal tunnel [German abstract]. *Handchir Mikrochir Plast Chir*, 22,203–205.

Redmond MD & Rivner D (1977). False positive electrodiagnostic tests in carpal tunnel syndrome. *Muscle Nerve*, 11,379–385.

Rider B & Linden C (1988). Comparison of standardized and non-standardized administration of the Jebsen Hand Function Test. *J Hand Ther*, 1(3),121–126.

Riley GP, Harrall RL, Constant CR, Cawston TE, & Hazleman BL (1994a). Glycosaminoglycans of human rotator cuff tendons: changes with age and in chronic rotator cuff tendinitis. *Ann Rheum Dis*, 53,367–376.

Riley GP, Harrall RL, Constant CR, Chard MD, Causton TE, & Hazeleman BL (1994b). Tendon degeneration and chronic shoulder pain: changes in the collagen composi-

tion of the human rotator cuff tendons in rotator cuff tendinitis. *Ann Rheum Dis*, 53,359–366.

Rodineau J (1991). Tendinitis and tenosynovitis of the wrist [French abstract]. *Rev Praticien*, 41,2699–2706.

Roos DB (1966). Experience with first rib resection for thoracic outlet syndrome. *Ann Surg*, 163,354–358.

Rothe T, Hanisch UK, Krohn K, Schliebs R, Hartig W, Webster HH, & Biesold D (1990). Changes in choline acetyltransferase activity and high-affinity choline uptake, but not in acetylcholinesterase activity and muscarinic cholinergic receptors, in rat somatosensory cortex after sciatic nerve injury. *Somatosens Mot Res*, 7,435–446.

Rothwell J (1995). Proprioceptors in muscles, joints, and skin. In *Control of Human Voluntary Movement* (pp. 86–126). New York: Chapman & Hall.

Rubin E & Faber JL (1988). *Pathology*. Philadelphia: Lippincott.

Rydevik B, Lundborg G, & Bagge U (1981). Effects of graded compression on intraneural blood flow. An in vivo study on rabbit tibial nerve. *J Hand Surg [Am]*, 6,3–12.

Rydevik B, McLean WG, Sjostrand J, & Lundborg G (1990). Blockage of axonal transport induced by acute, graded compression of the rabbit vagus nerve. *J Neurol Neurosurg Psychiatry*, 43,690–698.

Safran MR, Garrett WE, & Seaber AV (1988). The role of warm-up in muscular injury prevention. *Am J Sports Med,* 16(2),123–129.

Sainburg RL, Poizner H, & Ghez C (1993). Loss of proprioception produces deficits in interjoint coordination. *J Neurophysiol*, 70,2136–2147.

Sanders RJ & Haug CE (1991). *Thoracic Outlet Syndrome: A Common Sequela of Neck Injuries* (p. 34). Philadelphia: Lippincott.

Schmelzeisen H (1990). Evaluating histologic findings of the rotator cuff of the shoulder [German abstract]. *Aktuelle Traumatol*, 20(3),48–51.

Scott J & Huskisson EC (1979). Vertical and horizontal analog scales. *Ann Rheum Dis,* 38, 560.

Seddon H (1943). Three types of nerve injury. *Brain*, 66,237.

Seddon HJ (1954). *Peripheral Nerve Injuries* (pp. 1–15). London: Her Majesty's Stationery Office.

Sjolund BH & Eriksson MBE (1979). Endorphins, analgesia produced by peripheral conditioning stimulation. In JJ Bonica (Ed). *Advances in Pain Research and Therapy*, Vol 3 (p. 587). New York: Raven Press.

Sommerich CM, McGlothlin JD, & Marrar WS (1993). Occupational risk factors associated with soft tissue disorders of the shoulder: a review of recent investigations in the literature. *Ergonomics*, 36,697–717.

Spinner M (1970). The anterior interosseous nerve syndrome. With special attention to its variations. *J Bone Joint Surg Am*, 52,84.

Stone JH (1992). Sensibility. In J Casanova (Ed). *Clinical Assessment Recommendations* (2nd ed, pp. 71–94). Chicago: American Society of Hand Therapists.

Sunderland S (1978). *Nerves and Nerve Injuries* (2nd ed). London: Churchill Livingstone.

Szabo RM (1989). *Nerve Compression Syndromes: Diagnosis and Treatment*. Thorofare, NJ: Slack, Inc.

Szabo RM & Gelberman RH (1987). The pathophysiology of nerve entrapment syndromes. *J Hand Surg [Am]*, 12,881–884.

Tassler PL, Dellon AL, & Canoun C (1994). Identification of elastic fibres in the peripheral nerve. *J Hand Surg [Br]*, 19,48–54.

Thorson EP & Szabo RM (1989). Tendonitis of the wrist and elbow. In ML Kasdan (Ed). *Occupational Medicine: Occupational Hand Injuries* (pp. 419–431). Philadelphia: Homley & Belfus, Inc.

Tidball JG (1983). The geometry of actin filament-membrane associations can modify adhesive strength of the myotendinous junction. *Cell Motil Cytoskeleton*, 3,439–447.

Tinel J (1915). Le signe du "fourmillement" dans les lesions des nerfs peripheriques [the "tingling" sign in peripheral nerve lesions]. (EB Kaplan, Transl.) *Presse Medicale*, 23,388–389. In M Spinner (1978). *Injuries to the Major Branches of Peripheral Nerves of the Forearm* (2nd ed; pp. 8–13). Philadelphia: Saunders.

Travell JG & Simons DG (1983). *Myofascial Pain and Dysfunction, The Trigger Point Manual, Vol 1: The Upper Extremities*. Baltimore: Williams & Wilkins.

Turnbull BG & Rasmusson DD (1990). Acute effects of total or partial digit denervation on raccoon somatosensory cortex. *Somatosens Mot Res*, 7,365–389.

Turnbull BG & Rasmusson DD (1991). Chronic effects of total or partial digit denervation on raccoon somatosensory cortex. *Somatosens Mot Res*, 8,201–213.

Upton ARM & McComas AJ (1973). The double crush in nerve entrapment syndromes. *Lancet*, 2,359–362.

Vogel HC (1977). Mechanical and chemical properties of various connective tissue organs in rats as influenced by nonsteroidal antirheumatic drugs. *Connect Tissue Res*, 5,91–95.

Walker JL, Evans JM, Resig P, Guarneri S, Meade P, & Sisken BS (1994). Enhancement of functional recovery following a crush lesion to the rat sciatic nerve by exposure to pulsed electromagnetic fields. *Exp Neurol*, 125,302–305.

Walsh MT (1994). Therapist management of thoracic outlet syndrome. *J Hand Ther*, 7(2),131–144.

Warhold LG, Osterman AL, & Skirven T (1993). Lateral epicondylitis: how to treat it and prevent recurrence. *J Musculoskel Med*, 10(6),55–73.

Warren CG, Koblanski JN, & Sigelmann RA (1976). Ultrasound coupling media: their relative transmissivity. *Arch Phys Med*, 57,218–222.

Weber EH (1835). Ueber den Tastsinn. *Arch Anat Physiol Wissen Med Muller's Arch*, 1,152–159.

Weinstein S (1993). Fifty years of somatosensory research: from the Semmes-Weinstein monofilaments to the Weinstein enhanced sensory test. *J Hand Ther*, 6(1),11–22.

Wilgis S & Murphy R (1986). The significance of longitudinal excursion in peripheral nerves. *Hand Clin*, 2,761.

Wolf SL (1984). Neurophysiologic mechanisms in pain modulation: relevance to T.E.N.S. In JS Mannheimer & GN Lampe (Ed). *Clinical Transcutaneous Electrical Nerve Stimulation* (pp. 41–55). Philadelphia: Davis.

Woo S, Maynard J, Butler D, Lyon R, Torzilli P, Akeson W, Cooper R, & Oakes B (1987). Ligament, tendon, and joint capsule insertions to bone. In SL-Y Woo & JA Buckwalter (Eds). *Injury and Repair of the Musculoskeletal Soft Tissues* (pp. 133–166). Park Ridge, IL: American Academy of Orthopedic Surgeons.

Woo SL-Y (1982). Mechanical properties of tendons and ligaments: I. Quasi-static and nonlinear viscoelastic properties. *Biorheology*, 19,385–396.

Woo SL-Y, Matthews JV, Akenson WH, Amiel D, & Convery FR (1975). Connective tissue response to immobility. Correlative study of biomechanical and biochemical measurements of normal and immobilized rabbit knees. *Arthritis Rheum*, 18(3),257–264.

Wright IS (1945). The neurovascular syndrome produced by hyperabduction of the arms. The immediate changes produced in 150 normal controls, and the effects on some persons of prolonged hyperabduction of the arms, as in sleeping, and in certain occupations. *Am Heart J*, 29,1.

Wulle C (1993). Intersection syndrome [German abstract]. *Handchir Mikrochir Plast Chir*, 25,48–50.

Yamada H (1970). Strength of biological materials. In FG Evans (Ed). *The Biomechanical Responses to Tension in a Peripheral Nerve*. Baltimore: Williams & Wilkins.

Zachary RB (1954). Results of nerve suture. In HJ Seddon (Ed). *Peripheral Nerve Injuries* (pp. 354–388). London: Her Majesty's Stationery Office.

Zarzecki P, Witte S, Smits E, Gordon DC, Kirchberger P, & Rasmusson DD (1993). Synaptic mechanisms of cortical representational plasticity: somatosensory and corticocortical EPSPs in reorganized raccoon SI cortex. *J Neurophysiol*, 69,1422–1432.

Ziskin MC & Michlovitz SL (1986). Therapeutic ultrasound. In SL Michlovitz (Ed). *Thermal Agents in Rehabilitation* (pp. 141–176). Philadelphia: Davis.

Suggested Reading

Dale WA (1982). Thoracic outlet syndrome. Critique in 1982. *Arch Surg*, 117,1437.

Dellon AL (1981). *Evaluation of Sensibility and Re-Education of Sensation in the Hand*. Baltimore: Williams & Wilkins.

Eaton RG (1992). Entrapment syndromes in musicians. *J Hand Ther*, 5(2),91–96.

Elvey RL (1975). Treatment of arm pain associated with abnormal brachial plexus tension. *Aust J Physiol*, 32,224–229.

Frampton VM (1988). Management of brachial plexus lesions. *J Hand Ther*, 1(3),115–120.

Frykman GK (1993). The quest for better recovery from peripheral nerve injury: current status of nerve regeneration research. *J Hand Ther*, 6(2),83–88.

Gellman H (1992). Tennis elbow (lateral epicondylitis). *Orthop Clin North Am*, 23,75–82.

Greenspan JD & LaMotte RH (1993). Cutaneous mechanore-ceptors of the hand: experimental studies and their implications for clinical testing of tactile stimulation. *J Hand Ther*, 6(2),75–82.

Jiminez S, Hardy MA, Horch K, & Jabaley M (1993). A study of sensory recovery following carpal tunnel release. *J Hand Ther*, 6(2),124–129.

Jobe, CM (1990). Gross anatomy of the shoulder. In CA Rockwood & FA Matson (Eds). *The Shoulder*. Philadelphia: Saunders.

Johnson SL (1990). Ergonomic design of handheld tools to prevent trauma to the hand and upper extremity. *J Hand Ther*, 3(2),86–93.

King PB & Aulicino PL (1990). The postoperative rehabilitation of the learmonth submuscular transposition of the ulnar nerve at the elbow. *J Hand Ther*, 3(3),149–156.

Lowe C (1992). Treatment of tendinitis, tenosynovitis, and other cumulative trauma disorders of musicians' forearms, wrists, and hands . . . restoring function with hand therapy. *J Hand Ther*, 5(2),84–90.

Lundborg G (1993). Peripheral nerve injuries: pathophysiology and strategies for treatment. *J Hand Ther*, 6(3),179–188.

Lundborg G, Gelberman RH, Minteer-Convery M, Lee YF, & Hargens AR (1982). Median nerve compression in the carpal tunnel—functional response to experimentally induced controlled pressure. *J Hand Surg [Am]*, 7,252.

MacDermid J (1991). Accuracy of clinical tests used in the detection of carpal tunnel syndrome: a literature review. *J Hand Ther*, 4(4),169–176.

Manheim C & Lavett D (1989). *The Myofascial Release Manual*. Thorofare, NJ: Slack, Inc.

Marras WS (1993). Wrist motions in industry. *Ergonomics*, 36,341–351.

Mitchell J & Osterman AL (1991). Physiology of nerve repair. *Hand Clin*, 7,481–490.

Moberg E (1958). Objective methods of determining the functional value of sensibility of the hand. *J Bone Joint Surg Br*, 40,454.

Mumenthaler M & Schliack H (1991). *Peripheral Nerve Lesions: Diagnosis and Therapy*. New York: Thieme.

Nirschl RP (1980). Medial tennis elbow: surgical treatment. *Orthop Transact*, 4,298.

Novak CB, Mackinnon SE, & Patterson GA (1993). Evaluation of patients with thoracic outlet syndrome. *J Hand Surg [Am]*, 18,292–299.

Ochs S (1975). Axoplasmic transport. In DB Tower (Ed). *The Nervous System, Vol 1: The Basic Neurosciences*. New York: Raven Press.

Pecina MM, Krmpotic-Nemanic J, & Markiewitz AD (1991). *Tunnel Syndromes*. Boston: CRC Press.

Putz-Anderson V (1988). *Cumulative Trauma Disorders: A Manual for Musculoskeletal Diseases of the Upper Limbs*. Philadelphia: Taylor & Francis.

Rayan GM (1992). Proximal ulnar nerve compression. Cubital tunnel syndrome. *Hand Clin*, 8,325–336.

Renstrom PAFH & Leadbetter WB (Eds) (1992). *Tendinitis I: Basic Concepts* (11). Philadelphia: Saunders.

Renstrom PAFH & Leadbetter WB (Eds) (1992). *Tendinitis II: Clinical Considerations* (11). Philadelphia: Saunders.

Schmidt RF (1985). *Fundamentals of Neurophysiology* (3rd ed). New York: Springer-Verlag.

Shanthaveerappa TR & Bourne GH (1963). The perineural epithelium: nature and significance. *Nature*, 199,577.

Spinner M (1978). *Injuries to the Major Branches of Peripheral Nerves of the Forearm* (2nd ed). Philadelphia: Saunders.

Sunderland S (1991). *Nerve Injuries and Their Repair*. New York: Churchill Livingstone.

Terzis JK & Smith KL (1990). *The Peripheral Nerve: Structure, Function and Reconstruction*. New York: Raven Press.

Totten PA & Hunter JM (1991). Therapeutic techniques to enhance nerve gliding in thoracic outlet syndrome and carpal tunnel syndrome. *Hand Clin*, 7,505–520.

Willis WD Jr & Grossman RC (1973). *Medical Neurobiology*. St. Louis: Mosby.

Woo SL-Y (1986). Biomechanics of tendons and ligaments. In GW Schmid-Schonbein, SL-Y Woo & BW Zweifach (Eds). *Frontiers in Biomechanics* (pp. 180–195). New York: Springer-Verlag.

PART III

Risk Factors Related to
Cumulative Trauma Disorders
in Business and Industry

Chapter 6

Physiologic Risk Factors

Barbara J. Headley

The current dilemma presented by cumulative trauma disorders (CTDs) is twofold: CTDs require a better understanding of the risk factors involved both to enhance our ability to prevent the development of the disorders and to contain it effectively. To date, the development of ergonomically sound workstations has had an impact on lowering the incidence of CTDs. However, workstation design has had a less-than-expected impact on overall reduction of such injuries. According to the Bureau of Labor Statistics, CTDs rose 26% in 1992, accounting for some 281,800 reported injuries. Expenses associated with CTDs, including medical treatment, lost work time, and insurance compensation, approached nearly $100 billion (CTD News 1994).

The employee experiencing symptoms of CTD often presents with seemingly contradictory symptoms and behaviors. Many employees are clearly unable to do their job tasks, yet outside of work, they can be actively involved in functions that appear more demanding. For example, although employees' jobs may involve no heavy lifting, the repetitive or constant static loading sustained during work may not be tolerated. Traditional medical workup of these employees, including x-ray, magnetic resonance imaging, electromyography (EMG), diagnostic testing, and blood work sheds no light on the inability of these individuals to perform their job tasks. Additionally, subjective evaluation of fatigue presents an enigma not only for these employees but for those evaluating them. For many, fatigue is determined by employee rating of perceived fatigue and pain levels; hence, perceived fatigue during work tasks often appears out of proportion to their ability to perform other tasks.

Employees with CTDs often feel that their symptoms are questioned by coworkers and minimized by health care providers. As their motives are questioned, the relationship with their employer becomes adversarial. Anger and social isolation put additional stress on the coping response. An increasingly integral factor in maintaining or returning employees to their jobs is the examination of CTD risk factors that include how an employee interacts with the workstation. Worker characteristics now are accepted as critical elements in the ergonomics of work demands. Each employee has a set of acquired postures, habitual patterns of muscle use, lifting style, or psychosocial issues that influence how he or she interacts with the work environment (Middaugh et al. 1994). Exploration of the physiologic factors related to the resultant fatigue and to the failure of muscles to recover from fatigue is now providing insight into the inability of employees to perform tasks that they seem capable of doing.

Muscle recruitment patterns and their effect on pain or functional limitations have been studied by numerous authors (Wolf et al. 1979, 1982; Middaugh & Kee 1987). This work provides a framework to examine an employee's interaction with the workstation and offers a model by which performance may be modified if it is determined to be compromising muscle efficiency. Work by other researchers provides insight into what can be gained from further evaluation and intervention with employees in industry (Hagberg 1981; Hagberg &

Kvarnstrom 1984; Christensen 1986; Kilbom 1988; Westgaard 1988).

The capability of surface EMG (sEMG) for examining muscle activity allows for potential quantification of fatigue. This technique uses surface electrodes applied to the skin to collect a summation of motor unit action potentials beneath the site. Precise electrode placement using well-defined anatomic landmarks and carefully measured interelectrode distances provides valuable information about recruitment patterns of dynamic movement based on electrode activity at each site. Although integrated data offer easier interpretation of dynamic activity, raw data must be used to obtain a power spectrum (PS). This PS represents the frequencies (expressed in Hertz) that are the firing rates of the motor units (MUs) sampled by the surface electrodes.

Although subjected to predictable distortion by the tissue through which it passes, the PS provides a meaningful method of measuring muscle fatigue and recovery. The most commonly used parameter is the median frequency (MF). A symptomatic employee can be evaluated at an ergonomically correct workstation to determine how persistent muscle dysfunction is perpetuating inability to tolerate job demands. Using spectral analysis, work-rest cycles can be determined based on physiologic recovery of muscle. This evaluation structure provides a model for work-site injury prevention that also includes the physiologic risk factors and offers a new armamentarium with which to treat CTD.

Postural Mechanics

Work by Middaugh et al. (1994) examined two operator characteristics implicated in the development and perpetuation of chronic musculoskeletal pain in the upper quadrant: poor posture and inappropriate patterns of muscle use. These authors examined 20 normal, healthy college students who had good upper-body posture and were asked to perform a task in both appropriate and inappropriate postures. The students demonstrated that something as seemingly small as improper placement of a keyboard can promote posturing that results in significant muscle overuse. Factors such as forward head posture can lead to prolonged muscle contraction in the neck and shoulder girdle. These habitual patterns of muscle

overuse can continue during the rest portion of the work-rest cycles. Such findings confirm the benefits of developing good postural work habits that emphasize muscle efficiency rather than strength.

Middaugh et al. (1994) examined poor postural habits and the ability to change those habits, and reported that individuals with chronic postural dysfunction and pain often have poor kinesthetic awareness and voluntary control of key muscles in the symptomatic area. Flor et al. (1992) examined groups of individuals with pain and found that poor muscle tension discrimination also extends to areas not involved in the pain complaints. Therefore, these individuals may be using improper muscles to perform a task. The concept of muscle skill versus muscle strength has been discussed elsewhere (Headley 1991, 1993).

The importance of postural homeostasis, postural stability, and integration of sEMG for re-education has been examined by Taylor (1990) and Headley (1994). Proper training for many of these individuals comprises using "just enough" muscle activity to perform a task correctly. This training can be done at the work site, allowing the other environmental factors that can contribute to symptoms (i.e., noise, temperature, coworkers, space constraints, lighting, and pacing or work quotas) to be examined in the actual environment. Data loggers have been used to track muscle activity over an entire workday or during particular job rotations (Headley 1994). This capability provides an additional type of quantitative assessment of muscle activity in industry.

Fatigue

The examination of muscle fatigue requires an understanding of the multiple sites of fatigue, of the impact of central and peripheral phenomenon, and of differences imposed by a variety of exercise formats. The complexity and variety of human movement suggest an interactive sequence of events, any one of which may produce fatigue under certain circumstances. Bigland-Ritchie and Woods (1984) suggested that muscle failure can occur, due to fatigue in three possible areas. First, sites of fatigue may lie within the central nervous system (CNS) (Bigland-Ritchie & Woods 1984). Second, fatigue may occur at neural transmission sites linking the CNS to muscle. Third, sites within individual muscle fibers may be responsible. As activity continues, functional changes may occur in any or all potential sites. Although the measurement of force reduction (or decreased work capacity) has been used as a method of quantifying muscle fatigue, fatigue is also accompanied by many other measurable changes, such as a shift in the sEMG PS, slowing of muscle conduction velocity and contractile speed, and the accumulation of H+, lactate, and other metabolites. Major questions yet to be answered are which of these events determine performance and which are simply incidental by-products.

It would be unwise to consider muscle fatigue as a singular phenomenon. Exercise type, muscle selection, and the nature of a task must be considered, as sites of muscle fatigue may be dependent on these and other factors.

Localized Muscle Fatigue

Localized muscle fatigue (LMF) has been defined operationally as a transient decrease in working capacity that results from the failure of a muscle or group of muscles to develop or sustain a certain expected force or power. LMF is a self-protective mechanism against damage to the contractile elements (Nyland 1993). During muscle fatigue, the force-frequency ratio shifts toward the lower frequency range with the slowing of muscle contraction. This action allows all MUs to remain fully activated despite a substantial reduction in motoneuron discharge rate. This reduction probably guards against failure of neuromuscular transmission. It may also serve to optimize regulation of force by limiting rate of discharge to the range in which force production can be modulated.

Differences exist among various MUs according to the contractile properties of the individual constituent muscle fibers. Because these properties change with fatigue, a reflex regulatory mechanism may exist within the CNS to match the motoneuron discharge rates to the changing contractile speed of the MUs they supply (Bigland-Ritchie & Woods 1984). In discussing several of the sites of LMF, Nyland (1993) identifies how changes at these local sites may affect the sEMG PS. Reduction of blood flow, low intracellular pH, metabolite accumulation, and alterations in potassium concentrations all may

contribute to the PS shift to lower frequencies that occurs with fatigue.

Though decreased blood flow has been implicated clearly in muscle fatigue at high work levels (>30% maximum voluntary contraction [MVC]), it is not impaired sufficiently at low levels of static isometric work loads (<10% MVC) to be considered a contributing factor in the development of fatigue. Sjøgaard et al. (1986) state that it is not possible to assess the percentage at which MVC blood flow restriction causes fatigue, as intramuscular pressure may vary considerably within a muscle group and between various parts of the same muscle (Sjøgaard et al. 1988). This pressure can vary even more profoundly between different muscles, as the structure of muscle fibers and connective tissue may play an important role in determining tissue pressures. These authors' findings suggest that blood flow is sufficiently high to maintain homeostasis at contractions below 10% MVC, which corresponds to the approximate force needed to maintain the arms in a horizontal working position without holding any tools. These authors do suggest, however, that intramuscular changes may cause fatigue even though there is no compromise of blood flow to muscle. They report an increase in muscle water content of 10% after 1 hour at 5% MVC. The water then may stay in the interstitial space because there is no increased osmotic force within the muscle fibers to cause further flux into the fibers. They conclude that daily long-lasting edema in the upper-quadrant muscles may cause chronic morphologic changes that could impair transport mechanisms seriously.

Another clue to the fatigue seen in CTDs may be found in the potassium depletion discussed by Sjøgaard in another work (1986). He found that in healthy human subjects, the MVC had fallen to 88% of the initial level after holding a 5% MVC for 1 hour. The data indicate that fast-twitch fibers are not recruited during low-level contractions. There was a 16% decrease in potassium within those muscle fibers recruited during the 1 hour at 5% MVC. Such changes would not cause exhaustion but well may explain why the muscle could not perform the same MVC as under normal resting conditions. Potassium may not be restored quickly at rest, because of the low resting blood flow. The increased water content also may be a factor in the slow recovery.

These data suggest that although micropauses recommended for the prevention of muscle fatigue may delay the time to fatigue, these brief pauses result in only partial metabolic recovery. Different metabolic components recover at varying rates; therefore, time needed for full recovery may in fact be increased by the micropauses. Sjøgaard (1986) suggests instead that long resting periods may be needed after prolonged low-level contractions before homeostasis is restored with respect to intracellular potassium concentration. As discussed by Sjøgaard, excessive fluid in the muscle may alter its ability to function with the tendency toward more rapid fatigue.

Edwards (1988) has reported that fatiguing muscular activity can result in severe depletion of adenosine triphosphate in a small proportion of muscle fibers, though the average depletion (of the entire muscle) is less impressive. Such findings reinforce the concept of selective recruitment of muscle fibers based on the load demands, with subsequent fatigue developing in those selective fibers. Selective muscle fiber fatigue may be a factor in the seemingly contradictory activity abilities in individuals with CTD.

Seidel et al. (1987) studied four male subjects by sEMG to examine changes in the lumbar paraspinal muscles during fatiguing isometric contractions. They report that sEMG changes clearly depend on the level of force sustained, with different myoelectric symptoms of muscle fatigue occurring with varying force levels. These authors suggest that the "scope of recruitment" (i.e., the number of MUs recruited) varies within equal ranges of force, with less variation occurring at higher forces. They propose the possibility of "selective fatigue" following sustained isometric constant-force contractions. This concept refers to the selection of a certain pool of MUs that is subject to fatigue when recruited according to force needs. Sustained contractions of only approximately 20% MVC quickly induced a functional insufficiency of muscles, thus requiring compensatory recruitment patterns.

Several studies have examined the relationship of sustained, low-level contractions to muscle fatigue (Jorgensen et al. 1988). It has been shown that the endurance capability for sustained contractions is approximately 1 hour for 10% MVC and "indefinite" endurance at contractions below 15–20% MVC cannot be maintained. A 12% reduction in maximal force was seen with significant decreases in the MU firing rate after a 1-hour contraction sustained at only 5% MVC. These changes vary with muscle type.

The differences in muscle fatigue developed with isometric contractions at equivalent tension levels suggest that certain areas of the muscle are supplied inadequately with blood, or (as Sjøgaard reports) cannot transport effectively within the muscle even at these low contraction levels. These areas of LMF and ischemia may represent the conditions for myofascial trigger points described by Simons (1992) and Hong (1994). Pauses occurring with intermittent contractions, however, may allow sufficient transport of blood supply to these intramuscular areas (Jorgensen et al. 1988).

Central Component of Fatigue

Fatigue of central origin relates to failure of one or several mechanisms to maintain muscle activation. These mechanisms include the ability to generate a sufficient and appropriate central command for the task, faithful transmission of the command to the involved motoneuron pools, and sustained activation of the muscle by the motoneurons (Enoka 1995). In the CNS, there may be a modulation factor that facilitates recruitment in fatigued muscle by altering the rate of muscle fiber recruitment. By measuring the time course of the muscle twitch, Bigland-Ritchie et al. (1983) found that fatigued muscle actually contracted and relaxed more slowly, with the time to peak tension and half-relaxation time dramatically increasing. Such a change would allow the muscle to generate higher forces at lower frequencies to maintain a consistent force output. CNS modulation through a feedback mechanism may sense the muscle speed and drive it with the appropriate stimulation frequency. Presumably, such regulation would require some sensory feedback from the individual muscles innervated (Bigland-Ritchie & Woods 1984).

There may be a loss of force during fatigue of sustained human MVCs, due to failure of the CNS to maintain adequate muscle activation rather than to failure of muscle contractility. Changes in the patterns of neural drive may have a variety of influences on the force-generating capacity of muscle (Bigland-Ritchie & Woods 1984). In a study in which subjects were asked to sustain a contraction of the knee extensor muscles at a constant force (5% torque), the force was maintained although four different parts of the quadriceps femoris muscle were used during the

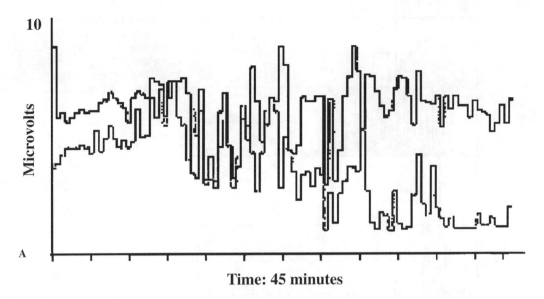

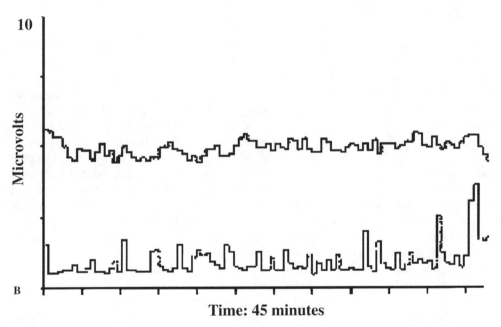

Figure 6.1. The upper trapezius muscles are monitored with a data logger while the person performs a bilateral, symmetric task at work. Each data-log collection period is 45 minutes in duration. **A.** The right upper trapezius, the symptomatic side, is working appropriately for the first 30 minutes but then begins to show some evidence of overload, dropping in amplitude. **B.** The right upper trapezius, 2 hours later, is inhibited in spite of stretching breaks every 15 minutes.

1-hour task (Sjøgaard et al. 1986). An increase in central drive may be seen when a synergistic or contralateral muscle is activated as the prime-mover fatigue. Central factors may be contributing to the "overload" phenomenon seen in monitoring the upper and lower trapezius fibers of a symptomatic employee at work, as shown in Figure 6.1.

Observations cited by Enoka (1995) suggest that the generation of a sufficient central command is not a trivial matter and that if a subject (or em-

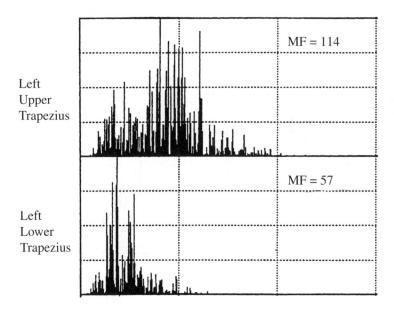

Figure 6.2. Median frequency (MF) values are calculated from the raw electromyographic data during a sustained isometric contraction. MF values are shown for the upper and lower trapezius muscles.

ployee) is not motivated, this lack of motivation will cause premature termination of a fatiguing task. Other factors, such as discomfort and tolerance of pain, cannot be ignored. Both of these factors may be influenced by a change in conditions under which the task is performed.

Fatigue Measurement

The use of amplitude sEMG values to assess muscle fatigue has several potential drawbacks. The relationship between force and amplitude is generally considered to be near linear but only when sEMG measurements are taken under strict adherence to isometric conditions, minimizing movement of the electrode site over the muscle fibers being sampled (Lieber 1992). Very careful consideration should be given to the collection methodology before conclusions are drawn when dealing with amplitude measures. Amplitude observations over only a short period may provide misleading clues regarding the degree of fatigue in a given muscle.

Changes in amplitude with fatigue generally assume changes in force production within the muscle. During LMF, the integrated sEMG signal (i.e., the amplitude) tends to increase two to five times in relation to the force of the muscle activation during "early" fatigue and decreases during "late" fatigue.

However, sEMG amplitude is of limited value as an objective method of LMF assessment, because it depends on the status of the contractile component and does not evaluate impaired excitation-contraction coupling as a possible fatigue mechanism.

sEMG amplitude has been reported to be less sensitive and reliable than the sEMG PS analysis in examination of LMF (Nyland 1993). The sEMG PS is examined through fast Fourier transformation of the raw EMG signal from the time domain to the frequency domain, an example of which is shown in Figure 6.2. The analysis of the EMG signal in the frequency domain involves measurements and parameters that describe specific aspects of the frequency spectrum of the signal (Basmajian & DeLuca 1985).

Certain general observations can be made about the behavior of the PS. A decrease in the firing rates of the MUs will contribute to a shift of the power density spectrum toward lower frequencies. Additionally, modification of the discharge characteristics of the MUs may also change the power-density spectrum because the cross-correlation terms will be affected. Factors such as synchronous discharge of MUs have a tendency to increase the energy in the part of the spectrum below 40 Hz. Any modification in the waveform of the MU action potentials will also be reflected in the Fourier transforms and thus in the power-density spectrum.

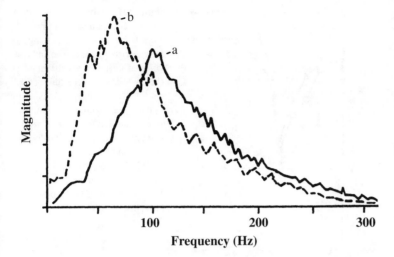

Figure 6.3. The median frequency in this case is shown before and after fatigue. The prefatigue value *(a)* is contrasted to the slower firing rate of the motor units after fatigue *(b)*. This shift in the power spectrum returns to normal after rest. (Reprinted with permission from JV Basmajian [1985]. *Muscles Alive* [5th ed, p 205]. Baltimore: Williams & Wilkins.)

The typical shift of the PS to the left with fatigue is shown in Figure 6.3. Tissue filtering effect determines the actual MU action potential's shape (Basmajian & DeLuca 1985; Nyland 1993). Peripheral factors that have also been reported to alter the sEMG PS distribution include muscle force level, muscle length, muscle fiber composition and distribution, skin and tissue impedance, electrode properties and geometry, muscle thickness, muscle fiber diameter, cross-talk between muscle, and various metabolic factors (Nyland 1993).

The study of healthy muscle reveals a pattern of recovery from fatigue that can, in part, be seen with the sEMG PS. Changes in the firing rates of active MUs have very little effect, if any, on the MF as long as the muscle does not develop fatigue. This fact adds to the value of using MF as a measure of fatigue and recovery (Solomonow et al. 1990). There is a consistency in the recovery process that is useful in examination of CTD, in spite of the fact that there are a number of sites of muscle fatigue and that different patterns of exercise are expected to effect muscle fatigue and recovery.

Studies of the flexor muscles by Krogh-Lund and Jorgensen (1992, 1993) demonstrate a basic recovery pattern that can be seen in several other studies. The flexor muscles of the elbow were studied at 30% MVC in both isolated and repetitive testing to examine changes in MF, conduction velocity, and amplitude. Changes in the sEMG PS with recovery are shown in Figure 6.4. In both the biceps and the brachioradialis muscles, the MF value dropped by 50%

of its original value by the time of exhaustion. After 1 minute of rest, there was an 85% increase in the MF value, with full recovery occurring within 5 minutes. The recovery and return to higher frequencies that occurred within the first minute almost totally eliminated the PS increase in the 8- to 40-Hz range.

Muscle Pain

Muscle pain, or myopain, includes a number of syndromes, such as myofascitis, fibromyalgia, regional muscle pain syndrome, muscular rheumatism, fasciitis, strains and sprains, trigger point myalgia, and the generic myofascial pain syndrome (Edwards 1988). The term *myopain* is used for pain originating in striated muscle, including fascia and tendinous insertions. Unlike nociception, pain does require conscious awareness (Mense 1993a).

The hypothesis of centrally driven factors in occupational muscle pain discussed by Edwards suggests that a disturbance in central control of postural MUs is the primary disorder underlying regional muscle pain syndromes. Headley (1994) has reported the clinical phenomenon of altered motor control strategies as a sequela and a perpetuating contributing factor in chronic myopain. Muscles that function normally as the prime mover in one task are absent in another.

The work by Mense would appear to support the sensitization of muscle nociceptors in the perpetuation of a lowered activation threshold of the noci-

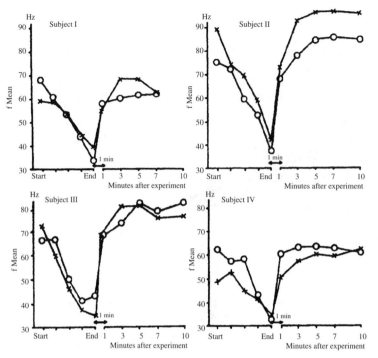

Figure 6.4. Median frequency data from the biceps muscles of four subjects is represented showing pre-exercise, postexercise, and rest values at 1, 3, 5, 7, and 10 minutes. The contractions were done at 60% and 50% (rest values) of maximum voluntary contraction. Two trials for each subject, collected 1 week apart, are plotted. (Reprinted with permission from I Kuorinka [1988]. Restitution of EMG spectrum after muscular fatigue. *Eur J Appl Physiol,* 57,313. Copyright © 1988, Springer-Verlag.)

ceptors. Preliminary results show that the behavior of human muscle nociceptors is indistinguishable from that of animal nociceptors studied. Nociceptors elicit pain regardless of the activating stimulus, although most receptors have a preferential sensitivity to a certain stimulus or combination of stimuli. The sensitivity of muscle nociceptors is not constant but can be increased easily by endogenous substances. The process of receptor sensitization occurs with all types of tissue lesions and is the main peripheral mechanism underlying the clinical symptoms of tenderness and hyperalgesia (Mense 1993a). Ischemic and inflamed muscle show increased sensitivity to activation, continued activation after the stimulus is withdrawn, and activation by mechanical stimuli not generally considered noxious. This peripheral sensitization may exist concurrent with central sensitization of dorsal horn cells, resulting in neuroplastic changes that would account for pain persisting in the absence of continued input.

Myofascial Pain Syndrome

A plethora of conditions have been referred to as myofascial pain syndrome (MPS), including chronic musculoskeletal pain syndrome, overuse syndrome, and occupational muscle pain, suggesting that similar or identical mechanisms may underlie these disorders. In this chapter, MPS is discussed as a type of myopain characterized by muscular trigger points, referred pain, and resultant changes in muscle activation.

The basic pathologic process underlying the formation of a trigger point appears to be a local disturbance in the muscle tissue, often a trauma due to overloading (Travell & Simons 1983; Mense 1993b). Trigger points may develop where there is a rupture of the sarcoplasmic reticulum and release of calcium from the intracellular stores. The increased calcium concentration causes sliding of the myosin and actin filaments, leading to a local physiologic contracture of myofilament activation without electrical activity. Actin and myosin filaments may remain shortened by the impairment of the calcium pump, resulting in palpable muscle fiber bands that feel hardened and tense. "Silent activation" is maintained until metabolic activity can be normalized or until stretching separates the actin and myosin filaments to facilitate relaxation of the muscle fibers (Simons 1988). Recent work points to the location of trigger points at the motor end plate (Simons 1996).

To differentiate active trigger points from other myopain, trigger point must be identified as very localized spot tenderness existing in a taut band with a resulting pain pattern that is recognized by the patient. The ability to elicit a local twitch response, another confirmation of an active trigger point, may be masked by the depth of the trigger point or limited by the skill of the examiner (Simons 1996).

Myofascial referred pain exhibits three levels of trigger point irritability. Trigger points that are highly irritable can produce severe pain even at rest. Active trigger points that are moderately irritable can cause referred pain when the involved muscle is stressed by activity. Mild irritability, seen in latent trigger points, is painful only when strong pressure is applied to the trigger point (Travell 1990; Simons 1993). The development of active trigger points may occur more easily in some individuals because of genetic predisposition. Taut bands may initially be pain-free until some stressor results in the formation of a latent trigger point. If further mechanical stress is imposed, the latent trigger point may become an active one. The location of these trigger points is remarkably consistent (Simons 1996).

The natural course of trigger points may include rapid remission with or without treatment. They may persist in a single muscle or, under the influence of one or more perpetuating factors, develop into a chronic MPS. The most common perpetuating factors seen in many industrial situations dealing with CTD may be continued performance of the same task that activated the trigger point initially and resulted in overload, the lack of sufficient variation in movement patterns, and a genetic predisposition to MPS. Additional factors may include the increasing tendency toward sedentary lifestyles that encourage little use of the muscle at its full range of motion, a generalized lack of strength-related tasks, and poor aerobic capacity. A number of additional perpetuating factors may result in persistent MPS in any population. Such factors include postural habits, previous history of prolonged pain, overuse, the number of muscle tension habits incorporated into lifestyle, current distress, stress or hassle index level, mood disorders (e.g., depression), sleep deprivation, vitamin inadequacies, concomitant joint dysfunction, inefficient motor control, learning and coping styles, and personality type (Travell & Simons 1983).

Referred Phenomenon

The referral of pain occurs most often in a central to peripheral direction (48% of the 147 trigger point patterns examined; Simons 1993). Several phenomena in addition to pain, such as burning, numbness, and tingling, may be referred by trigger points. Several trigger points may also create autonomic distress, such as dizziness, ipsilateral sweating, or blurred vision. The referred sensory phenomenon arising from trigger points is most likely related to the sensitization of muscle afferent nerves that include nociceptors. One possible reason for the referred pain is the inability of higher centers to identify the actual pain source because of the convergence of nociceptive dorsal horn neurons with inputs from various tissues. Referral of myopain may also reflect the formation or activation of CNS connections and could be another aspect of neuroplasticity (Mense 1993a). In their research on animals, the Mense group described the appearance of new receptive fields following noxious stimulation located in deep tissues (never in the skin). The majority of new receptive fields were located distal to the original sites (Hoheisel et al. 1993). Mense proposes two new components to the convergence-projection theory: (1) Convergent connections from deep tissues to dorsal horn neurons are present but "sleeping" and are activated by nociceptive input from skeletal muscle; and (2) referral to myotomes outside the lesion is caused by spread of central sensitization to adjacent spinal segments (Mense 1994). The patterns of referred pain are remarkably consistent across the population and can lead the clinician to the causative trigger point (Travell & Simons 1983).

The effect of trigger points on muscle activity may be one of hyperirritability or inhibition. Both have been demonstrated and reported (Headley 1990; Simons 1993). Both referred muscle dysfunction phenomena can be eradicated by deactivation of the causative trigger point. In this fashion, sEMG can be used to demonstrate changes in the level of irritability of trigger points in some individuals. These reflex motor effects of trigger points may prove to be an important factor in the development of muscle dysfunction in patients with MPS and occupationally related pain complaints. Ivanichev (1990) has also reported disturbance of coordination in a muscle with active trigger points that has been observed by this

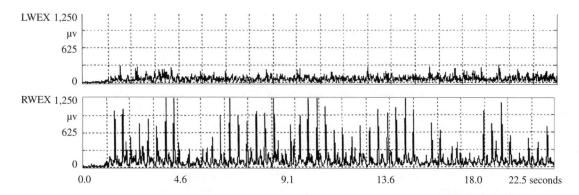

Figure 6.5. In a patient identified as having tennis elbow in the left arm, the forearm extensor muscle group was monitored bilaterally during rapid pronation and supination. Right wrist extensor muscle group (RWEX) recruitment is hyperactive and erratic. A trigger point was present in the right extensor carpi radialis longus. Tracing is 22 seconds in duration; peak amplitude is 1,250 μV. (LWEX = left wrist extensor muscle group.)

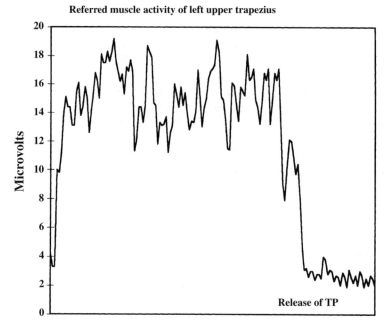

Figure 6.6. The patient is seated and relaxed, and an electrode is in place on the left upper trapezius muscle. The trigger point (TP) in the left long head of the triceps is stimulated for 20 seconds, and referred muscle activity in the left upper trapezius is recorded. Referred muscle activity drops quickly when the TP stimulation is stopped.

author as well (Simons 1993). An example is provided in Figure 6.5.

In the presence of trigger points, inhibition or referred spasm may originate in the same afferents and cause the referred pain. In Figure 6.6, the trigger point located in the long head of the triceps not only referred pain to the upper trapezius but created a localized spasm until the trigger point in the long head of the triceps was released.

Musculotendinous Junction

The musculotendinous junction (MTJ) plays a role in force transmission. Muscle fibers in this MTJ are often stiffer than other muscle fibers. In addition, when muscle fiber length is increased during growth, the addition of sarcomeres occurs in the region of the MTJ. The MTJ resembles load-bearing membranes with extensive folding and dense subsarcolemmal material. The membrane folding may perform three functions in reducing load: (1) decreasing the stress imposed by increasing the surface area, (2) aligning the membrane at very low angles relative to applied force vectors, and (3) placing an adhesive interface between tissue layers, increasing the cell-to-tendon junction (Noonan & Garrett 1992).

Two types of indirect muscle injury that may affect this region are delayed-onset muscle soreness and muscle strain. Muscle strain injury, often associated with CTD, demonstrates pathologic changes near the MTJ or near the tendon-bone junction. Strain injuries may occur in response to forcibly stretching a muscle passively or when the muscle is working eccentrically. Examination of cellular changes after MTJ injury has revealed that severe hypercontraction and some necrosis may exist, suggesting an ongoing, calcium-induced injury process. Damage is limited to a very small area, and such containment of injury may be an inherent property of the MTJ tissue (Noonan & Garrett 1992). When a muscle is held in an isometric contraction, strain is transmitted to the tendon. The amount of lengthening that occurs in the tissues to allow for sarcomere shortening in the central portion of the muscle reflects changes in loading absorbed through the MTJ (Lieber 1992).

Fatigue is considered to be a factor that predisposes a muscle to strain injury. When compared with nonfatigued muscle, fatigued muscle was observed to have decreased load, length, and energy absorbed before failure. The failure of muscle to recover from fatigue, as seen in CTD, may increase the risk factor for MTJ injuries as the time to return the muscle to a metabolically rested state is increased (Noonan & Garrett 1992).

Delayed-onset muscle soreness develops most often in muscles that are working eccentrically. A muscle that is required to perform work demands of unaccustomed intensity or duration is likely to be damaged physically. Eccentric contractions are characterized by external forces acting on the muscle greater than those produced by the muscle itself. Damage during eccentric work has been attributed to the fact that during negative work, a smaller number of MUs are active. Therefore, the mechanical stress to the Z bands in the sarcomeres and connective tissue is greater (Mense 1993b).

Middaugh et al. (1994) stress the importance of considering muscle overuse in relation to the accustomed range of generated tension, velocity, or working length for muscle in any given individual. When a muscle is accustomed to moderate levels of activity through only a moderate percent of its full excursion, muscle soreness can be elicited with activity levels that are only slightly more demanding. These factors emphasize the importance of maintaining active lifestyles outside the work environment, reducing functional limitation and injury both at home and in the workplace.

Often the MTJ is an area of marked tenderness in CTD patients and it must be treated to reduce symptoms and promote healing. Increased flexibility in muscle tissue appears to reduce the loading on the MTJ and may therefore contribute to injury reduction. The amount or type of stretching to reduce stress loading successfully cannot be determined easily.

Motor Control Strategies and Myopain

When muscles fatigue and reach overload or inhibition, compensatory recruitment patterns develop to allow an employee to continue performing job tasks. As a result of this compensation, new movement habits or motor control strategies evolve, making it easier to use the compensatory patterns. Should the inhibited muscle(s) become capable of functioning, motor control strategies may continue to exclude it. Compensatory motor programs add biomechanical stress to the system and create secondary symptoms.

The study of motor control examines posture and movements that are controlled by central commands and spinal reflexes. *Motor learning* refers to a set of processes associated with practice or experience that lead to relatively permanent changes in the capability for producing skilled action. Motor programs or strategies include information that specifies fixed relationships among muscles. These strategies are stored in memory and recalled to guide action (Montgomery & Connolly 1991).

The current status of motor program theory continues to be modified regularly. The original concept set forth by Keele postulated that a motor program was a "set of muscle commands that are structured before a movement sequence begins." Research supports the concept that many movements are preprogrammed with modifying influences to be considered. Increasing plasticity and flexibility have been included in the theoretic systems.

The concept of a generalized motor program suggests that entire motor programs are not stored but that algorithms defining classes of action are available, subject to internal and external cues to modify execution. The dynamic approach argues that characteristics such as timing, force, and amplitude of movement are emergent properties of the motor system as it interacts with the environment. The more current definition of a motor program, however, reflects the orders of actions, rather than their specific elements, and allows for the plasticity so evident in this system (Morris et al. 1994).

Myopain generally alters motor control strategies when muscle dysfunction reaches inhibition of muscle activity. Muscle inhibition alters movement mechanics, requires compensatory motor strategies, and increases strain on joints and soft-tissue structures. Overload of a muscle secondary to activation of a trigger point enhances the development of compensatory movement patterns. Fatigue-based compensatory movement generally begins proximally. When proximal muscle stability is compromised, biomechanics and forces generated by movement are altered.

If the body is asked to continue to perform a function, the plasticity of the human CNS allows development of a compensatory pattern to accomplish that request. Such capability initially works to the body's benefit, and a problem may evolve only if the compensatory activity continues for a prolonged period. Continued activity may lead to fatigue in the muscles asked to compensate. These "second-string" muscles increase their work load and contribute to altered biomechanical stresses. This compensation will continue unless the proximal muscles are treated for active trigger points interfering with normal movement, and the muscles then are re-educated and provided with work-rest cycles to maintain an adequate level of function without fatigue.

Of utmost importance in evaluating CTD is understanding how MUs are recruited to perform a specific task. It is important to recognize that overload fatigue may be occurring only in task-specific MUs that may not be reached in a traditional rehabilitation program. Task-specific fatigue characterizes the early stages of CTD. Caldwell et al. (1993) describe research on task-specific MUs in muscles controlling the elbow. Specificity of MU activity was found for torque directions of flexion or supination. Even muscles considered unifunctional were found to contain MUs that are recruited in a task-dependent manner. In later stages, when central fatigue fails to sustain muscle activation, an entire muscle may be removed selectively from one movement pattern (i.e., shoulder flexion) but continue to recruit normally in other movements. An example of such movement-specific fatigue in muscle recruitment is demonstrated in Figure 6.7; the lower trapezius is recruited as expected in flexion but shows significant inhibition in abduction. If the fatigue persists, the inhibition may become more global, and any motor plan that generally includes the fatigued muscle may be altered to exclude it from recruiting. This may result in a clinical picture of apparent weakness in that muscle. The use of strengthening programs that emphasize power will often contribute to failure in rehabilitation and return-to-work attempts when central inhibition is contributing to the global alteration of motor plans.

The concept of functional compartments within muscles has been discussed by Segal et al. (1991). Several muscles studied extensively were reported to yield EMG patterns from different regions within each muscle and related to direction of movement. If muscle regions were functionally independent, they would have to have some anatomically distinct partitions. Such partitions were found in all three muscles investigated. Segal et al. stressed the need to investigate both the architecture and innervation pattern that, in some cases, were not identical.

Physiologic Risk Factors and Interventions

Muscle dysfunction is generally considered a local phenomenon related to muscle fiber damage, muscle weakness, or disrupted innervation of the muscle fiber. The information on CTD emerging with sEMG indicates that muscles may test "within normal limits" during standardized manual muscle testing but not recruit appropriately during numerous functional tasks. The muscle does not show total inhibition but, rather, movement-specific functional inhibition. Motor control strategy changes may explain such inconsistencies. If these changes in motor planning could be identified as causative in generating discrepancies in movement patterns, it would challenge the tendency to label such inconsistencies as evidence of malingering, symptom magnification, or psychosocial in nature. In fact, motor control theory

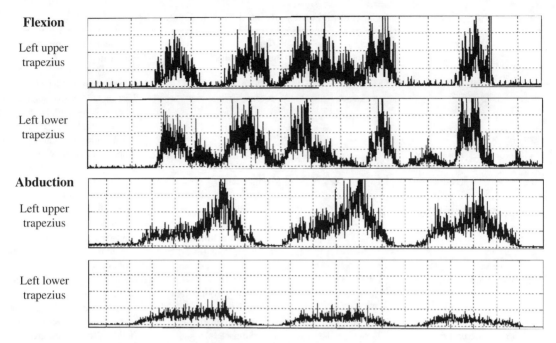

Figure 6.7. Monitored with four bilateral electrode sites, a patient with distal forearm complaints was asked to perform shoulder flexion and abduction through full range of motion. The upper and lower trapezius sites are shown, and a good recruitment pattern in flexion but significant inhibition of the lower trapezius in abduction are demonstrated. (Scale, 1–100)

stresses that such dysfunction in the recruitment of muscle must be related to central drive.

Proximal Instability to Distal Dysfunction

As upper-quadrant muscle fatigue progresses, influenced by both LMF and fatigue of central origin, compensatory muscle patterns change as synergistic or accessory muscles fatigue and cervical muscles are involved secondarily. Muscle dysfunction with accompanying soft-tissue changes continues to progress in one of several patterns. For some individuals, muscle dysfunction results in headaches becoming the primary complaint; for others, shoulder problems emerge as the primary source of symptoms. For those who may eventually develop CTS, the compensatory muscle patterns and trigger points proceed distally into the arm, forearm, and hand. The combination of trigger points and muscle dysfunction seen in muscle-related CTD suggests a causative relationship in proximal to distal CTD

between active trigger point development, muscle compensation, and fatigue.

Dynamic functional muscle testing using sEMG has provided insight into the muscle dysfunction and symptom complaints of static, low-load CTD problems. Standard protocols have been developed by the author, including testing of active, resisted, static, repetitive, and loaded tasks. In addition, a fatigue-testing format combines isometric testing of fatigue before the protocol, a dynamic movement protocol, and repeat fatigue isometric testing on completion of the protocol and after a standardized rest period. The results of these protocols demonstrate a significant difference between the clinically different patients and asymptomatic controls when scored quantitatively for types of muscle dysfunction (Headley 1996c). The failure of muscles to recover has also been reported as statistically significant in an examination of 55 patients with upper-quadrant CTD as compared with six control subjects (Headley 1996a).

The ability of the employee with CTD to recover function and reduce symptoms may be dependent

Table 6.1. Stages of Cumulative Trauma Disorder–Related Muscle Dysfunction

	Trigger Points	Muscle Dysfunction	Fatigue Characteristics*	Functional and Symptom Complaints
Stage 1	LTR, UTR	LTR ↓, UTR ↑, task-specific	Mild delay (2–3× normal) in recovery from fatigue	Pain between shoulder blades, UTR area; possible soreness when leaving work at end of day; no problem performing leisure activities; seldom recognized as an evolving CTD problem
Stage 2	LTR, UTR, levator, intraspinatus, SPS, scalene	LTR ↓, UTR ↓↑, scalene ↓, task-specific	Moderate delay (4–6× normal) in recovery from fatigue; fatigue failure is specific (i.e., limited to low load, static fibers)	Soreness that may persist to next morning; pain that might be eliminated only with rest; inability to do static tasks at home without pain but still able to perform other activities without symptoms
Stage 3	LTR, UTR, levator, infraspinatus, SPS, scalene, teres minor, posterior deltoid, FA flexors	LTR ↓, UTR ↓↑, scalene ↑, FA flexors ↓↑, dysfunction generalized to most tasks	Severe delay (8–12 hrs) in recovery from fatigue; fatigue failure more generalized, involving entire muscle(s)	Increasing fatigue during week; reported need for rest after work by midweek to continue working; use of weekend and holidays to recover; great difficulty maintaining a static work task
Stage 4	LTR, UTR, levator, infraspinatus, SPS, scalene, teres minor, posterior deltoid, FA flexors, FA extensors, SCM	LTR ↓, UTR ↓, scalene ↓, FA flexors ↓, FA extensors ↓↑, SCM ↓↑, generalized dysfunction	Profound delay (12–36 hrs) in recovery from fatigue; MF fails to show any recovery 1 full day after fatigue testing	Profound functional limitation in all daily activities; inability to do simple activities of daily living at home; poor prognosis for any work requiring static load on involved muscle groups

↑ = hyperactive; ↓ = inhibited; ↓↑ = either inhibited or hyperactive; LTR = lower trapezius; UTR = upper trapezius; CTD = cumulative trauma disorder; SPS = serratus posterosuperior; FA = forearm; SCM = sternocleidomastoid; MF = median frequency.
*Determined by surface electromyography and reflecting the power spectrum median frequency of LTR.
Note: This table reflects surface electromyography evaluations of more than 200 patients who had a CTD, using electrode sites overlying the LTR, UTR, scalene, SCM, and FA flexors and extensors. Dynamic functional muscle testing is standardized, as is the isometric fatigue testing for spectral analysis, done before and after fatigue and after specified rest periods.

on both his or her genetic predisposition and the stage at which intervention is attempted. The stages of CTDs are a combination of both chronicity (time) and severity (number of muscles involved). Four stages (Table 6.1) relate to individuals performing upper-quadrant static and repetitive tasks at very low loading (i.e., requiring muscle recruitment levels of less than 8% of their MVC).

Carpal tunnel symptoms may be seen in some patients as the end product of proximal to distal muscle dysfunction and fatigue failure. In the pop-

ulation that initially experiences proximal symptoms, symptoms similar to carpal tunnel may arise first from proximal trigger points and only in its chronic stage represent true carpal tunnel syndrome. Surgery to address the compression of the median nerve in the carpal tunnel space in this population subgroup will be seen as only partially successful, and patients will then turn their attention to early proximal symptoms that were not addressed.

The relationship of task specificity and its implications in CTD may be examined in work done by

Kilbom (1988). Two groups of employees were studied: The first group performed a variety of postures and exertions related to lifting and assembling automotive parts; the second group worked on the assembly of circuit boards, working only in a seated position and exposed mainly to postural static loads. This study examined the assumption that individuals with high muscle strength have a lower risk of anaerobic intramuscular compromise and fatigue than do those with low muscle strength. One-year longitudinal studies were done on these two employee populations with pre- and post-test measurements of MVC and static endurance. The static strength test was in the range of 20–50% MVC. The results showed that low muscle strength was a risk factor for development of shoulder-neck-arm disorders in those employees working in the automotive industry. No such relationship could be demonstrated in the assembly employees, however. Although both groups reported a high incidence of symptoms, the mechanisms of injury are likely to be different, given the differences in job tasks, measured predictors, and outcome findings. The tests may have favored measurement of the MUs most likely to be used in the automotive group, thereby showing a predictive pattern of symptoms related to lack of strength. In the assembly group, the pre- and post-tests may not have tested adequately the task-specific static loading requirements of these employees, thereby collecting data that did not correlate well with pretest expectations. The importance of low static loads in symptom development cannot be underestimated; adequate work-rest cycles, in addition to changes in muscle length (i.e., stretching), may be the critical factors in understanding prevention of low-load CTD injury.

Rest and Recovery Factors

The type of task performed by the scapular stabilizers is often static or one in which muscle excursion is limited as compared to its available range from lengthened to shortened position. The static load, in this sense, is the constancy of the position in which scapular stabilizers are allowing movement of more distal segments by maintaining a postural position that may not change for prolonged periods. However, in spite of such static postural positioning, it is rare to have muscles generate a continuous isometric contraction of the same amplitude. There will be some variation in amplitude if the distal segments are moved in any way. Therefore, the muscle activity generated by the postural stabilizers reflects dynamic work that is supported by a constant static load on the same muscles or portions thereof. In Figure 6.8, the upper and lower trapezius muscles are being monitored during a data-entry task in which the mouse is also used. The static load on the right upper trapezius muscles is obvious by the lack of descent to the baseline, probably because of the use of the mouse. Figure 6.9 demonstrates another variation of static and dynamic muscle activity. The forearm flexors and extensors are being monitored during a data-entry task. The mouse is being used by the right hand. After several minutes of using the mouse intermittently, the forearm extensor group fails to return to its earlier level of static loading, significantly increasing the fatigability of the forearm extensor group. It is the anticipatory nature of the mouse activity that apparently gives rise to the higher static load, as the employee continues to move back and forth from the mouse to the keyboard.

Jonsson (1988) describes a static load as a constant level of muscle contraction that exists because the muscle does not come to a full resting level despite changes in the dynamic work load. Having examined the sequencing of muscle recruitment by MUs and the constancy of that order of recruitment based on the work load imposed and motor strategy chosen, this underlying level of static load shown in Figure 6.10 becomes critical in the development of proximal scapular muscle fatigue.

Veiersted and Westgaard (1993) report similar findings on examining the development of trapezius myalgia in workers performing light manual work. New employees were examined every tenth week for 1 year. The development of symptoms to warrant classification of patient status was high (17 of 30 employees). The development of complaints throughout the week showed a slight but significant increase during the first 5 days of the week, decreasing on weekends and on holidays. The authors conclude that many new cases of nonchronic trapezius myalgia occur during the first year of employment, especially during the first 6 months, in a job with low static load. These findings suggest a delayed recovery during the week as compared to increased recovery from fatigue when the light static work load is not performed for 2 or more consecutive days.

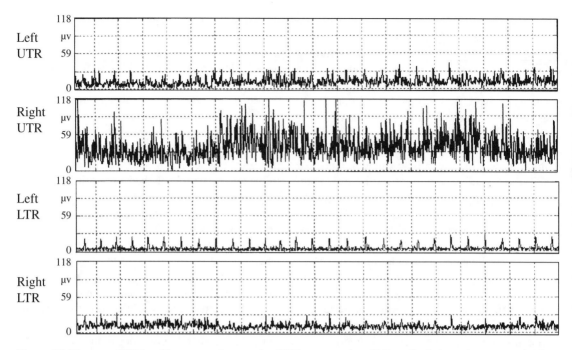

Figure 6.8. The upper (UTR) and lower trapezius muscles (LTR) were monitored bilaterally during a data-entry task. The UTR demonstrates a higher static level of activity with no return to the baseline throughout the task (8 minutes), even though the mouse was used only intermittently.

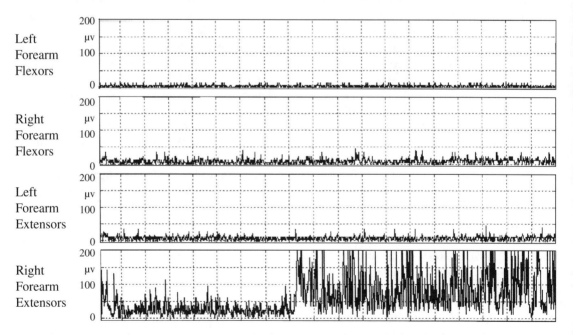

Figure 6.9. The forearm flexor and extensor groups are monitored during a data-entry task. Although the use of the mouse with the right hand is intermittent, the right extensor muscle group increases its activity level and does not decrease it when the hand returns to the keyboard. Overall, the static load on the right extensor group is significantly higher than that on the contralateral muscle group.

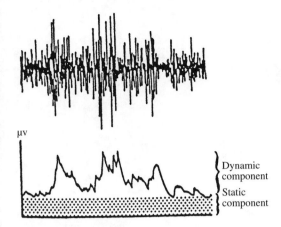

Figure 6.10. The raw and corresponding root mean square electromyographic signal for approximately 6 seconds of activity are shown. The muscular load may be subdivided into a static and a dynamic component. (Reprinted with permission from B Jonsson. Static load component in muscle work. *Eur J Appl Physiol*, 57,305. Copyright © 1988, Springer-Verlag.)

The suggested failure to recover discussed in the previous study was examined by Stokes et al. (1989), who examined the adductor pollicis muscle with both high- and low-frequency stimulation to fatigue. They found that at low frequencies, declines in force were greater during the second series despite similar changes in compound action potential amplitude. The low-frequency fatigue failure they describe reduced low- but not high-frequency fatigue resistance, suggesting that the impaired endurance of fatigued muscle during voluntary activity results primarily from peripheral changes at low frequency. The functional consequence of low-frequency fatigue is a reduced endurance capacity during subsequent voluntary activity.

Headley (1996a) examined 55 patients with muscle-related CTD in a prospective study. Muscle fatigue and recovery were examined using sEMG analysis of the PS. Bilateral lower trapezius electrode sites were monitored pre- and postexercise and after a 7-minute rest period. There was a statistically significant difference ($p < 0.05$) between the pre- and postexercise values, indicating that muscle fatigue did occur. When the pre-exercise MF value was compared with the recovery values, again a statistically significant difference ($p < 0.05$) was demonstrated, indicating that recovery

did not occur. An example of the failure to recover is shown in Figure 6.11, wherein the data of one of these patients are plotted in comparison to a control. Patients were no better after 7 minutes of rest than immediately after the fatigue test. These findings differ from normal muscle recovery expectations, when 70–90% of MF fatigue recovery is shown to occur within the first minute of rest (Solomonow et al. 1990; Krogh-Lund & Jorgensen 1992, 1993).

Using an amplitude probability distribution curve developed by Hagberg, Jonsson (1988) determined that the lowest level of muscular contraction during an entire work cycle represents the level below that which is considered constant "static work load." The amplitude probability can be expressed as a fraction of the total duration that the EMG signal measured is lower than or equal to the amplitude designated as $p = 0$. Without high-peak values being achieved by employees performing low-load static tasks, there are few criteria to represent adequately the load assumed by the musculoskeletal system when prolonged low loading occurs. For this reason, sEMG is seen as an important tool for detection of muscle loads in vocational situations. This method of analysis may enhance the ability to study fatigue using amplitude measures.

In a study by Christensen (1986), muscle activity was recorded in the deltoid, infraspinous, and trapezius muscles in 25 subjects performing monotonous and repetitive work. The author reported that those subjects who had increased pain or discomfort in the shoulder had a higher static level in the deltoid muscle (7.8% of the MVC) than did those subjects with no pain or discomfort (4.8% of the MVC). Symptomatic subjects were judged to have static levels that exceeded the levels recommended by Jonsson (1988). The high levels of activity in these muscles may account for the high incidence of discomfort and pain reported by the subjects in this study.

Delayed Latency

The concept of delayed latency refers to the time it takes a muscle to reduce muscle activity amplitudes fully after the command for relaxation has been given by the CNS. This lack of relaxation with a

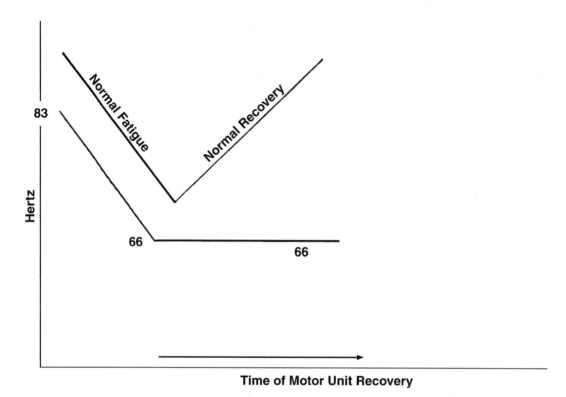

Figure 6.11. Subject's left lower trapezius muscle had an acceptable median frequency value initially. With exercise, the value dropped to 66 Hz, as one would expect with fatigue. However, after 7 minutes of rest, the muscle shows no recovery, a characteristic of this patient population with a cumulative trauma disorder.

long latency may eliminate relaxation between work tasks, even though the muscle is thought to be unloaded and relaxed. The contraction level nonetheless serves as a static load and contributes to muscle fatigue.

In a study by Elert and Gerdle (1989), the shoulder stabilizers of 20 healthy subjects were studied using sEMG and isokinetic testing. MVC data were collected at four velocities and 150 repetitions of maximal shoulder flexion. Measures of perceived fatigue were also collected. The authors found a marked drop in force and a corresponding reduction in mean power frequency of all four muscle groups monitored with sEMG. Another finding related to the repeated contractions was the difference in individual ability to relax between contractions. In examining the capacity of the muscle to rest during the passive extension phase, the presence of high sEMG levels in some individuals was associated with reduced force output.

Surface Electromyography Gaps

sEMG gaps reflect the amount of time a muscle does not demonstrate active sEMG signal from an electrode site. This gap is brief and involuntary. A study of lower-extremity muscles by Fugl-Meyer et al. (1985) concluded that the relative pauses (gaps) between repetitive concentric contractions make it possible for slow-twitch fibers to continue maximal contractions for a long time without decreased output. Inability to relax between concentric contractions, more closely resembling a static work load, results in poorer performance in the long run. Such continuous activity during all phases of work will overtax the low-threshold (slow-twitch) MUs.

Upper-quadrant muscles were examined in a prospective study by Veiersted and Westgaard (1993) for similar EMG gaps. This study of new employees examined the association between the level and pattern of muscle usage during the performance of a specific job and the development of symptoms in the trapezius muscle. The authors report that the analysis of all the EMG gap recordings, except the first, indicated that the risk of becoming a patient decreased by 6% for each additional gap per minute. Examination of the pattern of EMG gaps showed that there was no time trend, suggesting that they were a stable quality of the temporal activity pattern. The trend was found in nearly all subjects, supporting the benefits of using a multivariate approach to the examination of muscle related risk factors.

The effects of task-specific fatigue during repeated contractions leads to compensatory recruitment patterns if the activity is continued. Learning a movement pattern that occurs more easily at lower speeds might suggest that training for highly repetitive work should take place at a slower pace initially. The slower pace will improve the ability of the muscle to take advantage of short pauses that actually can exist during task performance. Progression in speed would have to be accomplished with respect to motor strategy training to ensure continued use of the proper motor plan as performance reaches expected levels for the job.

Job Rotation

Although job rotation to reduce the physical loading of muscles has been promoted for a number of years, it may affect only the dynamic component of the work load. The more proximal muscles may not be sufficiently relieved of their static load even though a variety of jobs has been performed. Jonsson (1988) recorded the right upper trapezius and used the amplitude probability model to demonstrate recruitment similarity. He found that job rotation for the purpose of reducing static muscular load in some cases may be of limited value in light work situations.

Multivariate Analysis

With a number of different analyses available for the examination of physiologic risk factors, using sEMG suggests that many methods are available for the examination of muscle rest and recovery factors. Examination of the raw data of symptomatic patients currently in treatment and controls (asymptomatic) performed by Headley (1996b) suggests that any test might not be discriminatory in identifying patients

versus controls. The multivariate approach was used in a pilot study for seven different parameters to identify clusters of risk factors that might be more consistently predictive of impending muscle-related CTD.

References

Basmajian JV & DeLuca CJ (1985). *Muscles Alive. Their Functions Revealed by Electromyography* (5th ed). Baltimore: Williams & Wilkins.

Bigland-Ritchie B, Johansson R, Lippold O, & Woods J (1983). Contractile speed and EMG changes during fatigue of sustained maximal voluntary contractions. *J Neurophysiol*, 50,313–324.

Bigland-Ritchie B & Woods J (1984). Changes in muscle contractile properties and neural control during human muscular fatigue. *Muscle Nerve*, 7,691–699.

Caldwell G, Jamison J, & Lee S (1993). Amplitude and frequency measures of surface electromyography during dual task elbow torque production. *Eur J Appl Physiol*, 66,349–356.

Christensen H (1986). Muscle activity and fatigue in the shoulder muscles of assembly-plant employees. *Scand J Work Environ Health*, 12,582–587.

CTD News (1994). Do you know the law? *CTD News*, 3(8),1.

Edwards RHT (1988). Hypotheses of peripheral and central mechanisms underlying occupational muscle pain and injury. *Eur J Appl Physiol*, 57,275–281.

Elert J & Gerdle B (1989). The relationship between contraction and relaxation during fatiguing isokinetic shoulder flexions. An electromyographic study. *Eur J Appl Physiol*, 59,303–309.

Enoka RM (1995). Mechanisms of muscle fatigue: central factors and task dependency. *J Electromyogr Kinesiol*, 5,141–149.

Flor H, Schugens MM, & Birbaumer N (1992). Discrimination of muscle tension in chronic pain patients and healthy controls. *Biofeedback Self Regul*, 17,165–177.

Fugl-Meyer A, Gerdle B, & Langstrom M (1985). Characteristics of repeated isokinetic plantar flexions in middle-aged and elderly subjects with special regard to muscular work. *Acta Physiol Scand*, 124,213–222.

Hagberg M (1981). Electromyographic signs of shoulder muscular fatigue in two elevated arm positions. *Am J Phys Med Rehabil*, 60,111–121.

Hagberg M & Kvarnstrom S (1984). Muscular endurance and electromyographic fatigue in myofascial shoulder pain. *Arch Phys Med Rehabil*, 65,522–525.

Headley BJ (1990). Evaluation and treatment of myofascial pain syndrome utilizing biofeedback. In JR Cram (Ed). *Clinical EMG for Surface Recordings*, Vol 2 (pp. 235–254). Nevada City: Clinical Resources.

Headley BJ (May 17, 1991). Strength or skill? *PT Forum*, 6–7.

Headley BJ (July 2, 1993). Assessing muscle skill. *PT Forum*, 23–24.

Headley BJ (1994). Chronic pain management. In SB O'Sullivan & TJ Schmitz (Eds). *Physical Rehabilitation: Assessment and Treatment* (3rd ed, pp. 577–602). Philadelphia: Davis.

Headley BJ (February 1996a). The failure of muscles to recover as a factor in upper quarter CTD. Presented at the American Physical Therapy Association—Combined Sections, Atlanta.

Headley BJ (February 1996b). Multivariate analysis of physiological risk factors related to CTD using surface EMG. Presented at the American Physical Therapy Association—Combined Sections, Atlanta.

Headley BJ (February 1996c). Muscle dysfunction: a comparison of symptomatic patients and controls. Presented at the American Physical Therapy Association—Combined Sections, Atlanta.

Hoheisel U, Mense S, Simons D, & Yu X-M (1993). Appearance of new receptive fields in rat dorsal horn neurons following noxious stimulation of skeletal muscle: a model for referred muscle pain? *Neurosci Lett*, 153,9–12.

Hong C-Z (1994). Considerations and recommendations regarding myofascial trigger point injection. *J Musculoskeletal Pain*, 2,29–59.

Ivanichev G (1990). *Painful Muscle Hypertonus* [in Russian]. Kazan: Kazan University Press.

Jonsson B (1988). The static load component in muscle work. *Eur J Appl Physiol*, 57,305–310.

Jorgensen K, Fallentin N, Krogh-Lund C, & Jensen B (1988). Electromyography and fatigue during prolonged, low-level static contractions. *Eur J Appl Physiol*, 57,316–321.

Kilbom A (1988). Isometric strength and occupational muscle disorders. *Eur J Appl Physiol*, 57,322–326.

Krogh-Lund C & Jorgensen K (1992). Modification of myoelectric power spectrum in fatigue from 15% maximal voluntary contraction of human elbow flexor muscles, to limit of endurance: reflection of conduction velocity variation and/or centrally mediated mechanisms? *Eur J Appl Physiol*, 64,359–370.

Krogh-Lund C & Jorgensen K (1993). Myo-electric fatigue manifestations revisited: power spectrum, conduction velocity, and amplitude of human elbow flexor muscles during isolated and repetitive endurance contractions at 30% maximal voluntary contraction. *Eur J Appl Physiol*, 66,161–173.

Lieber RL (1992). *Skeletal Muscle Structure and Function*. Baltimore: Williams & Wilkins.

Mense S (1993a). Nociception from skeletal muscle in relation to clinical muscle pain. *Pain*, 54,241–289.

Mense S (1993b). Peripheral mechanisms of muscle nociception and local muscle pain. *J Musculoskeletal Pain*, 1(1),133–170.

Mense S (1994). Referral of muscle pain. *APS Journal*, 3(1),1–9.

Middaugh S & Kee W (1987). Advances in electromyographic monitoring and biofeedback in treatment of chronic cervical and low back pain. In M Eisenberg & R Grzesiak (Eds). *Advances in Clinical Rehabilitation*, Vol 1 (pp. 137–172). New York: Springer.

Middaugh SJ, Kee WG, & Nicholson JA (1994). Muscle overuse and posture as factors in the development and maintenance of chronic musculoskeletal pain. In R Grzesiak & D Ciccone (Eds). *Psychological Vulnerability to Chronic Pain*. New York: Springer.

Montgomery PC & Connolly BH (1991). *Motor Control and Physical Therapy: Theoretical Framework and Practical Applications*. Hixson, TN: Chattanooga Group.

Morris ME, Summers JJ, Matyas TA, & Iansek R (1994). Current status of the motor program. *Phys Ther*, 74,738–752.

Noonan TJ & Garrett WE (1992). Injuries at the myotendinous junction. *Clin Sports Med*, 11,783–806.

Nyland J (1993). Relation between local muscular fatigue and the electromyographic signal with emphasis on power spectrum changes. *Isokin Exer Science*, 3,171–180.

Segal R, Wolf S, DeCamp M, Chopp M, & English A (1991). Anatomical partitioning of three multiarticular human muscles. *Acta Anat (Basel)*, 142,261–266.

Seidel H, Beyer H, & Brauer D (1987). Electromyographic evaluation of back muscle fatigue with repeated sustained contractions of different strengths. *Eur J Appl Physiol*, 56,592–602.

Simons DG (1988). Myofascial pain syndrome due to trigger points. In J Goodgold (Ed). *Rehabilitation Medicine* (pp. 686–723). St Louis: Mosby.

Simons DG (June 1992). Myofascial pain syndrome. Presented at the American Physical Therapy Association National Conference, Denver, CO.

Simons DG (1993). Referred phenomena of myofascial trigger points. In L Vecchiet, D Albe-Fessard, & U Lindblom (Eds). *New Trends in Referred Pain and Hyperalgesia* (pp. 341–357). Amsterdam: Elsevier.

Simons DG (1996). Clinical and etiological update of myofascial pain from trigger points. *J Musculoskeletal Pain*, 4,93–121.

Sjøgaard G (1986). Water and electrolyte fluxes during exercise and their relation to muscle fatigue. *Acta Physiol Scand Suppl*, 128,129–136.

Sjøgaard G, Kiens B, Jorgensen K, & Saltin B (1986). Intramuscular pressure, EMG and blood flow during low-level prolonged static contractions in man. *Acta Physiol Scand*, 128,475–484.

Sjøgaard G, Savard G, & Juel C (1988). Muscle blood flow during isometric activity and its relation to muscle fatigue. *Eur J Appl Physiol*, 57,327–335.

Solomonow M, Baten C, Smit J, Baratta R, Hermens H, D'Ambrosia R, & Shoji H (1990). Electromyogram power spectra frequencies associated with motor unit recruitment strategies. *J Appl Physiol*, 68,1177–1185.

Stokes M, Edwards R, & Cooper R (1989). Effect of low frequency fatigue on human muscle strength and fatigability during subsequent stimulated activity. *Eur J Appl Physiol*, 59,278–283.

Taylor W (1990). Dynamic EMG biofeedback in assessment and treatment using a neuromuscular re-education model. In J Cram (Ed). *Clinical EMG for Surface Recordings*, Vol 2 (pp. 175–193). Nevada City, CA: Clinical Resources.

Travell J & Simons D (1983). *Myofascial Pain and Dysfunc-*

tion. The Trigger Point Manual, Vol 1. Baltimore: Williams & Wilkins.

Travell JG (1990). Chronic myofascial pain syndromes. Mysteries of the history. In JR Fricton & EA Awad (Eds). *Myofascial Pain and Fibromyalgia. Advances in Pain Research and Therapy,* Vol 17 (pp. 129–137). New York: Raven.

Veiersted KB & Westgaard RH (1993). Development of trapezius myalgia among female workers performing light manual work. *Scand J Work Environ Health,* 19,277–283.

Westgaard RH (1988). Measurement and evaluation of postural load in occupational work situations. *Eur J Appl Physiol,* 57,291–304.

Wolf SL, Basmajian JV, Russe TC, & Kutner M (1979). Normative data on low back mobility and activity levels. *Am J Phys Med,* 58,217–229.

Wolf SL, Nacht M, & Kelly JL (1982). EMG feedback training during dynamic movement for low back pain patients. *Behav Ther,* 13,395–406.

Chapter 7

Biomechanical Risk Factors

Martha J. Sanders

As early as 1717, health care practitioners speculated on factors within the work environment that contribute to cumulative trauma disorders (CTDs). Ramazzini (1717) first identified "violent and irregular motions," "bent posture," and "tonic strain on the muscles" as contributing factors. Centuries later, researchers agree that force and awkward or static postures contribute in some way to CTDs (Armstrong 1986; Putz-Anderson 1988; Bullock 1990). However, our ability to quantify and determine the relative weight of each factor in the overall scheme of CTDs still remains limited. The following case exemplifies the juxtaposition of factors involved in CTDs and the difficulty in determining a precipitating event.

> Carl, a 64-year-old man who had been employed as a heavy equipment operator for 20 years, described a work history of jack hammering on road crews, welding, and wiring commercial buildings. Over a period of 2 years, Carl noticed that he could no longer sense the amount of pressure he was exerting on the controls and that he was dumping loads of gravel too quickly and "jerking" the heavy machinery dangerously. He stated that his fingers were numb by the end of the day and that his hands felt weak. In fact, Carl had increasing difficulty pulling himself into the cab. (He weighed 370 lb.) Once in his cab, he sat all day except during coffee breaks. Although he was close to retirement, he loved his job and planned on working as long as he was able.

Carl appeared to be developing signs and symptoms of carpal tunnel syndrome (CTS). However, determining which factor presented the greatest risk for the development of CTS is not straightforward. Was the repetitive grasping and manipulating of controls the source of the problem, or the fact that operation of the controls required high hand forces? Was Carl's sitting in a slumped posture all day the cause, or was Carl's history of jack hammering and electrical work to blame? How did Carl's weight affect the risk of CTS? Most likely, all factors played a role, although we cannot be certain which factor or factors played the primary role in Carl's situation.

Much current research in biomechanics as related to CTDs attempts to delineate both the relative weight of each risk factor and the task parameters that identify safe limits for individual workers. By definition, a *risk factor* is an attribute of or exposure to a situation that increases the probability of developing a certain disease or disorder. The greater the exposure to a risk factor, the greater the risk for developing a disorder; exposure to several factors substantially increases the risk. In Carl's case, his history of working with vibrating tools combined with his present job probably increased his risk for developing CTS, as compared to someone whose work involves varied tasks.

Researchers suggest that an interaction between risk factors may have a multiplicative rather than an additive effect (Armstrong & Ulin 1995). We remain uncertain about the extent to which parameters for each risk factor vary with respect to the individual worker, exposure, work style, and recovery times (Harber et al. 1993; American National Standards Institute 1994). Because research is inconclusive about which risk factor or combination of factors places a particular person at risk for developing CTDs, our best means of assessing the risk

129

of injury is to measure all factors. With this information, we can monitor individual workers as well as compile information from jobs that illustrate safe levels of risk (Putz-Anderson 1988; Joseph & Bloswick 1992; Armstrong & Ulin 1995).

In this chapter, we review seven biomechanical risk factors for CTDs in the workplace: repetition, force, awkward posture, static posture, vibration, mechanical stresses, and cool temperatures. Biomechanical principles that underlie each risk factor will be discussed, to aid the health care practitioner in understanding and critically analyzing the interaction of risk factors.

Repetition

Repetition refers to the performance of the same motions over and over within a given time period. Repetitive work became the hallmark of the industrial revolution as management attempted to increase manufacturing efficiency by eliminating and simplifying motions. Today, the Information Age continues this propensity toward repetition through computer use, instrument control panels, and service occupations. However, the musculoskeletal problems associated with repetitive work have become a concern to certain occupational groups such as supermarket checkers (Margolis & Kraus 1987), dental hygienists (MacDonald et al. 1988), workers in fish processing (Chiang et al. 1993), and telecommunications workers (Putz-Anderson et al. 1992).

The physiologic problems that arise from repetitive work or overuse of certain muscles, tendons, and soft-tissue structures have been addressed in terms of muscle fatigue (Sjøgaard et al. 1988; see Chapter 6 in this book), tissue density changes (Armstrong et al. 1984), and tissue strain (Goldstein et al. 1987; Rodgers 1987), among others. Tissue strain theory will be discussed and related to CTDs. The reader is referred to Armstrong et al. (1984) for a discussion of histologic changes in tissue density that result from repetitive work.

Tissue Strain and Repetition

Tissue strain from repetitive motion can be explained in terms of the material properties of tissues. All materials have certain intrinsic properties that

determine the manner in which the materials will respond to an external load or force. *Deformation* and *strain* are terms used to describe a change in the size or shape of a material in response to an external load (Leveau 1992; Norkin & Levangie 1992).

The properties of the materials will determine the extent of the deformation. *Elastic materials* rapidly deform or change shape when an outside force is applied and then return immediately to the original shape when the force is removed. Examples of elastic materials are elastic tubing, rubber bands, or springs. *Viscoelastic materials* deform slowly when a load is applied and then slowly return to the original shape once the load is removed. Thermoplastics and most body tissues, such as tendons, ligaments, and muscles, are composed of viscoelastic materials (Leveau 1992).

The relationship between load (forces applied) and deformation (change in material shape) is described by *Hooke's law*, which states that deformation increases proportional to the load applied, or the strain (deformation) increases in proportion to the stress resisting the load (Serway 1983). In other words, the amount of deformation depends not only on the magnitude of the external load but also on the ability of the material to resist the load. For example, steel and bone are very stiff materials and therefore deform minimally if one applies a heavy outside force. The twig of a branch, however, will bend or deform significantly with very little force because the twig itself offers little resistance.

The *stress-strain curve* describes the total load-deformation relationship. This curve reflects the response of materials to successive loading. Figure 7.1 indicates that in the initial stages of loading, the material returns to its original shape after the load is applied and removed (elastic range). However, over a period of time, the material reaches a certain point at which the material does not return to its original shape (elastic limit) and becomes permanently deformed. Beyond this point, further deformation occurs with very little increase in load (plastic range). The ultimate strength is represented by the highest point on the curve; the rupture or breaking point is the point at which the material fails (Leveau 1992; Norkin & Levangie 1992).

Materials may fail because of mechanical fatigue or creep. *Mechanical fatigue* refers to cyclic loading of a material past its point of endurance (such as stress fractures). *Creep* refers to prolonged or

Figure 7.1. Stress-strain curve. (A = elastic range; E = elastic limit; B = plastic range; U = ultimate strength; R = rupture or breaking point.) (Redrawn with permission from BF Leveau [1992]. *Williams's & Lissner's Biomechanics of Human Motion* [3rd ed]. Philadelphia: Saunders.)

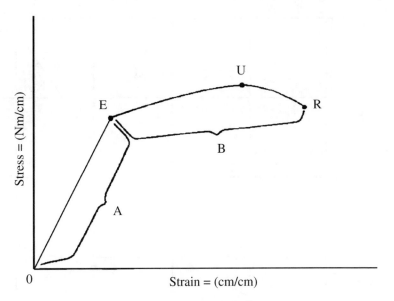

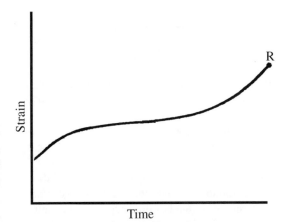

Figure 7.2. The concept of creep. Prolonged loading of tendons causes strain or deformation over time. (R = rupture or breaking point.) (Redrawn with permission from BF Leveau [1992]. *Williams's & Lissner's Biomechanics of Human Motion* [3rd ed]. Philadelphia: Saunders.)

dons during repetitive work will elongate the tendon and create microtears in the tissue. Initially, these viscoelastic tendons recover, repair, and return to their original length (elastic range). This mechanism allows the worker to function with no apparent problem. However, if external loads are applied too often or too quickly, leaving inadequate time for complete recovery, a residual strain develops in the tendons. Over time, tendons accumulate strain that may weaken, deform, or create a chronic inflammatory response in the tendon (Chaffin & Andersson 1984). The worker may begin to feel pain while performing the usual tasks.

At a certain point (such as during overtime or excessive work for several weeks), the accumulation of strain and the magnitude of the load supersede the ability of the tissues to repair. The worker is unable to keep up the work pace. The tissue becomes permanently deformed (plastic range) and thereafter needs less force or load to break or rupture. This model may explain why workers seem to report one particularly stressful event prior to seeking medical help, although the client may have performed repetitive work for years. It may also explain why workers seem to have a lower tolerance to repetition when returning to work after a CTD than when they originally started the job.

To more fully understand the relationship of accumulated tissue strain (referred to as *creep*) to repetitive work, Goldstein et al. (1987) studied the strain in tendons during repetitive pinching activities at submaximal loads. Researchers subjected the finger flexor tendons of cadavers to various workloads

constant submaximal loading of a material, causing increased strain or deformation over time (Leveau 1992; Figure 7.2). (Refer to Chapter 5 for a discussion of mechanical properties of tendons.)

Although human tissue differs from other materials in its healing properties, this stress-strain model has important implications for the etiology of CTDs and the musculoskeletal problems associated with repetitive work (Chaffin & Andersson 1984; Goldstein et al. 1987; Dobyns 1991). External loads applied to ten-

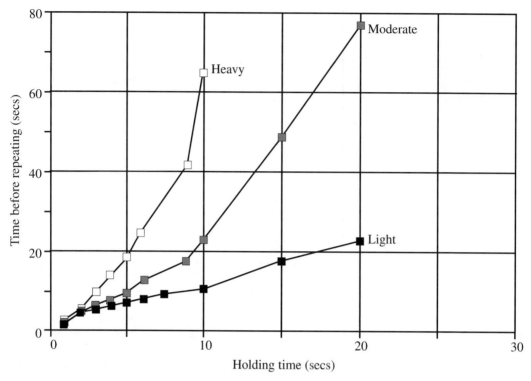

Figure 7.3. Work-recovery times for static work. The total cycle time (time before repeating, *y* axis) is a function of the effort duration (or holding time, *x* axis) and the effort intensity (graphed curves). (Reprinted with permission from S Rodgers [1987]. Recovery time needs for repetitive work. *Semin Occup Med*, 2[1],19–24.)

and frequency cycles and then measured the strain accumulated within the tendons. Results indicated that the frequency cycles (or work-rest cycles) were correlated significantly with tendon strain. In a 2-second work cycle followed by a 9-second recovery period, no significant change in tendon strain was noted after 500 cycles. However, when work time was increased to 8 seconds and recovery time decreased to 2 seconds, the accumulated strain in the tendon was equivalent to an 80% increase in load after 500 cycles. Goldstein et al. (1987) contend that the recovery time between successive loads is the greatest indicator of tendon strain in repetitive work.

Fatigue Model

Clearly, recovery time plays an important role in repetitive work. The concept of work and recovery cycles was introduced by Rohmert (1973) and developed by Rodgers (1987, 1988, 1994) in relation to CTDs in industry. Rodgers (1987) noted that industry standards for repetitive tasks were based solely on the amount of time necessary to complete a motion, without regard for the amount of effort involved or recovery time needed. When workers were required to perform heavy tasks at the same rate as light tasks, they clearly fatigued much more quickly. Rodgers proposed that work cycles in industry (the total time required to perform a task and recover from the task) incorporate muscular effort as well as effort duration, allowing for longer recovery times for heavy, repetitive work.

Rodgers (1987, 1988) proposed the fatigue model, which identifies the interaction between the effort duration or time of continuous effort, the effort intensity, the frequency of repeating the actions, and the total cycle time. Figure 7.3 identifies the effort duration (or continuous effort) (*x* axis), effort intensity (graphed curves), and total cycle time necessary to perform a task (*y* axis). The effort intensity corresponds to the percentage of a person's

Table 7.1. Relationships Between Intensity of Effort (Expressed as Maximum Capacity for Muscle Contraction or Aerobic Activity) and Duration of Static Muscular or Aerobic Activity

Percent of Maximum Capacity	Duration of Static Muscle Effort	Duration of Aerobic Work
100	6 secs	6 mins
85	12 secs	12 mins
70	20 secs	20 mins
50	1.0 mins	1 hr
40	2.5 mins	2 hrs
33	4.0 mins	8 hrs
15	7.5 mins	16 hrs

Sources: Compiled from S Rodgers (1988). Job evaluation in worker fitness determination. *Occup Med: State of the Art Reviews*, 3(2), 219–239; Eastman Kodak Company (1983). *Ergonomic Design for People at Work*, Vol 1. New York: Van Nostrand Reinhold; and W Rohmert (1973). Problems in determining rest allowances: I. Use of modern methods to evaluate stress and strain in static muscular work. *Appl Ergon*, 4,91–95.

maximum voluntary capacity (MVC) in that working posture or aerobic work capacity. Effort intensity can be measured as a function of perceived exertion (Rodgers 1987, 1988) such as light (30%), moderate (50%), and heavy (80%), because direct measurements are not always possible. Effort intensity can also be related to particular muscular activities identified in the model (Rodgers 1994).

Table 7.1 summarizes the relationship between the effort intensity for static muscle strength (percent of MVC) or cardiovascular endurance and the maximal time that a muscle group (or person) may spend in static contraction or aerobic activity before fatiguing. If the duration of work activity without adequate recovery exceeds these times, cardiovascular or muscular energy will decrease, indicating fatigue.

Recovery time is calculated in Figure 7.3 by subtracting the effort duration or continuous holding time from the total cycle time. For example, a light-effort task that requires a 10-second continuous holding time will require a 12-second cycle, which allows 2 seconds for recovery. However, if the task requires heavy effort, a 10-second holding time will necessitate a cycle time of 65 seconds to allow for a 55-second muscle recovery period.

The fatigue model can assist the health care practitioner in predicting the potential for muscle fatigue in certain jobs, in evaluating physical job demands, and in solving problems in job design. For example, by using the model one can determine whether the amount of recovery time for the worker's effort is sufficient to avoid fatigue or whether the effort should be reduced to sustain the cycle time (Rodgers 1987). Rodgers (1988) also has introduced a functional description based on the model that helps prioritize which jobs need to be modified. See Rodgers 1988 for a thorough discussion and case application.

Research on Repetition and Cumulative Trauma Disorders

Research has attempted to isolate risk factors. This task, however, is extremely difficult because several risk factors usually occur together in work environments. In industry, Silverstein et al. (1987) attempted to document repetition and force and then to identify the risk of developing a work-related CTD on the basis of exposure to these factors. In a cross-sectional study, researchers examined the prevalence of CTS among 652 workers in 39 different jobs, as related to force and repetitive hand use on the job. All workers were observed, videotaped, and classified into four groups on the basis of their exposure to force and repetition in the workplace. The four groups were low force–low repetition, high force–low repetition, low force–high repetition, and high force–high repetition. A sample of workers from each job underwent a structured interview and physical examination to determine the presence of symptoms associated with CTS.

Results indicated that the prevalence of CTS was 5.6% in the high force–high repetition group and 0.6% in the low force–low repetition group (Silverstein et al. 1987). Odds ratios indicated that the risk of developing CTS was 15 times greater in the high force–high repetition group than in the low force–low repetition group. The low force–high repetition jobs presented a slightly higher risk than the high force–low repetition jobs; therefore, repetition was considered to be a greater risk factor in the analysis than was force. Deviations in posture and use of vibrating tools were not controlled in the study.

Other investigators argue that group comparison of job-related characteristics and prevalence does not present an accurate assessment of individual exposure or the specific motions under study (Harber et al. 1993). Harber's group investigated the relationship between individual exposure to specific motions and individual symptoms in supermarket checkers. The investigators interviewed and videotaped 50 supermarket checkers three times during busy and routine work hours. The videotapes were analyzed according to the motions performed and grip used. Each subject was classified as positive or negative according to the presence or absence of reported upper-extremity symptoms.

Results indicated that repetitive wrist flexion and extension appear to be related to checkers' hand-wrist symptoms and symptoms specific to CTS (such as burning pain). Repetitive forearm pronation also was related to hand-wrist symptoms. There were associations among duration (years checking), intensity (hours checking per week), and the presence of symptoms. Further analysis demonstrated a relationship between posture of the lumbar spine and distal hand-wrist symptoms (Harber et al. 1993).

This study supports previous research on the role of repetitive motion in CTDs. Investigators (Harber et al. 1993) further demonstrate a study design that examines individual exposure, work style, and posture, a method that is highly relevant to predicting individual health outcomes and implementing ergonomic changes.

Measurement

Repetition has been measured in a number of ways. Health professionals tend to focus on the number of similar movements in a given time period, whereas engineers focus on the work quantity (expressed as the amount of time to complete a task) (Armstrong 1986). It would appear that as work quantity increases, so does the repetition. However, the repetition increases only if all the motions in the task involve similar muscle groups. Hence, one must carefully examine the actual repetitive nature of the job in order to determine whether repetition indeed increases.

Silverstein et al. (1987) developed a method by which to categorize jobs into low- or high-repetition groups on the basis of the estimated cycle time for a job task and the percentage of time performing the same fundamental cycle. *Cycle time* refers to the amount of time necessary to complete a task. Within a cycle, there may be a series of steps or movements that are repeated. These movements are referred to as *fundamental cycle* (Silverstein et al. 1987). According to the method of Silverstein et al., jobs are classified as *low repetitive* if the cycle time is more than 30 seconds and if less than 50% of the cycle time involves performing the same kind of fundamental cycle. (In other words, similar movements are repeated less than 50% of the time.) A job is considered to be *high repetitive* if the cycle time is less than 30 seconds or more than 50% of the cycle time involves performing the same kind of fundamental cycle. This classification has been used widely in research studies (Silverstein et al. 1987; Chiang et al. 1993).

Other approaches measure the repetition *rate*, the average number of motions performed within a unit of time, such as motions per shift (Putz-Anderson 1988). Hammer (1934) measured repetition in terms of the number of manipulations per hour and concluded that more than 2,000 manipulations per hour, or 30–40 manipulations per minute, were considered to be repetitive.

Although cycles and repetition rates attempt to quantify job repetitiveness, these systems consider only the speed at which the worker performs the movements rather than the quality of movements. Armstrong and Ulin (1995) introduced a qualitative scale that rates the degree of repetition as related to the worker's ability to keep up with the work. Work is rated as follows:

- *Very high:* The worker's body parts are in rapid, steady motion; the worker has difficulty keeping up with the pace.
- *High:* The worker's body parts are in steady motion; any difficulty causes the worker to fall behind.

- *Medium:* The worker's body parts are in steady motion, but he or she is able to keep up, with time for brief pauses or rest.
- *Low:* The worker has no difficulty keeping up; there are frequent pauses during work to wait for another job or machinery cycle.
- *Very low:* The worker is inactive most of the time but occasionally uses his or her hands.

Armstrong and Ulin note that, using this scale, jobs with vastly different productivity standards can be compared. For a complete discussion of this scale, the reader should see the original publication (Armstrong & Ulin 1995).

Force

Nearly all activities require some degree of force to stabilize the body, resist gravity, and move loads. *Force* can be defined as a "push or pull produced by the action of one body against another" (Leveau 1992, p. 308) or "the mechanical effort to accomplish a specific movement or exertion" (American National Standards Institute 1994).

Two types of forces addressed in biomechanics are external and internal forces. *External forces* are the loads exerted on the surface of the body during work-related activities such as lifting, pushing, or grasping objects. *Internal forces* refer to the tension generated within the muscles, tendons, and ligaments that resist external loads. External loads are more readily measured and tend to be the reference point for industry. In industry, force is commonly expressed as the amount of effort required by a worker to overcome external loads through pushing, pulling, grasping, or handling objects.

Force has been implicated as a factor in CTDs, especially when combined with other risk factors. Investigators suggest that the risk of CTDs increases with an increase in force (Armstrong & Chaffin 1979; Armstrong et al. 1984; Silverstein et al. 1987). However, as discussed previously, parameters for acceptable forces in industry have not been established.

Researchers suggest that the body's ability to generate and sustain muscle forces varies with body posture, body orientation, frictional forces of materials, and the wearing of gloves.

Frictional Forces

Frictional forces are forces that develop when one surface slides over another surface. Frictional forces that develop between two surfaces can play an additional role in the total force needed to move an object. The amount of force needed to produce motion of one surface relative to the other depends on how tightly the surfaces are pressed together and the texture of each surface (Leveau 1992).

Coefficient of Friction

The *coefficient of friction* refers to the slipperiness between two objects or the effect of the texture of the materials on the overall force needed to move an object. Coefficient of friction is expressed as a value from 0 to 1 or greater. Surfaces with a low coefficient of friction glide easily over each other; examples are greased metal on metal and joint surfaces bathed by synovial fluid. Surfaces with a high coefficient of friction resist movement yet provide greater stability between the two objects. Examples of surfaces with a high coefficient of friction include rubber crutch tips on a wooden floor and sandpaper on skin (Buchholz et al. 1988; Leveau 1992).

Clearly, friction is an important factor in the ability to grip and manipulate objects. Objects with a low coefficient of friction tend to slide out of the hand and require higher grip forces to grasp and hold. For example, it is more difficult to open a jar with wet hands than with dry hands because the jar slips. It is also more difficult to turn pages of a book with dry hands rather than wet hands because the pages tend to "slip" away.

A higher coefficient of friction provides stability and requires lower hand forces to move the surfaces. Use of a rubber pad to open a jar will increase the coefficient of friction between the jar and the fingers and thus make the task easier. Comaish and Bottoms (1971) suggest that individuals sense frictional forces between objects and adjust grip forces accordingly.

Research

Knowledge of the coefficient of friction is relevant to the design of tool handles, controls, and assembly jobs. Buchholz et al. (1988) studied both the effects of the coefficient of friction on pinch forces for common materials and the changes in the coef-

Table 7.2. Coefficients of Friction for Common Materials Against Human Skin

Material	Dry (n = 42)	Moist (n = 42)	Combined (n = 84)
Sandpaper (no. 320)	—	—	0.61 + 0.10
Smooth vinyl	—	—	0.53 + 0.18
Textured vinyl	—	—	0.50 + 0.11
Adhesive tape	0.41 + 0.10	0.66 + 0.14	—
Suede	0.39 + 0.06	0.66 + 0.11	—
Aluminum	—	—	0.38 + 0.13
Paper	0.27 + 0.09	0.42 + 0.07	—

Sources: Adapted from TJ Armstrong (1990). Ergonomics and cumulative trauma disorders of the hand and wrist. In JM Hunter, EJ Mackin, & AD Callahan (Eds). *Rehabilitation of the Hand: Surgery and Therapy* (3rd ed). Philadelphia: Mosby; and B Buchholz, LJ Frederick, & TJ Armstrong (1988). An investigation of human palmar skin friction and the effects of materials, pinch force, and moisture. *Ergonomics*, 31,317–325.

Table 7.3. Effects of Wrist Angle on Power Grip Strength

Wrist Angle (Degrees)	Percentage of Power Grip
Neutral	100
Flexion 45	60
Flexion 65	45
Extension 45	75
Extension 60	63
Ulnar deviation 45	75
Radial deviation 25	80

Source: Adapted from S Rodgers (1987). Recovery time needs for repetitive work. *Semin Occup Med,* 2(1),19–24.

ficient of friction for materials against moist and dry skin. These investigators found that pinch forces increase when materials with a low coefficient of friction are grasped (such as aluminum in moist hands). Pinch forces decrease when moist hands rather than dry hands grasp porous materials such as suede, adhesive tape, and paper. This increased coefficient of friction requires lower pinch forces. The researchers recommend that adhesive tape and suede be used in industrial environments for handling materials with high moisture or heat indices, due to their high frictional properties (Buchholz et al. 1988). Armstrong (1990) summarizes that approximately 53% more hand force is required to hold a tool when the skin is dry rather than moist. (See Chapter 8 for further discussion on tool handles.) Table 7.2 outlines the coefficient of friction for human skin against common materials.

Posture and Force

Posture or position greatly affects the ability of muscles to generate power. Overall, muscles generate optimal forces for the desired movement when the extremity is positioned in neutral—that is, roughly halfway between the beginning and ending ranges of motion for an extremity (Chaffin & Andersson 1984; Leveau 1992). In this position, the moment arm about the joint is longest and the muscle is at the best biomechanical advantage for work. When muscles generate forces in a deviated position, the muscles must generate higher internal forces to accomplish the same task. (In the next section, we further discuss biomechanics and posture.)

Table 7.3 demonstrates this concept relating hand-grip strength to hand posture. In a neutral position, one's grip strength is 100%. However, when the wrist flexes to 45 degrees, for example, the grip strength is only 60% of its entire strength. That figure drops to 45% when the wrist flexes to 65 degrees (Rodgers 1987). In this position, the individual must work more than twice as hard to accomplish the same task. Three to four more times the force is required to exert the same force level in a pinch versus a power grip (Tichauer 1978; Armstrong 1986).

Haselgrave (1991) found that the maximal force that workers generated for a job varied with the workers' positions—standing, kneeling, or lying on their backs. Haselgrave suggested that the variability in force was due to changes in the workers' abilities to use their body weight, to brace their feet or shoulders against a surface (thus providing joint stability), and to use stronger muscle groups to accomplish the job.

Silverstein et al. (1987) discussed the combined risk of high force and high repetition as related to CTDs (see preceding section). Armstrong and Chaffin (1979) studied the effects of hand size and work methods on the presence of CTS in two groups of female production sewers, one group with a history of CTS and the other group with no such history. These researchers found no correlation between hand size and CTS. However, individuals with a history of CTS were found to use higher hand forces and more frequent pinch grips during work than individuals with no history of CTS. Although we cannot be certain whether the use of higher forces and pinch grips is the cause or effect of CTS, it appears that force may play a role in CTDs in this group of workers.

Two recent case-control studies also support the contention that high forces may contribute to CTDs. One study compared the work practices of dental offices with and without claims for CTS. Results indicated that dental hygienists' hand pain was related more to heavy prehension forces used during scaling (removing plaque) than to repetition of the task (Strong & Lennartz 1992).

A study by Ekberg et al. (1994) investigated the relationship between neck and shoulder pain in workers and the physical, organizational, and psychosocial aspects of the job. Researchers found that workers who performed light lifting were 13.6 times more likely to develop neck and shoulder symptoms than were those who performed no lifting. Interestingly, those who reported ambiguity in the work role were 16.5 times more likely to develop neck and shoulder pain. This report demonstrates the continued relationship between physical and psychosocial variables.

Gloves

Most research suggests that gloves increase grip force requirements because gloves interfere with the tactile and proprioceptive feedback necessary to determine the appropriate grip force; therefore, individuals grip harder than is necessary to accomplish a task (Armstrong 1990). Hertzberg's study of airline pilots (1955) found that pilots exerted 25–30% more force to overcome the bulkiness of the gloves. Tichauer (1978) explains that use of bulky gloves may lead to inadequate control of the hands when operating tools or dials and difficulty sustaining objects in the hand. Buchholz et al. (1988) suggest that gloves often re-

duce the coefficient of friction between the hand and the surface and thus require higher grip forces. Certainly, properly fitting gloves are key to effective use.

Measurement

Force can be measured or estimated in a number of ways. Most job analyses estimate the external forces needed to accomplish a given task by identifying the weight of an object, the location of an object, the distance carried, and the duration of the action. This approach identifies the external force that a worker must generate, and can be compared to norms for the worker's age and occupation. However, this method does not indicate the exertion perceived by the individual worker.

Psychophysical methods have been used to identify workers' perceptions of acceptable lifting load limits (Ciriello et al. 1990) and to predict overexertion injury at work (Herrin et al. 1986). Studies often associate the lifting activity with Borg scales of perceived exertion, to rate the degree of discomfort or force associated with the task. Armstrong and Ulin (1995) suggest that worker ratings be used similarly to assess forceful exertions or torque on a tool. Workers may rate their perception of forces used on a scale, in an effort to determine acceptable force levels.

Another method of analyzing force involves placing a pressure-sensitive gauge at the point of contact of the force. To measure hand or finger forces, small pressure-sensitive devices are attached to the hands or gloves while the individual performs a task. This allows for direct measurement of the forces on the hands or fingers (Joseph & Bloswick 1991).

Finally, the internal forces (or the actual muscle requirements of the job) can be measured using surface electromyography (sEMG). (See Chapter 6 for a discussion of sEMG.) sEMG measures the muscle activity or, more specifically, the motor unit potential of twitching muscle fibers. Surface electrodes are placed on the muscles involved, and these record the sum of all motor unit potentials reaching the electrode (Chaffin & Andersson 1984).

Posture

Posture is one of the most frequently cited risk factors for CTDs (Armstrong 1986; Pheasant 1991). Al-

Table 7.4. Work Postures to Avoid for Long Durations

Body Part	Posture to Avoid
Neck	Forward flexion ≥20 degrees
Shoulder	Flexion or abduction ≥30 degrees (elbow above midchest)
	Extension and internal rotation (down and behind)
Elbow	Extreme elbow flexion
	Extreme supination and pronation with grasp
Wrist	Extreme flexion
	Extreme extension
	Ulnar or radial deviation with grasp
Fingers	Pinching or pressing with the fingertips
	Thumb extension

Sources: Compiled from V Putz-Anderson (Ed) (1988). *Cumulative Trauma Disorders: A Manual for Musculoskeletal Diseases of the Upper Limbs.* Philadelphia: Taylor & Francis; E Grandjean (1988). *Fitting the Task to the Man* (4th ed). London: Taylor & Francis; T Luopajarvi (1990). Ergonomic analysis of workplace and postural load. In M Bullock (Ed). *Ergonomics: The Physiotherapist in the Workplace.* New York: Churchill Livingstone; and TJ Armstrong (1986). Ergonomics and cumulative trauma disorders. *Hand Clin,* 2,553–565.

though the influence of good posture on employee health and productivity is recognized widely in ergonomic and manufacturing circles, a clear definition of what constitutes good posture remains elusive.

Norkin and Levangie (1992) discuss static and dynamic posture in biomechanical terms, noting that very little effort is required to sustain an upright, static posture. The motor control necessary to maintain dynamic posture, however, is very complex, dependent on tactile, articular, and proprioceptive feedback mechanisms. Optimal posture, in biomechanical terms, is that in which body segments are aligned vertically, and the center of gravity passes through all joint axes. The compression forces of body segments in optimal posture are distributed evenly over weight-bearing surfaces, with *no excessive tension exerted on the ligaments and muscles.* Although this definition is imprecise, it provides a basis for examining posture in any part of the body.

Corlett (1981) addresses posture in functional terms relative to the task being performed. Among the principles Corlett offers for workplace design that promotes good posture during work are upright head and neck positions for visual tasks, sitting or standing options, equal distribution of weight while standing, use of joints in midrange, work performed "below the level of the heart," and the ability of the worker to assume several safe and varied postures throughout the day.

Grandjean (1988) and Chaffin & Andersson (1984) present recommendations for specific body positions during work. Those positions listed in Table 7.4 should be avoided if they will have to be maintained for long periods. These researchers suggest that the head and neck should be positioned at 10–15 degrees of neck flexion during visual work; shoulders should flex or abduct no more than 30 degrees; elbows should flex to no more than 90 degrees; and other joints should be positioned in neutral for execution of tasks. Unfortunately, much of what has been touted as good posture in industry is derived from laboratory experiments that rarely simulate actual work settings.

Haselgrave (1994) sought to bring functional and biomechanical aspects of posture together in a model influenced by Corlett (1981). This model proposes that individuals adopt a posture during work tasks according to the functional demands of the tasks and the individuals' anthropometric capabilities. This posture is modified by the physical and spatial constraints within the working environment. Haselgrave (1994) explains that workers first position themselves according to the primary demands of the task. For example, sewing machine operators must view the material closely and therefore work in extremes of neck and trunk flexion and shoulder abduction. Because visual demands are the greatest priority, neck and trunk flexion postures take precedence over other body postures.

The primary demands of the task are also the primary points of interaction between the worker and the workplace. When the task demands (e.g., high precision and high speed) are in conflict, the worker assumes a position of compromise between the least body discomfort and the quickest manner in which to perform the task, which may also be the most hazardous. Haselgrave (1994, p. 785) summarizes that "posture therefore arises from the functional demands of vision, reach, manipulation, strength, and endurance, and is constrained by the geometric relationship between the person's own anthropometry and the layout of the workplace." (See Haselgrave 1994 for a complete discussion of this model.)

Research indicates that several aspects of posture may be related to CTDs. Static postures involve maintaining the same position for relatively long periods of time; awkward postures involve working in a position that is deviated from neutral.

Awkward Postures

Work in awkward postures can be harmful when movements extend tissues beyond the normal range of motion, causing a tear or strain. Work is especially harmful when awkward movements are combined with force. Posture as it affects muscle strength will be discussed from two perspectives, physiologic and biomechanical. Each perspective supports the need for health care professionals to identify and promote optimal postures for workers in all industries.

The *length-tension relationship* describes the ability of a muscle to generate tension and exert force on a bony lever. Norkin and Levangie (1992) explain that there is a direct relationship between the tension developed within the muscle and the length of the muscle. This relationship is based on muscle physiology. Contraction of a muscle occurs when the smallest components of a muscle fiber, actin and myosin filaments, bind together to form a *cross-bridge*. The cross-bridge is considered the basic unit of active muscle tension. When the muscle is at its resting length (usually in midrange or neutral), actin and myosin filaments form the maximum number of cross-bridges and thus develop the maximal amount of muscle tension. When a muscle is lengthened, there is less overlap of the filaments and fewer cross-bridges form. Thus, only moderate tension develops within the muscle in its lengthened position. When the muscle is shortened, the cross-bridges have already been formed, so the muscle develops less tension. Therefore, as stated, use of a muscle in a lengthened or shortened position will require greater internal muscle forces than would be required to use a muscle in neutral (Chaffin & Andersson 1984; Leveau 1992; Norkin & Levangie 1992).

From a biomechanical standpoint, posture affects muscle force through concepts related to lever systems and torque throughout the body. Torque (T, or rotational force about a joint) is a function of the internal muscle force (F) multiplied by the perpendicular distance $(\perp D)$ between the joint axis and the

application of the muscle force ($T = F \times \perp D$). This perpendicular distance is also known as the *moment arm* ($T = F \times MA$). When two bony segments are in neutral (such as the elbow at 90 degrees), the moment arm is longest, and therefore the muscle produces the most torque. Figure 7.4 demonstrates that as two bony segments rotate from neutral into full flexion or extension, the moment arms become smaller. Thus, less torque is developed and less rotational force is executed in the direction of the segment (Chaffin & Andersson 1984; Leveau 1992; Norkin & Levangie 1992).

Neck and Shoulders

Individuals unconsciously develop awkward neck and shoulder postures as a result of poor workplace ergonomics and personal work style (Barry et al. 1992). Typical neck and shoulder postures are forward flexion of the neck and protraction and internal rotation of the shoulders. These postures may cause localized pain as well as symptoms in the distal extremity.

Maeda et al. (1980) examined the relationship between upper-extremity postures and musculoskeletal symptoms of 179 female keyboard operators and salespeople. The keyboard operators worked in a seated position with their necks flexed and rotated to the left for visual and inputting tasks. The salespeople spent each work day walking, standing, and bending down. Results of a survey indicated that the keyboard operators complained of stiffness and pain in the lumbar area and left side of the neck, as well as arm and hand pain (more so on the dominant side). Salespeople complained predominantly of torso and low-back pain. This study noted the effect of neck posture and static sitting on musculoskeletal complaints (Maeda et al. 1980).

Dental hygienists also report a high prevalence of neck and shoulder pain during clinical work. In fact, up to 68% of all dental hygienists report painful neck and shoulder conditions that emanate from static, flexed postures throughout the day (Osborn et al. 1990; Oberg & Oberg 1993). When Oberg (1993) analyzed the ergonomic factors that influenced one dental hygienist's pain, he found that a work position of 45-degree neck flexion and 30-degree lateral flexion to the right was associated with neck and shoulder pain. Biomechanical computation revealed that twice the muscle force was needed to support the head in forward flexion (50

A   B   C

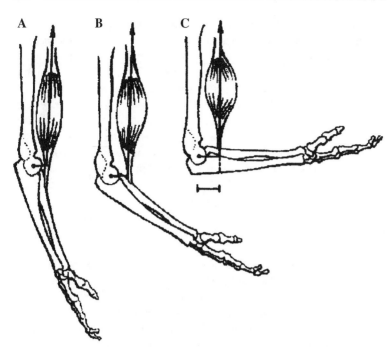

Figure 7.4. Moment arm of the biceps (perpendicular distance from the tendon insertion to the joint axis) changes with elbow position. **A.** The elbow is extended and moment arm is small; compressive forces are greater than rotational forces. **B.** At 45 degrees, compressive and rotational forces are equal. **C.** At 90 degrees, the moment arm is longest; rotational forces are greatest. (Redrawn with permission from BF Leveau [1992]. *Williams's & Lissner's Biomechanics of Human Motion* [3rd ed]. Philadelphia: Saunders.)

N) than in a neutral, upright position (26.7 N). The total muscle force needed to support a position of 90-degree shoulder abduction and 60-degree elbow flexion during work is 186.7 N (Oberg 1993).

Shoulder Elevation

Workplace factors that may cause a worker to elevate his or her shoulders regularly during work include tasks that require overhead reaching, unsupported use of the hands away from the body, or a chair height that is too low. The use of shoulders elevated in flexion or abduction has been associated with localized fatigue and tendinitis in the biceps and supraspinatus muscles, as well as with decreased productivity (Tichauer 1978; Hagberg 1981; Putz-Anderson 1988).

Hagberg (1981) demonstrated that workers who used their arms in a position exceeding 90 degrees of abduction rapidly develop fatigue in the upper trapezius muscle and compensatory muscle patterns. Chaffin (1973) examined the relationship between muscle fatigue and arm abduction angle in healthy men and found that subjects fatigued in 15 minutes when using the arms at 90 degrees of abduction and in 30 minutes when using the arms at 60 degrees but did not fatigue after an hour when the arms were abducted to only 30 degrees.

When Tichauer (1978) examined the relationship between chair height and shoulder abduction angle, similar problems of fatigue and decreased efficiency were noted. Chair height that was 3 in. too low for the worker produced an arm abduction angle of 45 degrees and excessive shoulder movements in an effort to place the hand. Several hours of work in this position reduced workplace efficiency by as much as 50%.

Results of these studies indicate that workers should maintain a position of less than 30 degrees of shoulder flexion or abduction during work activities.

Elbow

Figure 7.4 demonstrates the position of the biceps muscle with the elbow at 90 degrees and with the elbow extended. When Tichauer (1978) studied the effect of various elbow positions on the elbow "soreness" of 38 workers who performed constant screwdriving exertions, the workers who used their elbows in at least 130 degrees of elbow extension reported 23 complaints of elbow pain, whereas workers who used the elbow in no more than 85 degrees flexion reported no pain. Tichauer explained that the elbow-extended position incites excessive compressive forces within the joint that ultimately cause the pain.

Tichauer (1978) noted that during rotational tasks, such as clockwise screwdriving, the biceps act to supinate the forearm and should therefore be positioned in neutral. To maximize the rotational forces of biceps during supination, the elbow should be positioned in 90 degrees of flexion.

Wrist

Work that incorporates extremes of wrist flexion and extension and radial and ulnar deviation may cause problems, especially when combined with grasp. During extreme wrist flexion and extension, the nerves and structures within the carpal canal are displaced against the carpal bones and the flexor retinaculum. Constant stretching and compression of the nerves against adjacent tissues may contribute to CTS. De Krom et al. (1990) found this to be the case in a study identifying the risk factors for CTS. These researchers found CTS to be associated with exposure to activities with flexed or extended wrists. The risk ratio increased four to five times for those subjects engaged in such activities for more than 20 hours per week.

The effects of wrist deviation on hand force and symptom development have been widely studied. Tichauer (1978) studied the outbreak of de Quervain's disease in wiring operators at a Western Electric plant and found the outbreak to be associated with the use of needle-nosed pliers. When Tichauer redesigned the pliers to include a bent handle, the prevalence of tenosynovitis dropped considerably. Only 10% of the new workers who used the bent-handled tool developed tenosynovitis after 12 weeks of work, whereas 60% of those workers who used the traditional pliers developed tenosynovitis after 12 weeks.

Similarly, Armstrong et al. (1982) found that poultry workers were developing CTS-like symptoms at an alarming incidence rate of 17.4 cases per 200,000 hours (the plant average was 12.8). A job evaluation revealed that workers were using a straight-handled knife to cut poultry thighs vertically, which demanded extremes of wrist flexion and ulnar deviation. Further, high forces were used to hold and cut the thighs. Researchers recommended a pistol-grip knife design with a wraparound handle to neutralize the wrist posture and allow the hand to relax between exertions.

Results of these studies indicate that the wrist should be used in neutral position whenever possible. Table 7.4 lists the postures that place workers at risk for developing a CTD.

Static Postures

The impact of static muscle loads on musculoskeletal pain has come to the forefront, particularly in precise, sedentary, or repetitive work that requires proximal low-level muscle tension or constrained work postures over long periods. The preceding section highlighted the integral relationship between static postures and awkward, repetitive work. Recently, investigations have focused on this phenomenon (Luopajarvi 1990; Milerad & Erickson 1994).

Although static work would appear less fatiguing than dynamic work, the opposite is actually true. *Dynamic work* involves a rhythmic contraction and relaxation of the muscle that enables an exchange of blood flow, nutrients, and muscle wastes (Grandjean 1988). *Static work* involves a prolonged state of contraction during which no apparent work is being performed. During static contractions, the internal pressure of muscle tissue compresses blood vessels and reduces blood flow to that muscle so that the oxygen and energy supply to the muscle is decreased. The waste products from the muscle accumulate, causing muscle fatigue and, eventually, pain. The blood flow is constricted in proportion to the exertion and duration of forces (Grandjean 1988; Luopajarvi 1990).

Maximal Holding Time

Researchers use the terms *maximal holding time* or *holding time* to refer to the duration that a static posture can be maintained continuously before fatigue sets in (Rodgers 1987, 1988). The maximal holding time varies with the muscle effort required of the most highly loaded muscle groups.

There is no consensus yet as to what constitutes high, moderate, or light effort. Many investigators express the muscle effort as a percentage of the MVC of a muscle (Romhert 1973; Rodgers 1987). Rodgers (1994) defines effort for each body part according to the posture of the extremity (close or away from the body) and the forces exerted on the extremity as well as a measurement of an individual's force (such as grip strength) compared to that of the available work force (Rodgers 1988).

The maximal holding time of a muscle has been the subject of many research studies. Grandjean (1988) and Chaffin & Andersson (1984) contend that muscles cannot sustain static contractions of 15–20% MVC for more than a few minutes before interruptions of blood flow and muscle fatigue ensue. Luopajarvi (1990) recommends that no more than 5–6% of the MVC be sustained for work lasting more than 1 hour. Rodgers (1988) integrated maximal holding time and effort intensity to better identify the factors involved (see Table 7.1).

In a more recent study, Sjøgaard et al. (1988) studied the muscle fatigue that occurs during isometric contractions such as in static work. The effect of isometric exercise on blood flow, blood pressure, and intramuscular pressure was examined in exercising muscles. Both intermittent and continuous contractions were performed at 5–50% of the subjects' MVC. Results indicated that although the blood flow was sufficient to maintain the muscle at low-level contractions (10% MVC), intramuscular changes (such as changes in water content or potassium depletion) caused muscle fatigue even at prolonged low levels. Impaired blood flow appeared to be the cause of fatigue at sustained high levels of effort (>30% MVC). Researchers further proposed that the impaired transport of nutrients during prolonged edema formation may be related to fatigue (Sjøgaard et al. 1988; see Chapter 6).

Examples of high-static components inherent in some types of work are fine manipulations performed away from the body, the holding of objects in the arms, placement of body weight on one leg while a pedal is operated with the other, extension or flexion of the head for long periods of time, and standing in one place for long periods (Grandjean 1988).

An ergonomic study of 88 occupations in Helsinki identified jobs with high static components. Those occupational groups with a high level of static work in the arms were dentists, transport personnel, hospital attendants, and installation workers. Static and forceful work was found among home care personnel, kitchen workers, and installation workers (Luopajarvi 1990).

Posture Assessment

The primary means of assessing posture are observation and recording of workers through direct contact or through the use of videocamera equipment. Once postures are observed, various schemes have been developed to record and describe workers' postures for clinical and research purposes. In most schemes, joint angles, duration times, and frequency of efforts are measured. Rodgers (1988) suggests that several workers, including highly skilled and less skilled workers, should be videotaped when one is assessing the physical components of a job, to determine variability in work methods.

Posture Targeting.   Posture targeting is an assessment method developed by Corlett et al. (1979) and used in numerous studies in Scandinavia (Oberg & Oberg, 1993). As demonstrated in Figure 7.5, this method uses a body diagram with 10 prearranged concentric circles or targets placed alongside the body parts. The individual is observed, and the posture for each body part is recorded as 45, 90, or 135 degrees from the target center. The postures are estimated from the standard, anatomic position provided by the body diagram. Movements in the sagittal plane (forward or backward) require a mark along the vertical axis; movements to the side of the body are marked along the horizontal axis. Changes in the postures of specific body parts can be documented throughout the duration of a shift. The reader is referred to Corlett (1990; also Corlett et al. 1979) for complete discussions of this approach.

Fine-Detailed Work Action and Posture.   Fine-detailed work action and posture (FWAPS) is a system developed by Judith Farrell in Australia for recording motions and postures in the workplace. The system documents the speed, frequency, posture, and duration of actions so that a record can be kept and compared across jobs. FWAPS has potential use for simulating job demands in work-hardening programs and for identifying relationships between work actions, postures, and injuries (Farrell 1992).

Self-Analysis Checklist.   Luopajarvi (1990) notes that workers themselves need to be more involved with the identification and correction of postures in the workplace. Self-analysis checklists have been developed for typists, data operators, and cashiers as part of an informational booklet that describes the optimal work environment, ergonomic recommendations, and advice on how to improve the existing

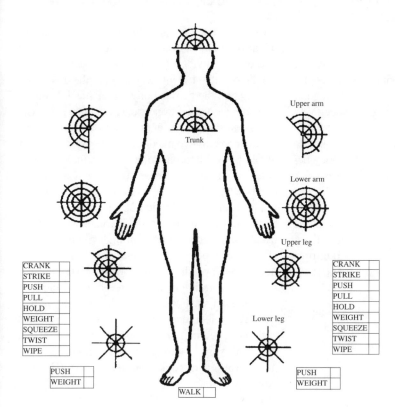

Figure 7.5. Posture-targeting diagram. Targets adjacent to each body part are used to record deviations from the standard position. (Reprinted with permission from EN Corlett, SJ Madeley, & I Manenica [1979]. Posture targeting: a technique for recording working postures. *Ergonomics*, 22,357–366.)

work situation. The purpose of the booklet is to encourage both the worker and the supervisor to collaborate in making improvements in the workplace.

Healthcam System.   A relatively new option for health care professionals is the use of Polaroid film with a grid background to document and compare worker postures. The Healthcam (Polaroid, Sammons Preston Inc, Bolingbrook, IL) offers a reliable method for measuring posture at specific joints, using a grid as a point of reference. Health care practitioners should photograph workers from several angles and several times throughout the shift as one picture does not reflect a worker's posture for the entire shift.

Computerized Motion Analysis System.   Advanced methods of computerized motion analysis, such as the PEAC system (PEAC Technologies Corp, Wheat Ridge, CO), offer both computerized recording of actions and frequency through use of videotaped processing and computerized data recording and processing.

Vibration

Prolonged exposure to vibration from vibrating hand tools or surfaces has been known to affect workers' overall health and to contribute to hand-arm vibration syndrome (HAVS) in an average of 50% of all workers who use vibrating tools (National Institute of Occupational Safety and Health [NIOSH] 1989). *Human vibration* refers to vibration experienced by the human body as a result of vibratory surfaces (Bruel & Kjaer Instruments 1993). Although conditions such as vibration white-finger syndrome and Raynaud's phenomenon are clearly related to vibration exposure, methods to assess and reduce vibration exposure are still being developed (Radwin & Armstrong 1985; Hampel 1992; Bruel & Kjaer Instruments 1993). In this section, we will review the basic physical concepts of vibration, discuss the effects of vibration on the human body, and provide recommendations to decrease workers' exposure to vibration.

Physical Concepts of Vibration

Vibration is described as an oscillating motion of a body about its resting position. Vibration can be understood as a series of waves that oscillate at regular or irregular intervals in distinct patterns specific to the body or vibration source (Chaffin & Andersson 1984; Grandjean 1988). Vibration, when applied to the human body, causes oscillations in the body tissues and produces a bodily response. The response depends on a number of factors including the frequency, direction, intensity, acceleration, and point of application of the vibration and the posture of the body at the point of vibration contact. The following terms specifically define vibration qualities (Bonney 1981; Chaffin & Andersson 1984; Grandjean 1988; NIOSH 1989):

- *Frequency* is the number of complete cycles of oscillations or repetitions of a vibrating body per unit of time. Frequency is measured in Hertz, or cycles per second.
- *Direction* is the course or path of the vibration. Vibration is measured in three orthogonal, bicentric axes: front to back *(x),* side to side *(y),* and up and down *(z).*
- *Amplitude* is the maximum displacement of a resting body from the original resting point.
- *Acceleration* is the change in velocity according to time.

Frequency and acceleration are commonly used to measure and define the vibrational wave form in meters per seconds squared. Acceleration is equated with the vibrational load or vibrational energy in a body; frequency and acceleration combine to produce a level of discomfort in the human body (Chaffin & Andersson 1984; Grandjean 1988; NIOSH, 1989).

Vibration sources can be broadly classified into two categories, free and forced vibration. *Free vibration* refers to the internal, natural oscillations of any body with elastic properties, such as human tissue. *Forced vibration* refers to the external, vibrating forces that are introduced to a body through sources such as vibrating tools or heavy vehicle seats. If an external vibrating force is applied to a body at or near its own natural frequency, the body will *resonate*, or vibrate at a higher amplitude than the original vibrating force applied. If vibration is applied to the body at other frequencies, the body will absorb or reduce the intensity of the vibration.

This occurrence is called *damping* or *attenuation* (Chaffin & Andersson 1984). Clearly, the frequencies of forced vibrations, such as those imposed by hand tools, that fall into the range of the natural frequencies of the human body are of special concern to health care practitioners and safety specialists.

Classifications for human exposure to vibration are divided into two major categories, segmental and whole-body vibration. Some sources include a third category, motion sickness (Bruel & Kjaer Instruments 1993). *Segmental vibration* (or hand-arm vibration) refers to vibration of a specific part of the body such as a hand or arm. Segmental vibration is usually associated with use of high-frequency (≥50-Hz) power tools such as pneumatic drills, grinders, nut-runners, or chain saws. *Whole-body vibration* refers to vibration of the entire body. Whole-body vibration may be transmitted to the body through the buttocks or feet, depending on whether a person is sitting or standing. Whole-body vibration is associated with very low-frequency (≤4-Hz) oscillations, as are found in trucks, buses, or cars (Eastman Kodak Company 1983; Grandjean 1988). *Motion sickness* occurs as a result of travel in many types of transportation including boats, planes, and cars. Motion sickness is associated with vibration of less than 1 Hz and affects individuals differently depending on age, visual acuity, and the vestibular system.

Effects of Vibration on the Body

As mentioned, human body parts oscillate at different natural frequencies and therefore react differently to various external, forced vibrations. Certain low-level vibrations simulate the natural frequency of the neck and trunk and therefore resonate to other parts of the body. For example, frequencies from 4 to 8 Hz cause resonance in the head and trunk and amplify vibrational load to other body parts by more than 200%. Vibrations at higher frequencies are dampened by local body tissues, causing the vibrational energy to stay localized. Grandjean (1988) summarizes the reaction of body parts to the following vertical vibrations:

- 2.5- to 5.0-Hz resonance in the neck and lumbar region
- 4.0- to 6.0-Hz resonance in the trunk, neck, and shoulders

- 20- to 30-Hz resonance between the head and shoulder
- Greater than 30-Hz resonance in the arms, hands, and fingers
- 60- to 90-Hz resonance in the eyeballs
- 100- to 200-Hz resonance in the lower jaw

When vibration is applied to a specific muscle belly or tendon, a reflex contraction of the muscle occurs, called the *tonic vibration reflex* (TVR). The TVR reaches a plateau and is maintained after approximately 30 seconds of the application of vibration. Thereafter, the muscle contracts as long as the muscle is in contact with the vibrating source. Radwin et al. (1987) suggest that workers may use higher grip forces to accomplish a job because of the influence of the TVR and decreased tactile sensation in the fingers as a result of prolonged exposure.

Physiologic Effect

Although each person reacts differently, somatic complaints due to vibration seem to be frequency specific and related to the resonance produced in specific body parts. Vibration at very low frequencies (≤ 1 Hz) tends to produce feelings of seasickness. Frequencies between 1 and 4 Hz may cause difficulty breathing, whereas frequencies between 4 and 12 Hz may cause chest pain, back pain, and severe discomfort. Impairment in the visual field, headaches, and eye strain are most prominent between 10 and 30 Hz (Grandjean 1988).

CTS and tendinitis are of great concern to workers using vibrating hand tools. Vibrational forces cause peripheral vascular and neural changes in the tissues affected by the vibration that may or may not return to normal, depending on the duration and intensity of the exposure. Reduced tactile sensitivity and the tonic vibration reflex combine to contribute to the use of high grip forces during repetitive manual tasks, which further increases the risk of chronic tendon and nerve disorders (Radwin et al. 1987).

Hand-arm vibration syndrome (sometimes called *secondary Raynaud's phenomenon* or *vibration white-finger syndrome*) is the term for chronic disorders most specifically associated with vibration

exposure. HAVS involves peripheral neurovascular changes in response to long-term or intense vibration exposure. The vibration causes damage to the blood vessels in the affected area. The damage becomes particularly apparent during cold temperatures, when blood vessels have difficulty reopening after constricting. This chronic constriction of blood flow causes numbness and tingling in the fingers, blanching of the fingers on exposure to cold, pain following the eventual return of circulation, and reduced grip strength and finger dexterity.

These symptoms disappear initially when the hands are warmed and vibration exposure is reduced. However, finger pain, loss of sensitivity, and progressive loss of function remain potential threats if the condition is left untreated (Armstrong et al. 1987; NIOSH 1989). Timber workers in Canada are an example of workers who are at risk for permanent damage to the hands from prolonged use of chain saws and heavy, repetitive work in the cold.

Symptoms of HAVS, primary Raynaud's phenomenon, and CTS can be difficult to differentiate because of the similarities of loss of tactile sensitivity and peripheral changes in all three conditions. Although the vascular signs and symptoms of HAVS are similar to those of Raynaud's phenomenon, the distribution of HAVS is usually asymmetric, whereas primary Raynaud's phenomenon is symmetric (NIOSH 1989). The occurrence of HAVS may be affected by numerous variables, including the level of acceleration (vibrational load), frequency and duration of tool use per day and cumulatively per month and year, and the ergonomics of tool use itself (NIOSH 1989).

Research

Research has demonstrated a strong relationship between the use of vibrating tools and the occurrence of CTDs, including HAVS and Raynaud's phenomenon. NIOSH (1989) reports that in studies comparing the prevalence of HAVS in exposed workers versus a control group, the exposed workers demonstrate a 40% higher prevalence rate of the disorder in more than half of the studies examined.

Cannon et al. (1981) studied factors contributing to CTS in 30 airplane assembly workers as compared with 90 matched controls. Researchers found

CTS to be most highly correlated with the use of vibrating hand tools at 10–60 Hz.

Radwin et al. (1987) examined the relationship among tool vibration, tool weight, and grip force. In 14 subjects, these researchers investigated the effect of hand-tool vibration and tool weight on grip force and the effect of hand-tool vibration on the contraction of hand flexor muscles and extensor muscles during grip force. Results indicated that average grip increased from 25.3 N without vibration to 32.1 N at 40 Hz (27% increase) and to 27.1 N (7% increase) at 160 Hz. The TVR was found to be associated with activation of forearm muscles at specific grip forces.

Finally, Dimberg et al. (1989) studied the relationship between neck and upper-extremity symptoms and work-related factors in 2,814 industrial workers. These investigators found that neck and upper-extremity symptoms were twice as prevalent in workers who used vibrating hand tools. Researchers suggested that the use of vibrating tools may also be associated with awkward hand positions, edema from the vibration, and reduced sensation, all of which necessitate increased grip force to hold the tool. (See NIOSH 1989 for a complete summary of recent research.)

Measurement

Assessment of vibration exposure is difficult because of the differences in hand-tool vibration frequencies, varied techniques among operators, and the problems of measuring vibration duration. Radwin et al. (1987) assert that vibration exposure must include not only the vibrational load from the tool itself but also the duration of the exposure and the worker's posture assumed while operating the tool. One must distinguish further between impact and nonimpact tools and include measurements of the vibration quantities along the three orthogonal axes.

Piezoelectric accelerometers are commonly used to measure vibration associated with handheld tools (Radwin & Armstrong 1985; NIOSH 1989; Bruel & Kjaer Instruments 1993). The vibrational measurement is taken at the point of contact with the body by placing sensors on the body part. The vibration oscillations impinge on the piezoelectric accelerometer and move a small mass against a crystal element. This crystal element produces an electrical current, the voltage of which is proportional to the acceleration of vibration. An amplifier may be used to overcome signal loss problems (NIOSH 1989).

Once the vibration acceleration is determined, researchers can determine the daily exposure dose and the length of time after which a certain percentage of workers will demonstrate symptoms of HAVS. Recommendations for safe exposure limits calculate the duration of the exposure and the dose (acceleration in meters per second squared) energy equivalents as a logarithmic function. Charts that display acceleration limits as a function of frequency and exposure are found in the references provided.

NIOSH (1989) has not issued specific exposure limits but recommends strict medical monitoring to prevent the occurrence of HAVS or CTDs. NIOSH suggests that vibrational measurements should be based on a time-corrected, 4-hour equivalent to facilitate comparison of data between studies.

Recommendations to Decrease Vibration Exposures

Recommendations for decreasing vibration exposure involve engineering controls, workplace practices, protective clothing, and worker training (NIOSH 1989). The following suggestions have been gleaned from Bonney (1981), NIOSH (1989), Brown (1990), and Hampel (1992).

Engineering controls

- Keep machines well maintained. Imbalanced tools or loose fittings may increase vibration.
- Reduce tool vibrational load to the lowest level possible for efficient operation of the task.
- Provide counterbalances to reduce the forces needed to hold and manipulate the tool.

Protective equipment

- Use damping materials in floor mats, seats, and handgrips to reduce the transmission of vibration to the body. Closed-cell foam most effectively isolates vibration; silicone and elastomers are also used for damping.
- Wear gloves with damping materials incorporated into the palms and fingers.
- Wear proper clothing to maintain body temperature and prevent vasoconstriction of the fingers induced by cold temperatures.
- Ensure that gloves fit properly.

Workplace practices

- Alternate work tasks to reduce vibration exposure.
- Reduce the number of hours per day and days per week that a worker uses vibrating tools.
- Reduce grip force necessary to operate the tool.

Worker training

- Train workers about the sources of vibration exposure and means of transmission to the body.
- Train workers to recognize the early signs of HAVS, CTS, or Raynaud's phenomenon and to understand the long-term effects.
- Review use of protective clothing, tool maintenance, and proper tool use.
- Reinforce the need to warm the hands before starting a job and to keep the body warm thereafter.

Mechanical Stresses

Mechanical stresses placed on human tissue from tool edges, tool handles, or equipment can contribute to tendon and soft-tissue injuries over a prolonged period (Tichauer 1966; Armstrong 1986). During tool use, grip forces are transmitted to the soft-tissue structures underlying the tool. If a tool edge is sharp, pointed, or blunt, the forces will be concentrated and transmitted to a small surface area, thus hastening pain and tissue damage to that area.

Common conditions that result from direct pressure on tissues are tenosynovitis and trigger finger. Tools such as short-handled pliers place pressure on the thenar eminence and may compress median nerve branches. Tools with ridged handles place pressure on the finger pulley system at the metacarpophalangeal and distal phalangeal joints. This pressure may cause irritation as the finger tendons move beneath the compressed pulleys.

Finger loops on tools such as scissors or tin cutters place direct pressure on the digital nerves lateral to the fingers. Prolonged pressure may cause localized paresthesias and tenderness. Gloves with elasticized wrists and expandable wristwatch bands place direct pressure on the median nerve at the carpal tunnel. Finally, leaning one's wrists or elbows on a table edge can also cause direct pressure to superficial structures.

Recommendations for decreasing mechanical stresses on soft-tissue structures include the following:

- Use handles with round edges.
- Cover the handle with a compliant rubber coating.
- Extend tool handles through the palm of the hand to distribute forces over a large surface area.
- Use loop handle designs with spring openings and plastic coating.
- Pad surfaces when hammering or pounding.

See Chapter 8 for a complete discussion of tool use and CTDs.

Cool Temperatures

The primary problems associated with industrial work in cool temperatures are local discomfort in the hands and feet and decreased manual dexterity after several hours of exposure (Parsons 1981; Eastman Kodak Company 1983). More severe problems such as frostbite, reduced circulation, and decreased tactile sensitivity may occur after prolonged exposure to very cold temperatures (Fox 1967; Parsons 1981; Armstrong 1986).

Workers' exposures to cold temperatures commonly occur in the following working conditions: work in refrigerated or cold-storage units; construction work in poorly heated buildings; outdoor maintenance, service, or construction work in cold climates; and cleaning with cold water (Eastman Kodak Company 1983). Additionally, fingers and distal extremities may be cooled as a result of manipulating cold materials (such as meat), using tools with cold handles, working in a cool environment (such as a cool office), or being exposed to cool-air exhaust from air-powered tools.

Cool temperatures have been demonstrated to affect tactile sensitivity, manual dexterity, reaction time, and the ability to perform complex tasks (Fox 1967; Eastman Kodak Company 1983). Studies indicate a strong relationship among ambient temperature, finger numbness, and tactile discrimination (Grandjean 1988). Researchers found that after several hours of exposure to cold at 15.5°C, workers' hands began to lose flexibility and dexterity; after exposure to cold at 7°C workers lost up to 20% dexterity in manual tasks (Eastman Kodak Company 1983). Fox (1967) discusses a critical hand skin temperature (HST) above which performance is relatively unaffected and below which there is a severe decline in performance. For tactile sensitivity, the critical HST is near 8°C; for manual dexterity, the critical HST is higher, between 12 and 16°C.

Clinically, individuals report subjectively increasing their muscle tension and contracting muscles in the cold. This behavior may increase the forces involved in task performance. Investigators further note the psychological stress that cold exposure produces, which might distract individuals during task performance. Fox (1967) discusses that the effects of both temperature and wind velocity (known as *windchill*) must be taken into account when addressing the hand surface temperatures. Wind velocity may be a more important factor than air temperature in decreasing the tactile sensitivity of outside workers.

In general, hand temperatures of less than 10–15°C are usually uncomfortable, although they do not produce injury. To date, there are no standards for temperatures in work environments; however, it is recommended that temperatures be maintained above 25°C to promote workers' comfort and good performance (Armstrong 1986).

Recommendations for minimizing the effects of cold temperatures include the following (Parsons 1981; Eastman Kodak Company 1983; Armstrong 1986):

- Wear well-fitting gloves.
- Use tool handles with low thermal conductivity.
- Work in an area not directly affected by exhaust air.
- Maintain a warm core body temperature; wear sufficiently layered clothing.
- Work in an area free from local drafts.
- Use windproof gloves or clothing if wind velocity is high.
- Maintain dry gloves and clothing; change garments as needed. Moisture from sweating will reduce the effects of insulated gloves or clothing.
- Warm hands and feet on an ongoing basis; do not wait until numbness sets in.

References

American National Standards Institute (July 14, 1994). Control of work-related cumulative trauma disorders: I. Upper extremities. ANSI Z-365. Working draft.

Armstrong TJ (1986). Ergonomics and cumulative trauma disorders. *Hand Clin*, 2,553–565.

Armstrong TJ (1990). Ergonomics and cumulative trauma disorders of the hand and wrist. In JM Hunter, EJ Mackin, & AD Callahan (Eds). *Rehabilitation of the Hand: Surgery and Therapy* (3rd ed). Philadelphia: Mosby.

Armstrong TJ, Castelli WA, Evans G, & Diaz-Perez R (1984). Some histological changes in carpal tunnel contents and their biomechanical implications. *J Occup Med*, 26,197–201.

Armstrong TJ & Chaffin DB (1979). Carpal tunnel syndrome and selected personal attributes. *J Occup Med*, 21,481–486.

Armstrong TJ, Fine LJ, Raduin RG, & Silverstein BS (1987). Ergonomics and the effects of vibration in hand-intensive work. *Scand J Work Environ Health,* 13,286–289.

Armstrong TJ, Foulke JA, Joseph BS, & Goldstein SA (1982). Investigation of cumulative trauma disorders in a poultry processing plant. *Am Ind Hyg Assoc J*, 43,103–115.

Armstrong TJ & Ulin SS (1995). Analysis and design of work-related upper limb disorders. In JM Hunter, EJ Mackin, & AD Callahan (Eds). *Rehabilitation of the Hand: Surgery and Therapy* (4th ed). Philadelphia: Mosby.

Barry RM, Woodhall WR, & Mahan M (1992). Postural changes in dental hygienists: four-year longitudinal study. *J Dent Hyg*, 65,147–150.

Bonney RA (1981). Human responses to vibration: principles and methods. In EN Corlett & J Richardson (Eds). *Stress, Work Design and Productivity*. New York: Wiley.

Brown AP (1990). The effects of anti-vibration gloves on vibration-induced disorders: a case study. *J Hand Ther*, 3(2),94–100.

Bruel & Kjaer Instruments (1993). *Good Vibrations? Instrumentation for Human Vibration Measurements*. Naerum, Denmark: Bruel & Kjaer.

Buchholz B, Frederick LJ, & Armstrong TJ (1988). An investigation of human palmar skin friction and the effects of materials, pinch force, and moisture. *Ergonomics*, 31,317–325.

Bullock MI (Ed) (1990). *Ergonomics: The Physiotherapist in the Workplace*. New York: Churchill Livingstone.

Cannon LJ, Bernacki EJ, & Walter SD (1981). Personal and occupational factors associated with carpal tunnel syndrome. *J Occup Med*, 23,255–258.

Chaffin DB (1973). Localized muscle fatigue—definition and measurement. *J Occup Med,* 15,346–354.

Chaffin DB & Andersson G (1984). *Occupational Biomechanics*. New York: Wiley.

Chiang H, Ko Y, Chen C, Yu H, Wu T, & Chang P (1993). Prevalence of shoulder and upper-limb disorders among workers in the fish-processing industry. *Scand J Work Environ Health*, 19,126–131.

Ciriello VM, Snook SH, Blick AC, & Wilkinson PL (1990). The effects of task duration on psychophysically determined maximum acceptable weights and forces. *Ergonomics,* 33,187–200.

Comaish S & Bottoms E (1971). The skin and friction: deviation from Amonton's laws and the effects of hydration and lubrication. *Br J Dermatol,* 84,37–43.

Corlett EN (1981). Pain, posture and performance. In EN Corlett & J Richardson (Eds). *Stress, Work Design and Productivity.* New York: Wiley.

Corlett EN (1990). Static muscle loading and the evaluation of posture. In J Richardson & EN Corlett (Eds). *Evaluation of Human Work: A Practical Ergonomics Methodology.* London: Taylor & Francis.

Corlett EN, Madeley SJ, & Manenica I (1979). Posture targeting: a technique for recording working postures. *Ergonomics,* 22,357–366.

De Krom MC, Kester AD, Knipschild PG, & Spaans F (1990). Risk factors for carpal tunnel syndrome. *Am J Epidemiol,* 132,1102–1110.

Dimberg L, Glafsson A, Stephansson E, Aagard H, Odén A, Andersson GBJ, Hansson T, & Hagert C (1989). The correlation between work environment and the occurrence of cervicobrachial symptoms. *J Occup Med,* 31,447–453.

Dobyns JH (1991). Cumulative trauma disorders of the upper limb. *Hand Clin,* 7,587–595.

Eastman Kodak Company (1983). *Ergonomic Design for People at Work,* Vol 1. New York: Van Nostrand Reinhold.

Ekberg K, Bjorkvist B, Malm P, Bjerre-Kiely B, Karlsson M, & Axelsdon O (1994). Case-control study of risk factors for disease in the neck and shoulder area. *Occup Environ Med,* 51,262–266.

Farrell J (1992). Selectively detailed analysis of work actions and posture. *Work,* 2(3),50–63.

Fox WF (1967). Human performance in the cold. *Hum Factors,* 9(3),203–220.

Goldstein SA, Armstrong TJ, Chaffin DB, & Matthews LS (1987). Analysis of cumulative strain in tendon and tendon sheaths. *J Biomech,* 20(1),1–6.

Grandjean E (1988). *Fitting the Task to the Man* (4th ed). London: Taylor & Francis.

Hagberg M (1981). Workload and fatigue in repetitive arm elevations. *Ergonomics,* 24,543–555.

Hammer A (1934). Tenosynovitis. *Med Record,* 140,353–355.

Hampel GA (1992). Hand-arm vibration isolation materials: a range of performance evaluation. *Appl Occup Environ Hyg,* 7,441–452.

Harber P, Bloswick D, Beck J, Pena L, Baker D, & Lee J (1993). Supermarket checker motions and cumulative trauma risk. *J Occup Med,* 35,805–811.

Haselgrave CM (1991). Consequences of variability in posture adopted for handling tasks. In M Kumashiro & ED Megaw (Eds). *Towards Human Work.* London: Taylor & Francis.

Haselgrave CM (1994). What do we mean by working posture? *Ergonomics,* 37,781–799.

Herrin GD, Jaraiedi M, & Anderson CK (1986). Prediction of overexertion injuries using biomechanical and psychophysical models. *Am Indust Hyg Assoc J,* 47,322–330.

Hertzberg HTE (1955). Some contributions of applied physical anthropology to human engineering. *Ann N Y Acad Sci,* 63,616–629.

Joseph BS & Bloswick DS (1991). Ergonomic considerations and job design. In M Kasdan (Ed). *Occupational Hand and Upper Extremity Injuries and Diseases.* Philadelphia: Hanley & Belfus.

Leveau BF (1992). *Williams's and Lissner's Biomechanics of Human Motion* (3rd ed). Philadelphia: Saunders.

Luopajarvi T (1990). Ergonomic analysis of workplace and postural load. In M Bullock (Ed). *Ergonomics: The Physiotherapist in the Workplace.* New York: Churchill Livingstone.

MacDonald G, Robertson MM, & Erickson SA (1988). Carpal tunnel syndrome among California dental hygienists. *Dent Hyg,* 62,322–328.

Maeda K, Hunting W, & Grandjean E (1980). Localized fatigue in accounting-machine operators. *J Occup Med,* 22,811–816.

Margolis W & Kraus JF (1987). The prevalence of carpal tunnel syndrome symptoms in female supermarket checkers. *J Occup Med,* 29,953–956.

Milerad E & Erickson MO (1994). Effects of precision and force demands, grip diameter, and arm support during manual work: an electromyographic study. *Ergonomics,* 37,255–264.

National Institute of Occupational Safety and Health (1989). *Occupational exposure to hand-arm vibration* [DHHS pub no. 89-106]. Cincinnati: US Department of Health and Human Services.

Norkin CC, & Levangie PK (1992). *Joint Structure and Function: A Comprehensive Analysis.* Philadelphia: Davis.

Oberg T (1993). Ergonomic evaluation and construction of a reference workplace in dental hygiene. *J Dent Hyg,* 67,262–267.

Oberg T & Oberg U (1993). Musculoskeletal complaints in dental hygiene: a survey study from a Swedish county. *J Dent Hyg,* 67,257–261.

Osborn JB, Newell KJ, & Rudney JD (1990). Musculoskeletal pain among Minnesota dental hygienists. *J Dent Hyg,* 63,132–138.

Parsons K (1981). Human responses to thermal environments: principles and methods. In EN Corlett & J Richardson (Eds). *Stress, Work Design and Productivity.* New York: Wiley.

Pheasant S (1991). *Ergonomics, Work, and Health.* Gaithersburg, MD: Aspen.

Putz-Anderson V (Ed) (1988). *Cumulative Trauma Disorders: A Manual for Musculoskeletal Diseases of the Upper Limbs.* Philadelphia: Taylor & Francis.

Putz-Anderson V, Doyle GT, & Hales TR (1992). Ergonomic analysis to characterize task constraint and repetitiveness as risk factors for musculoskeletal disorders in telecommunication office work. *Scand J Work Environ Health,* 18(Suppl 2),123–126.

Radwin RG & Armstrong TJ (1985). Assessment of hand vibration exposure on an assembly line. *Am Ind Hyg Assoc J*, 46,211–219.

Radwin RG, Armstrong TJ, & Chaffin DB (1987). Power hand tool vibration effects on grip exertions. *Ergonomics,* 30,833–855.

Ramazzini B (1717). De Morbis Artificum Diatriba. In W Wright (Trans, 1940). *The Diseases of Workers.* Chicago: University of Chicago Press.

Rodgers S (1987). Recovery time needs for repetitive work. *Semin Occup Med*, 2(1),19–24.

Rodgers S (1988). Job evaluation in worker fitness determination. *Occup Med,* 3(2),219–239.

Rodgers S (July 8, 1994). Ergonomics: work, rest, leisure—an occupational therapy perspective. Presented at the American Occupational Therapy Association, Canadian American Conference, Boston.

Rohmert W (1973). Problems in determining rest allowances: I. Use of modern methods to evaluate stress and strain in static muscular work. *Appl Ergon,* 4,91–95.

Serway RA (1983). *Physics for Scientists and Engineers with Modern Physics.* Philadelphia: Sanders College Publishing.

Silverstein BA, Fine LJ, & Armstrong TJ (1987). Occupational factors and carpal tunnel syndrome. *Am J Ind Med,* 11,343–358.

Sjøgaard G, Savard G, & Juel C (1988). Muscle blood flow during isometric activity and its relations to muscle fatigue. *Eur J Appl Physiol*, 57,327–335.

Strong DR & Lennartz FH (1992). Carpal tunnel syndrome. *Cert Dent Assist Journal*, 20(4),27–39.

Tichauer E (1966). Some aspects of stress on forearm and hand in industry. *J Occup Med,* 8,63–71.

Tichauer ER (1978). *The Biomechanical Basis of Ergonomics.* New York: Wiley.

Chapter 8

Ergonomic Risk Factors

Martha J. Sanders

Successful employee health programs involve both preparing the worker for the job and providing a safe, comfortable work environment. Medical therapies, rehabilitation programs, job training, pre-employment testing, and fitness-for-duty programs fit the worker to the job: That is, these programs traditionally match or increase the capacities of a worker to meet the job demands.

The focus of ergonomics, on the other hand, is the fitting of the job to the worker. Ergonomic approaches strive to design a work environment that is efficient, safe, and comfortable for every worker. Ergonomics encompasses the design of workstations and equipment, the identification and elimination of tasks that are potentially unsafe or dangerous, the control of environmental factors, and the concern for factors within the organization that may affect the ability of the worker to perform the job (Pheasant 1991).

As the work force becomes increasingly diverse with larger numbers of older, female, and disabled workers comprising the work force, ergonomic programs are challenged to design a work environment for the so-called limited user, the individual who does *not* fall within the size or capacity norms but who *can* perform the job functions (Pheasant 1991). Thus, the need for properly sized and designed equipment is increasingly vital to work efficiency and productivity today (Morse & Hinds 1993).

This chapter is an overview of selected ergonomic factors that may contribute to cumulative trauma disorders (CTDs), including anthropometrics, workstation design, tools, lighting, and job design. The references listed at the end of the chapter are an additional source for more in-depth discussion.

Anthropometrics

Anthropometrics refers to the study of human dimensions or body size. Human dimensions include height, limb length, and limb girth, as well as physical capacities such as lifting, carrying, and grasping (Pheasant 1991). Anthropometrics is fundamental to ergonomics in that it applies workers' body dimensions to the design of jobs, workplaces, equipment, tools, and personal protective equipment. Health care practitioners should be familiar with the basics of anthropometrics to make recommendations that minimize worker fatigue and the overall risk for CTDs.

Initial steps in applying anthropometric data to ergonomic design include identifying both the user population and the criteria that "will provide a satisfactory match between the user and the product" (Pheasant 1991, p. 122). For example, if a machine shop's management team decides to buy chairs for all the shop's machinists and assembly persons, the purchaser must identify *who* will be using the chairs (two distinct groups, machinists and assembly persons) and *which criteria* will constitute a good chair for each group. Among the criteria to be considered may be comfort, support, ability to get close to the machine, and general preference. It is important to remember that the criteria will not be the same for the two user groups. Therefore, one generic chair style will rarely fit the needs of all workers.

Clearly, to achieve optimal ergonomic design, anthropometric data should be specific to the work force (Bullock 1990; Sunderland 1995). However, normed anthropometric data can be applied to an industrial population by recognizing such factors as gender, nationality, age, and occupation of the workers (Pheasant 1991).

Originally, anthropometric data were derived from a sample of military personnel in the 1950s and so represented a select population of young, presumably fit, men. Recently, data have been added from military female and older working populations. However, individuals with disabilities and persons of certain ethnic backgrounds may continue to be under-represented in anthropometric charts (Morse & Hinds 1993). Nevertheless, experts suggest that anthropometric norms can be applied to the industrial population by increasing the frequency and ranges of extreme body measurements (Eastman Kodak Company 1983).

Anthropometric charts are used in the following manner to design the optimal workstation. First, anthropometric measurements are gathered from a large sample population and are analyzed statistically to identify a range and frequency distribution of workers' sizes or capacities. Anthropometric data are then communicated in percentiles for men and women according to age. From these data, designers determine the necessary clearance, reach, and optimal location of controls for the majority of the population. For example, in Figure 8.1, for the dimension of seated functional overhead reach (see line 16, Figure 8.1), the ninety-fifth percentile indicates that 95% of the population will have a reach span of 54.8 in. or less; 5% will have a reach span of less than 43.6 in.

Ideally, the workstation should be designed to fit each worker. However, with a changing work force, manufacturers are likely to design a workstation that will accommodate most workers, including the largest man (ninety-fifth percentile) and the smallest woman (fifth percentile) for reasons of cost-effectiveness. The chosen cut-off percentiles are called *design limits* (Pheasant 1991).

Body measurements gathered for anthropometric charts include static and dynamic dimensions (Bullock 1990). *Static* or structural dimensions, similar to goniometry, are measurements of specific anatomic structures such as limb length, width, and circumference. These measurements are applied to the design and size specifications of workstations or tools. *Dynamic* or functional dimensions refer to measurements taken for daily activities such as lifting, grasping, or reaching objects that relate directly to the job. Dynamic dimensions are more difficult to document and measure because of the wide variety of individual movement patterns. These measurements are especially important for designing jobs, identifying the work flow, conducting employment screenings after a job has been offered, selecting the most appropriate tools for the job, or adapting workstations for a varied population.

Four main categories of anthropometric criteria are used in ergonomic design:

- *Clearance*, referring to headroom, legroom, elbowroom.
- *Reach*, referring to the location of controls, storage materials, and the need to reach over an object to perform a task.
- *Posture*, referring to body positions relative to the height of the work surface and controls.
- *Strength*, referring to grip strengths and muscle strength related to lifting or carrying weighted loads.

The major concern with postural criteria is avoiding static loads on the neck and shoulder musculature (Pheasant 1991).

Generally, ergonomic consultants are interested in the limited user—that is, the user whose body size or capacities are outside the design limit norms. Individuals in this category will be most sensitive to design deficiencies. To accommodate the limited user, clearances should always be designed for the largest user (ninety-fifth percentile), whereas reaches should always be designed for the smallest user (fifth percentile; Pheasant 1991).

Figures 8.1 and 8.2 provide normative data for anthropometric information related to sitting, standing, and reaching. Figure 8.3 summarizes anthropometric information relative to hand-tool and equipment design. The referenced dimensions include data from both men and women combined, for the fifth, fiftieth, and ninety-fifth percentiles.

Workstation Design

The efficient design of a workstation is critical to workers' productivity and energy level throughout

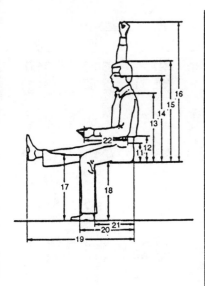

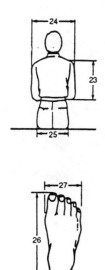

Measurement Number and Description	Percentile		
	5	50	95
11. Thigh clearance height	4.3	5.3	6.5
12. Elbow rest height	7.3	9.3	11.4
13. Mid-shoulder height	21.4	23.6	26.1
14. Eye height	27.4	29.9	32.8
15. Sitting height, normal	32.0	34.6	37.4
16. Functional overhead reach	43.6	48.7	54.8
17. Knee height	18.7	20.7	22.7
18. Popliteal height	15.1	16.6	18.4
19. Leg length	37.3	40.5	43.9
20. Upper-leg length	21.1	23.0	24.9
21. Buttocks-to-popliteal length	17.2	19.1	20.9
22. Elbow-to-fist length	12.6 (11.4)	14.5 (13.8)	16.2 (16.2)
23. Upper-arm length	12.9 (12.1)	13.8 (13.8)	15.5 (16.0)
24. Shoulder breadth	14.3	16.7	18.8
25. Hip breadth	12.8	14.5	16.3
26. Foot length	8.9	10.0	11.2
27. Foot breadth	3.2	3.7	4.2

Figure 8.1. Anthropometric data (in inches) for men and women seated. Statistics in parentheses represent an industrial population. (Reprinted with permission from SA Falkenburg & DJ Schultz [1993]. Ergonomics for the upper extremity. *Hand Clin,* 9[2],268.)

the day. The workstation design influences a worker's postures, work patterns, and sequence of actions for the job. A well-designed workstation should minimize the worker's static work patterns and provide several ergonomically correct positions that the worker may assume throughout the day (Putz-Anderson 1988).

Many workers will modify their workstations independently with makeshift arrangements such as pillows or cardboard boxes. Health care workers

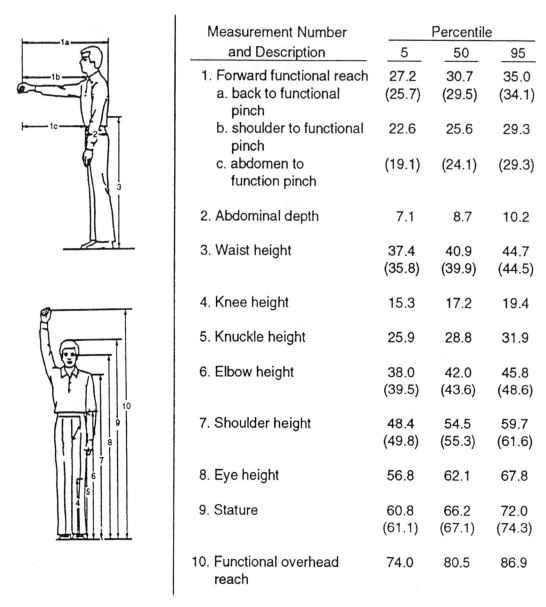

Measurement Number and Description	Percentile		
	5	50	95
1. Forward functional reach	27.2	30.7	35.0
a. back to functional pinch	(25.7)	(29.5)	(34.1)
b. shoulder to functional pinch	22.6	25.6	29.3
c. abdomen to function pinch	(19.1)	(24.1)	(29.3)
2. Abdominal depth	7.1	8.7	10.2
3. Waist height	37.4	40.9	44.7
	(35.8)	(39.9)	(44.5)
4. Knee height	15.3	17.2	19.4
5. Knuckle height	25.9	28.8	31.9
6. Elbow height	38.0	42.0	45.8
	(39.5)	(43.6)	(48.6)
7. Shoulder height	48.4	54.5	59.7
	(49.8)	(55.3)	(61.6)
8. Eye height	56.8	62.1	67.8
9. Stature	60.8	66.2	72.0
	(61.1)	(67.1)	(74.3)
10. Functional overhead reach	74.0	80.5	86.9

Figure 8.2. Anthropometric data (in inches) for men and women standing. Statistics in parentheses represent an industrial population. (Reprinted with permission from SA Falkenburg & DJ Schultz [1993]. Ergonomics for the upper extremity. *Hand Clin*, 9[2],267.)

should examine carefully each worker's modifications to gain insight into the worker's perceived discomfort and his or her solutions to the problem.

For the purposes of this discussion, a workstation includes the work surface, sitting or standing area, objects (or controls) manipulated and, in some cases, a visual display area. The following guidelines apply to all workstations: The area should be *large enough* to permit the full range of movements required for the task. The workstation should provide *proximal support* for the seated worker, a *prop* for rest for the standing worker, and *padded or rounded edges* for the work surface, and it should allow use of the extremities in a *neutral position*. The design should be *specific* to the task being performed. Finally, the equip-

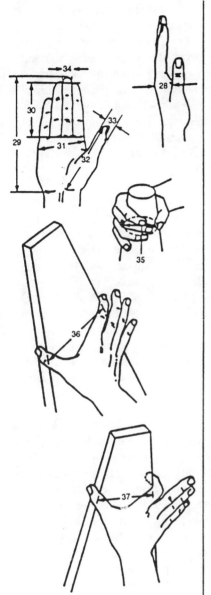

Measurement Number and Description	Percentile		
	5	50	95
28. Hand thickness, metacarpal III	1.0	1.2	1.4
29. Hand length	6.7	7.4	8.0
30. Digit two length	2.3	2.8	3.3
31. Hand breadth	2.8	3.2	3.6
32. Digit one length	3.8	4.7	5.6
33. Breadth of digit one's interphalangeal joint	0.7	0.8	1.0
34. Breadth of digit three's interphalangeal joint	0.6	0.7	0.8
35. Grip breadth, inside diameter	1.5	1.8	2.2
36. Hand spread, digit one to two, first phalangeal joint	3.0	4.3	6.1
37. Hand spread, digit one to two, second phalangeal joint	2.3	3.6	5.0

Figure 8.3. Anthropometric data (in inches) for hand dimensions. Men and women are represented equally. (Reprinted with permission from SA Falkenburg & DJ Schultz [1993]. Ergonomics for the upper extremity. *Hand Clin,* 9[2],269.)

ment must be *easily adjustable* to accommodate all workers (Grandjean 1988; Putz-Anderson 1988; Pheasant 1991).

The height of the work surface is critically important. A work surface that is too high may cause increased shoulder fatigue, whereas a work surface that is too low may cause low-back problems. The proper work height is determined by both the worker's height and the task requirements of the job. Precise work requires a higher work surface to provide proximal stabilization. Heavier work requires a lower work surface to increase the muscle forces available. These principles apply to work done while seated or standing. (See the sec-

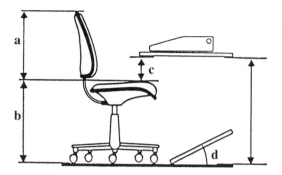

Figure 8.4. Recommended guidelines for a seated workstation. (a = backrest: 18–20 in. [48–50 cm]; b = seat height: 15–22 in. [38–54 cm]; c = leg clearance: minimum 7 in. [17 cm]; d = footrest angle: 10–25 degrees.) (Reprinted with permission from E Grandjean [1988]. *Fitting the Task to the Man* [4th ed]. London: Taylor & Francis.)

tion on standing workstations for specific measurement guidelines.)

Ideally, the workstation should combine both sitting and standing positions. In the early twentieth century, the majority of workers stood while they were working and moved about frequently on the job. Today, an estimated three-fourths of all workers are sedentary and remain seated for prolonged periods. Although sitting requires decreased physiologic effort and provides greater stability for the worker, sitting also increases spinal compression forces and the potential for static loading on the neck and shoulders (Grandjean 1988; Pheasant 1991). The following discussion highlights general guidelines for seated and standing workstations and workstation layout.

Seated Workstations

A most important aspect of a seated workstation is the chair design and fit. A good chair design can minimize long-term neck, back, and even leg problems when adjusted properly. Grandjean (1988) points out that chairs have historically been a status symbol, with the chief occupying the ceremonial stool or throne. Although an elegant chair sends a message of authority and prominence even today, the importance of chair design on everyday productivity and comfort is often overlooked. A good ergonomic chair can cost as little as $220 and as much as $1,100.

Researchers emphasize that sitting is not a static activity (Pheasant 1991). If one observes seated workers for an extended period of time, one will note that individuals shift regularly from side to side, lean forward and backward, and stretch their legs throughout the day. The dynamic nature of sitting therefore requires a chair design that offers options for adjustment. The following are guidelines for designing a seated workstation (compiled from Grandjean 1988; Pheasant 1991; Eastman Kodak Company 1983):

- *Adjustable chair height:* Chair seat height should be equal to or slightly lower than knee height to allow for adequate leg clearance and to allow the feet to be flat on the floor. For light tasks, the work surface should be slightly below the elbow (2–4 in.; Figure 8.4).
- *Seat pan:* The seat pan depth should measure from the buttocks to the knee and be wide enough to provide thigh support. A seat pan that is too deep causes the user to sit forward and lose contact with the backrest. A seat pan that is too short causes pressure under the knee or thighs. The edges should be rounded and the seat upholstered.
- *Seat angle:* A seat angle of 100–110 degrees is a good compromise between minimizing disc pressures and allowing for use of the hands. The seat angle should be adjustable forward and backward by 5 degrees and have a locking device.
- *Backrest:* A backrest should support the lumbar and midthoracic spine for the greatest postural support. For office workers who lean back, the chair should have a high backrest with a lumbar pad. For industrial workers who work upright, the chair should have at least a lumbar support, with adequate space for the buttocks between the backrest and the seat pan.
- *Footrest:* Footrests are necessary to relieve pressure on the thigh and low back, particularly if the feet are not flat on the floor. Rings on high work chairs may or may not accommodate a short person if the rings do not adjust. Inexpensive footrests can be purchased or made from wooden crates.
- *Armrest:* Armrests are recommended when the arms are held in the same position, particularly *away* from the body, for much of the task. Armrests can be part of the chair or clamped to

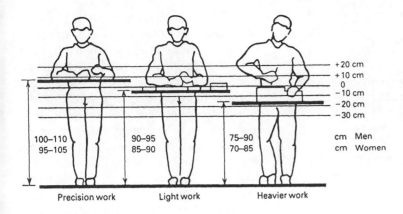

Figure 8.5. Recommended heights for standing workstations. Height varies with type of work performed. (Reprinted with permission from E Grandjean [1988]. *Fitting the Task to the Man* [4th ed]. London: Taylor & Francis.)

the front edge of the desk. Armrests should swivel and tilt as needed to relieve the static loading of the neck and shoulders and provide the proper work position. Edges should be padded and round.

- *Upholstery:* A contoured seat pan and good padding will help to distribute the pressure of the ischial tuberosities. Seat material should be porous, stain-resistant, and compressible to approximately 1–2 in. The material should reduce static electricity and avoid heat transfer.
- *Base*: The chair base should have five points or casters for the greatest stability.

Standing Workstations

Standing is very efficient and places only low-level static forces on the lower extremity. However, many workers complain of leg pain after standing for long periods. Such complaints are related to increased venous pressure on the lower extremity while standing and the lack of venous return to the heart. The result is pooling of the blood in the legs, an actual increase in leg volume, and a feeling of discomfort or heaviness in the lower extremity (Pheasant 1991).

Standing has also been associated with low-back and foot problems. Foot pain, particularly plantar fasciitis and "heel spurs," have been associated with prolonged standing on a hard surface. A hard surface such as concrete does not promote the subtle muscular contractions in the feet and legs that pump blood to the heart. Further, the foot musculature becomes stressed by constant pounding on a hard surface. In terms of low-back pain, individuals tend to

assume positions that increase the lumbar lordosis. However, there is no consensus regarding the relationship between lumbar lordosis while standing and low-back pain (Pheasant 1991).

Despite these problems, standing workstations may be the best option for jobs that require higher forces, extended reaches, or frequent movement between several workstations (Eastman Kodak Company 1983). A small prop seat, leaning area, or stool must be provided for workers who continually work while standing.

Workers and health care practitioners must also pay attention to the visual and manipulative demands of a task. Invariably, the placement of visual displays and objects that must be manipulated determines the position of the head and neck. According to Grandjean (1988), visual display monitors should be angled approximately 0–15 degrees below eye level (see Chapter 16).

Finally, health care practitioners must also recognize that standing still is not a static activity. Observations of standing workers indicate that workers sway slowly back and forth and from side to side, similar to seated workers. The body's center of gravity alternately shifts from over the ankles to slightly behind the hip joints (Pheasant 1991).

The following are guidelines for the design of standing workstations:

- *Proper work height* depends on the height of the person and the type of task performed. Unless specified, the elbow should be flexed to approximately 90 degrees, the shoulders abducted or flexed less than 20–25 degrees, and the neck slightly flexed (Figure 8.5).

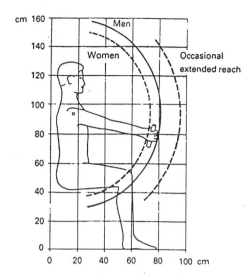

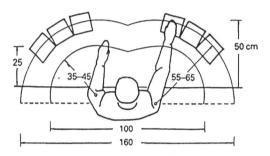

Figure 8.6. Recommended vertical (top) and horizontal (bottom) distances for reaching and grasping from a seated workstation (in centimeters). Reach distances are measured from the shoulder to hand; grasp distances are measured from the elbow to hand. Values include men and women from the fifth percentile. (Reprinted with permission from E Grandjean [1988]. *Fitting the Task to the Man* [4th ed]. London: Taylor & Francis.)

- For *precise or delicate work*, the work surface should be approximately 2–4 in. (5–10 cm) above the elbow.
- For *light assembly work,* the work surface should be approximately 2–4 in. (5–10 cm) below the elbow.
- For *heavy work,* the work surface should be approximately 4–5 in. (10–15 cm) below the elbow (Putz-Anderson 1988).
- *Work surface edges* should be rounded or padded to avoid mechanical stresses to underlying structures.

- *Hard floor surfaces* (such as concrete) should be cushioned with antifatigue mats or rubber matting to decrease the stress on the legs and low back. Specific floor mats are available for most industries.
- *Shoes* worn by the worker should have adequate instep support and a slip-resistant sole. A polyurethane or viscoelastic polymer insert will help cushion and absorb the forces from walking or standing on a hard surface.
- *Footrests* are necessary to relieve stress on the low back and to provide a change of position for the legs. Options include a foot rail, a low-inclined stool, or footrests similar to those for seated work.

Frequently Used Equipment and Controls

Work equipment or controls that are used on a regular basis should be located within comfortable reach for the worker. Putz-Anderson (1988) advocates that frequently used supplies and equipment be kept within an area that can be easily reached by a "sweep of the forearm" when the upper arm is in neutral. Although an individual's reach can be extended by standing, moving forward, leaning, or flexing the trunk, a worker will fatigue if the reach is overextended for long periods of time.

Individual reach capabilities can be envisioned as a three-dimensional semicircular shell in front of the worker (Eastman Kodak Company 1983). Figure 8.6 indicates that the reach distance in front of the body is approximately 17–18 in. depending on the person's body size and whether he or she is standing or sitting. The reach distances to the side will be slightly less than those for the front. Reach distances should be reduced by 2 in. (5 cm) for tasks that require hand grasp (Eastman Kodak Company 1983).

A reach distance for repetitive use should be nearly half the maximum distance from the shoulder to the extended fingers. The worker should not reach above shoulder height or behind the back on a frequent basis.

Workplace Layout

Well-designed workplaces are efficient because there is no wasted effort on the part of the workers.

Workers are able to establish a "flow" or natural working rhythm that follows the natural movement of extremities and a logical sequence for the task. Although most workplaces are laid out well initially, over time the job might expand and the work area might become personalized (with pictures, pen holders, flowers, etc.) such that a logical work flow is interrupted. Experience has shown that most workers will acknowledge workplace clutter but do not realize the impact clutter has on their job tasks or postures.

Overall, the most important principle for workplace layout is to decrease static loading on muscles, because such loading eventually leads to pain and muscle fatigue. Loading on the muscles of the neck and shoulder is the most obvious concern. Grandjean (1988) suggests that static effort should be reduced to not more than 15% of an individual's maximum voluntary capacity for short durations and to 8% for tasks of longer duration. Other researchers concur that even at 10% maximum voluntary capacity, the muscle will fatigue over time (Sjøgaard et al. 1988; see Chapter 6).

Static grasping and holding of equipment should also be examined and minimized whenever possible. Problems of decreased blood flow and injury to underlying tissue become problematic with prolonged tool or equipment use. (See the next section on tools for a complete discussion).

The following guidelines (compiled from Grandjean 1988; Putz-Anderson 1988; Pheasant 1991) are reminders for those health care consultants well versed in biomechanics or motion-time measurements. For consultants just entering occupational ergonomics, the guidelines provide an additional checklist of areas to consider.

- Store items used most often in the most accessible location.
- Group items that are used together in the same location and best sequence.
- Perform frequently repeated tasks within an arm's length in front of oneself and avoid reaching above shoulder height or behind the body.
- Perform manipulative work with the elbows flexed to 90 degrees and held close to the body.
- Keep motions symmetric or opposite during work tasks, to reduce static loads on the trunk.
- Minimize work performed with the trunk flexed and the extremities in awkward positions.

- Avoid maintaining the arms outstretched for long periods. This posture will cause muscle fatigue rapidly and will reduce the accuracy of fine hand and arm movements.
- Alternate between sitting and standing workstations.
- Position work at a height that is optimal for the worker's visual acuity, to prevent neck and eye strain.
- Create a natural rhythm for the work, using curvilinear rather than straight-line motions to accomplish tasks.

Tool Design

Despite automation, workers continue to use tools on a daily basis for assembly and precision tasks that require careful monitoring or expertise (Cochran & Riley 1986). Workers' use of tools has evolved from the use of varied tools throughout the day to reliance on specific tools for extended periods of time (Tichauer 1966). As the demand for precision and high productivity continues, the potential for cumulative trauma to the hand and forearm because of improper tool design and use remains high. This discussion elucidates for the health care practitioner basic issues of hand biomechanics, prehension, and tool design to define the relationship between tool use and CTDs.

Prehension Patterns

Basic to a discussion of tools is a common language or classification system for the grasps used to describe tool handling. Napier (1956) proposed a simple yet clear distinction between power and precision grasps that has been globally accepted. A *power* (or cylindrical) grasp refers to clutching an object in the palm of the hand with the thumb wrapped around the object. Figure 8.7 demonstrates that to perform a power grasp, the wrist must assume a position of ulnar deviation to align the index finger and thumb with the longitudinal axis of the forearm and tool (Napier 1956; Fraser 1989).

A *precision* grasp refers to holding an object between the thumb and opposing fingers. This grasp allows for sensory input to the fingers and active manipulation of objects. To perform a precision grasp,

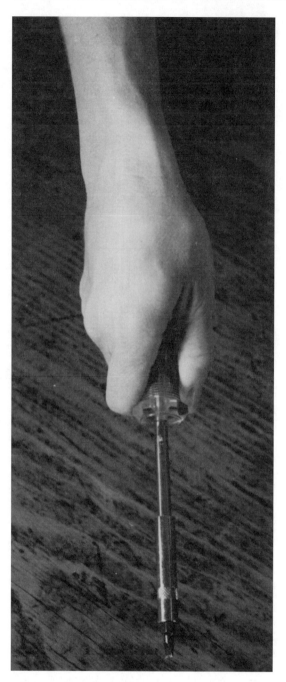

Figure 8.7. A power grasp. The object is held firmly in the palm of the hand. The wrist is deviated ulnarly in order to align the hand with the longitudinal axis of the tool.

named a *three-jaw chuck* or *tripod*; see Figure 8.8), *pincer* (Figure 8.10), and *spherical grasps* (Figure 8.11). A hook grasp does not include the thumb. The lateral pinch grasp is the strongest of all precision grasps. When a precision grasp is needed, a modified palmar grasp is used 75% of the time.

Although this classification distinguishes between grasps, the power and precision grasps are rarely used independently of each other. In a combined grasp such as knitting, the ulnar fingers secure the object (in this case, needles) in the palm while the thumb and index fingers are free to manipulate (Napier 1956; Figure 8.12). While performing a given task, the operator may combine or switch grasps on a tool, depending on the purpose. For example, when using a screwdriver to hang a picture, an individual may initiate the project with a precision grasp to set the screw but will most likely switch to a power grasp to embed the screw in the surface. Similarly, when opening a bottle, one will use both power and precision grasps.

Principles for Hand and Tool Use

The relationship between the type of grasp, the position of the hand, and hand anatomy is integral to proper tool use. The following biomechanical principles (compiled from Tichauer 1966; Rodgers 1987; Spaulding 1989; Hunter et al. 1990; and Jenkins 1991) for hand and tool use will assist managers, health care consultants, and workers in understanding the implications for using and choosing tools.

Biomechanical considerations

- A power grasp is four times stronger than a precision grasp. Use a power grip whenever possible.
- Maximal grip strength is generated at 0–15 degrees of wrist extension.
- Wrist deviation reduces the grip force available. At 45 degrees of wrist extension, grip strength is 75% of maximal; at 45 degrees of flexion, grip strength is reduced to 60% of maximal. With the wrist deviated, workers must generate significantly more force to accomplish the task.
- Intrinsic muscles provide optimum stability for grasping at midrange between full finger flexion and extension.

the wrist is positioned in slight extension, and the thumb and fingers are partially flexed and opposed around the object (Figure 8.8). Types of precision grasps include *lateral* (Figure 8.9), *palmar* (also

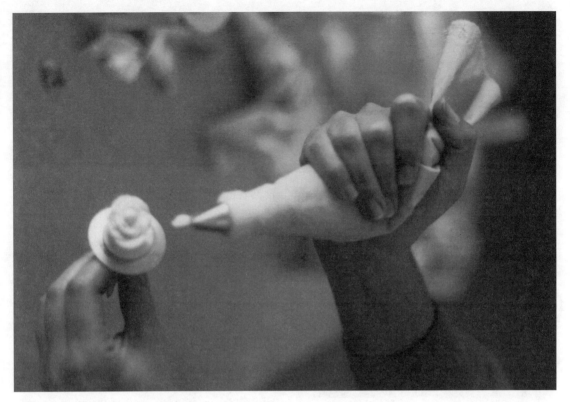

Figure 8.8. Power and precision grasps. The palmar pinch (left) is a type of prehension grasp in which the thumb opposes an object with both the index and middle finger.

Neurovascular considerations

- The median nerve is superficial in the palm of the hand and at the base of the thumb.
- The radial digital nerves and arteries run lateral to each finger and are unprotected by fat pads.
- The ulnar nerve passes between the medial epicondyle and the olecranon at the elbow and just deep to the pisiform bone at the ulnar border of the wrist.

Musculoskeletal considerations

- Elbow extension should be combined with pronation, and elbow flexion should be combined with supination, for synergistic action of arm musculature.
- All hand grasping requires isometric contractions of the wrist extensor muscles to position the wrist. Repetitive grasping causes microtears in the wrist extensors. Stronger grasping requires stronger muscle contractions.

- Grasping combined with wrist deviation places added stress on wrist musculature and the median nerve.
- Lateral pinch combined with wrist deviation stresses the abductor pollicis longus and extensor pollicis brevis tendons.
- Digital creases are not protected by fat pads. Consequently, the finger pulley systems underlying digital creases are prone to direct or repetitive trauma.

Tool Design

Today, industry consultants and managers must consider not only the most appropriate tool for the specific job but also the range of tool sizes necessary for a diverse work force. Most obviously, tools that are balanced and sized for men with larger muscle mass will demand more force from female

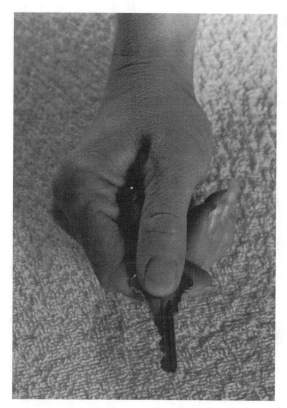

Figure 8.9. A lateral pinch. The thumb is adducted against the ulnar border of the index finger. The lateral pinch is the strongest of all pinches.

users with smaller hand mass. Conversely, the operation of precision tools that are balanced and designed for a smaller hand (such as dental hygiene instruments) will cause excessive strain for men with larger hand mass.

As Meagher (1987) explained, "One size does *not* fit all." Tools must be sized to fit the worker, and consideration must be given to the normal biomechanics of the hand. Further, workers should "try out" the tools before committing to their long-term use. Meagher (1987) argues that the most important elements of tool design with regard to human usage are handle size, shape, and texture, ease of operation, shock absorption, and weight.

Handle Size

The handle size refers to either the diameter of the tool handle, for cylindrical tools (such as a hammer or pneumatic tools), or the span between handles,

for crimping tools or tools with two handles (such as pliers, scissors, or clippers). The correct tool handle size allows the worker to generate optimal strength for the job without straining the flexor tendons or intrinsic muscles.

Cylindrical Tools. To generate the maximum grip strength, the flexor digitorum superficialis and flexor digitorum profundus provide flexion forces while the intrinsic muscles stabilize the tool in the hand. When a power grasp is used on a tool with a cylindrical handle, the proximal and distal interphalangeal joints should be in midflexion; the distal joint of the middle and ring fingers should overlap the distal joint of the thumb. The optimal diameter for a cylindrical tool is 1.5 in. (4 cm) with ranges from 1.25 to 2.00 in. (3–5 cm), depending on the individual's hand size (Figure 8.13; Eastman Kodak Company 1983; Cochran & Riley 1986; Meagher 1987). Gripping can be enhanced with finger stops or a thumb stall to reduce slippage (Robinson & Lyon 1994).

Two-Handled Tools. The span between handles for crimping tools or double-handled tools should be 2.5–3.5 in. (6.5–9.0 cm) at the application of force (Eastman Kodak Company 1983). The maximal flexor force should be leveraged at the proximal interphalangeal joint to use the stronger flexor digitorum superficialis tendons for flexion. Crimping tools should have a spring opening so as not to injure the dorsal structures of the hand against the handle when opening the jaws of the tool. The spring should open the handles no more 3.5–4.5 in. (9.0–11.5 cm) to prevent stretching the thumb collateral ligaments (Figure 8.14.)

Precision Tools. Most precision tools require some type of a modified palmar or tripod grasp. To allow better control and manipulation, precision tools should have a small diameter and a smooth front end. The optimum diameter for precision tools is 0.45 in. (12 mm), the acceptable range being from 0.3 to 0.6 in. (8–16 mm; Figure 8.15; Eastman Kodak Company 1983; Robinson & Lyon 1994).

Inappropriately Sized Tools. If a tool's handle diameter is not appropriately sized, the hand muscles and ligaments become strained and easily fatigued when using the tool. For example, if the tool diameter or span between handles is too large,

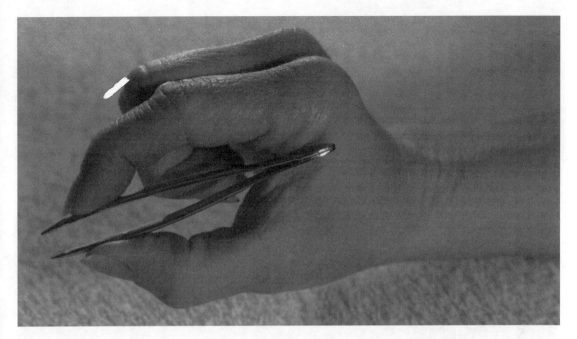

Figure 8.10. A pincer grasp. Opposition is performed using the tip of the thumb and index fingers.

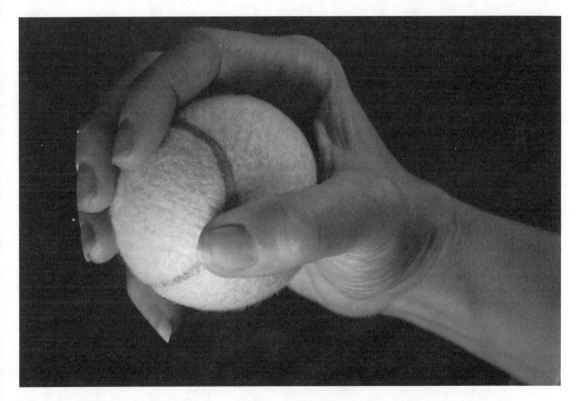

Figure 8.11. A spherical grasp. The object is held in the palm, and fingers are abducted securely around the object.

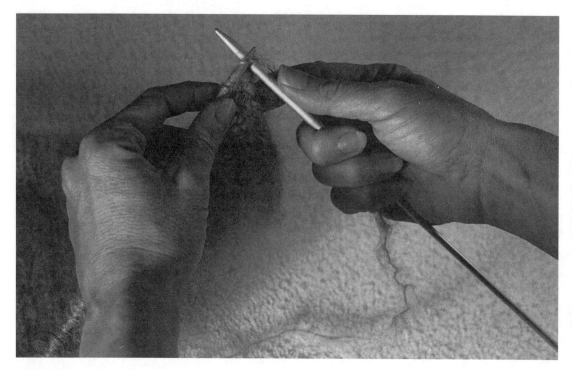

Figure 8.12. Both power and precision grasps are used simultaneously in many activities. Knitting requires use of a pincer grasp to manipulate the yarn and a power grasp to hold the needle in the palm of the hand.

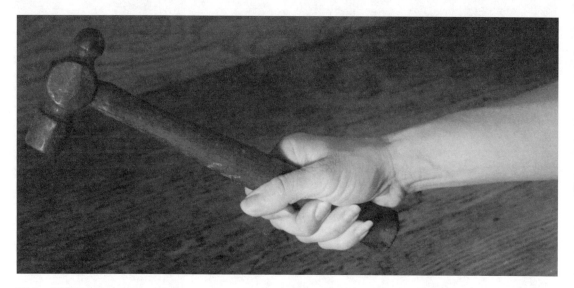

Figure 8.13. Handle size for a cylindrical tool. Both distal interphalangeal and proximal interphalangeal joints should be in midflexion.

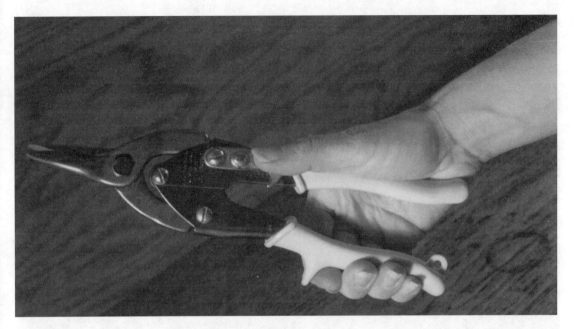

Figure 8.14. Handle size for a two-handled tool. Proximal interphalangeal joints should be in midflexion at the application of force.

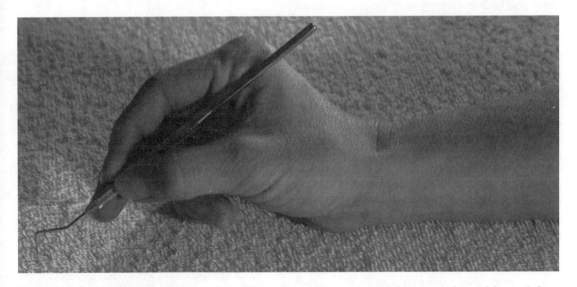

Figure 8.15. Handle size for precision tools. A modified palmar or tripod grasp is used commonly for precision work. Precision tools have a small diameter and smooth tip for accurate work.

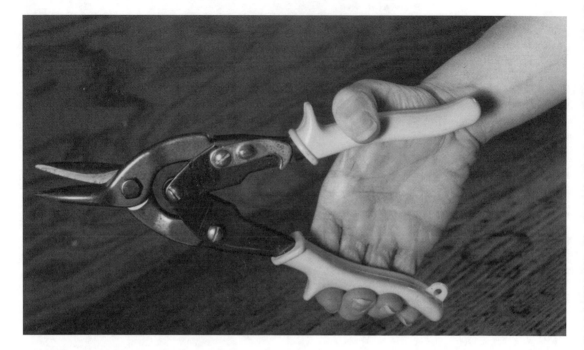

Figure 8.16. Overly wide handle openings. Excessive stress is placed on the collateral ligaments of the thumb carpometacarpal and metacarpophalangeal joints when handle openings are too wide. Force is applied at the distal interphalangeal joint rather than at the proximal interphalangeal joint.

the force is applied at the distal phalanx. The weaker flexor muscle, the flexor digitorum profundus, becomes the primary flexor. When force is applied at the distal phalanx, the tendon force is two to three times greater than when forces are applied at the middle phalanx. Handle openings on crimping tools that are too wide also place excess stress on the collateral ligaments of the thumb carpometacarpal and metacarpophalangeal joints (Figure 8.16).

If the handle is too small, the finger flexors and intrinsics must generate more force because the muscles are already contracted maximally and thus are at a mechanical disadvantage. The intrinsics must generate added force to maintain the position (Johnson 1990).

Handle Contour

The shape or contour of a tool's handle should follow the transverse arch of the hand to use the stronger ulnar musculature and to permit an even application of force between all fingers. The handle should rest on the thenar and hypothenar eminences

to prohibit compression of the neurovascular bundles between the fingers (Meagher 1987). Most tool handles are cylindrical in shape, although a slightly curved or cone shape better facilitates gripping by following the transverse arch (Fraser 1989).

Optimal Shape. Studies regarding the relationship between handle shape and muscle force suggest that the optimal shape for a tool relates to the direction of the forces exerted. Studies by Cochran and Riley (1986) suggest the following:

- Triangular or rectangular handles are superior for forward push-pull forces or for using the wrist in extremes of wrist flexion or extension.
- Circular or rectangular handles or handles that are circular with two flat sides should be used for sideways or orthogonal forces such as are used for slicing meat.
- Circular or square handles are best for use in tasks that demand lower forces for longer periods of time.

The shape and size of tools are very much related and should be evaluated by the individual worker.

Digital Separators.   Digital separators or finger recesses present both biomechanical and neurovascular problems. Separators force the fingers into abduction, which strains the intrinsics and flattens the hypothenar eminence. Further, the separators may apply pressure to neurovascular bundles (the digital arteries and nerves) lateral to each finger. Although the separators were originally designed to promote handle control, the separators actually limit a worker's options for moving or adjusting the tool in his or her hand (Tichauer 1966; Eastman Kodak Company 1983).

Finger Rings.   Finger rings pose the same problem as do digital separators in terms of compressing the neurovascular bundles lateral to each finger. The finger loops (as in scissors or tin snips) place pressure on a small surface area and can injure dorsal or volar structures below the loops. Loop-design scissors allow for a more even distribution of pressure in the hand (Figure 8.17).

Handle Orientation

A tool handle that is not well oriented to the body causes the worker to assume awkward postures during work tasks and to use more force to accomplish the task. Workers often compensate for wrist deviation by elevating the elbows and abducting the shoulders, thus transferring stresses to another area of the body. Many tools, such as hammers or pliers, necessitate positioning the hand in ulnar deviation to accomplish a task (Robinson & Lyon 1994).

Tichauer (1978) found a high incidence of tenosynovitis among workers performing wiring operations at an electronics manufacturing plant. When the traditional straight-handled pliers were replaced with bent-handle designs, the incidence of tenosynovitis decreased from 60 to 10% for those using the bent-handle design. The adage, "Bend the tool, not the hand," signifies that a neutral wrist position is optimal for tool use. Handle curves are recommended for tools that require the hand to be positioned in ulnar deviation during use, such as hammers, pliers, and saws. For most tools, at least a 20-degree curve positions the hand in neutral and, thus, decreases ulnar deviation (Tichauer 1966; Schoenmarklin & Marras 1989). Novice workers seem to derive more benefit from handle curves than do experienced workers. Today, tools such as hammers, pliers, scissors, and knives with curved handles can be purchased.

Curved handles are most effective when all work is performed on the same plane. However, the proper handle orientation also depends on the work surface being used. In-line cylindrical tools can be used for drill work being performed on a horizontal surface, such as a workbench, whereas a pistol grip is effective for work performed on a vertical surface. Figure 8.18 demonstrates the improved position for the wrist when using a pistol grip on a knife. For pistol grips, the angle of the handle in relation to the longitudinal axis should be 70–80 degrees (Robinson & Lyon 1994). Tools such as paint rollers, paintbrushes, hoes, and garden equipment can be adapted with pistol grips (Johnson 1990).

Handle Length

Sufficient length of a tool is necessary to distribute the pressure of forces evenly across the hand and to prevent direct pressure on the median nerve in the palm of the hand or at the base of the thumb. A tool handle should be long enough to extend proximal to the thenar eminence and permit adequate freedom of movement on the handle (Putz-Anderson 1988). A short tool handle (Figure 8.19A) may injure not only the superficial median or ulnar nerves but also the tendon sheaths, causing trigger finger and digital neuritis. Figure 8.19B shows a more even distribution of forces on the thenar eminence structures.

Anthropometric data suggest that the range of palm width is 2.8–3.6 in. (Eastman Kodak Company 1983). The minimum tool length recommended for most tasks is 4 in. (10 cm), although a length of 5 in. (13 cm) is preferred. When gloves are to be worn during tool use, an additional 0.5 in. (13 mm) should be added to the tool's length (Putz-Anderson 1988).

Handle Texture and Materials

The texture of the tool handle directly affects the transfer of force from the worker to the tool. A tool handle must allow for insulation against heat and for shock absorption, and it must provide some friction for ease of grasping the handle. Wood has traditionally offered such advantages, but wood has low resistance in that it eventually cracks or separates from the metal component. New polystyrene and stain-resistant plastics have

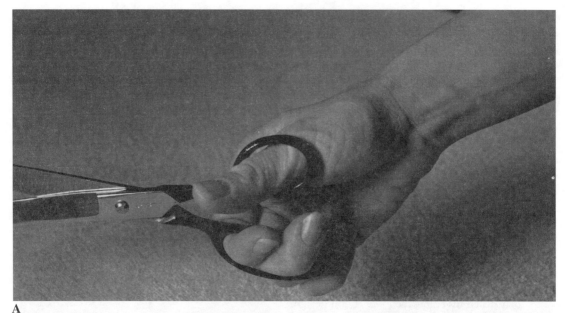

A

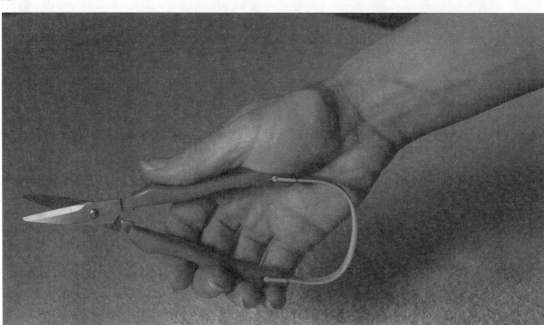

B

Figure 8.17. Handle contour. **A.** Finger loops on scissors may compress the digital neurovascular bundles lateral to the thumb and index fingers. **B.** Loop-design scissors distribute pressure evenly across the thenar eminence and fingers.

replaced wood. However, these materials should be covered with rubber, leather, or synthetic layers of material for comfort and ease of grasping the tool (Fraser 1989). A tool handle with a lightly compressible surface or a thin rubber coating pro-

vides good proprioceptive feedback, friction, and moisture for gripping.

Slipperiness.   The *coefficient of friction* refers to the slipperiness of an object and has been calculated

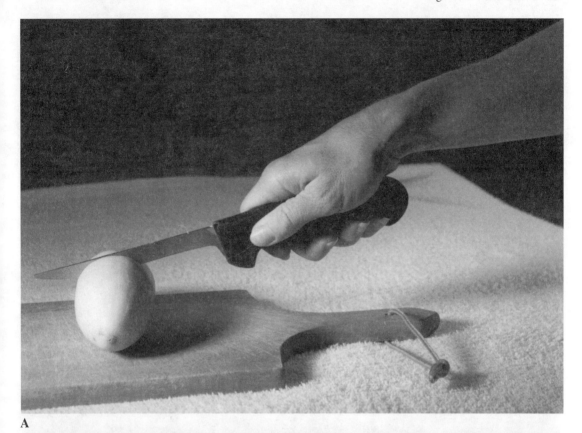

A

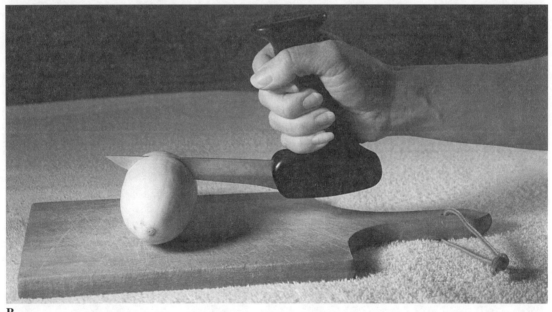

B

Figure 8.18. Handle orientation. **A.** A straight-handle design causes the wrist to deviate ulnarly once force is applied. **B.** A pistol-grip design promotes a neutral wrist position and use of arm musculature to accomplish the task.

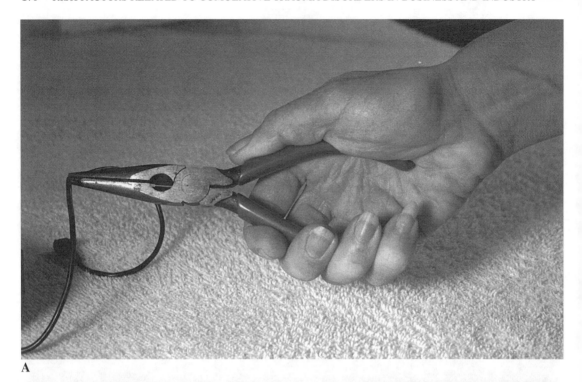

A

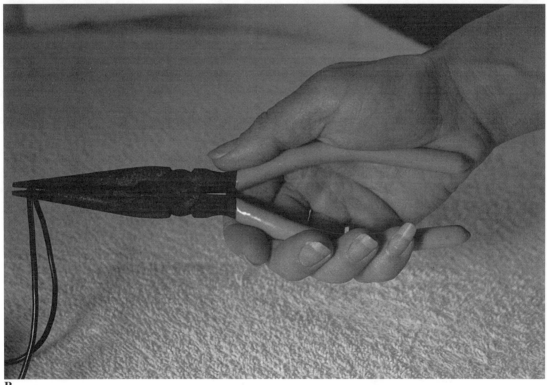

B

Figure 8.19. Handle length. **A.** A short handle may injure superficial structures in the thenar eminence, such as the median nerve. **B.** Handles should extend proximally through the thenar eminence to distribute the pressure.

for many surfaces (see Chapter 7). A tool handle that is too slippery or too dry will require extra force to maintain the tool in the hand. Poultry workers develop CTDs in part because of the excessive force needed to grasp and cut slippery poultry carcasses.

Generally, a higher coefficient of friction will improve the ability to grip and thus lower the grip force requirements. Tool handles should have the ability to maintain frictional forces when moist, as many workers develop sweaty palms during the day. Buchholz et al. (1988) studied the effects of material type and moisture on pinch forces. Buchholz's group identified that porous materials such as cloth-based tapes and suede had a higher coefficient of friction when wet and would therefore be good choices for tool handles in environments with much moisture. Rubber coating is a good all-around choice for wet or dry environments. Clearly, materials with a very high coefficient of friction, such as sandpaper, may cause abrasion and should be avoided.

Surface Pattern.   Tool surfaces should not be perfectly smooth because the tool will rotate or slip in the hand during use. However, tools handles that are too coarse or knurled can lead to discomfort or skin irritation and therefore decrease work efficiency (Fraser 1989). Handles should not have deep fluted edges or ridges that may injure underlying hand structures.

Fraser (1989) suggests a dull roughening or distinctive surface pattern to provide sensory input and to assist the user in maintaining grip. Greenberg and Chaffin (1977) suggest that patterns in the tool handle should be perpendicular to the force exerted to avoid slippage and improve surface friction. For push-pull loads, circumferential ripples are advantageous; for twisting or rotational forces (screwdrivers), longitudinal grooves are preferable. A study of instrumentation among dental hygienists revealed a preference for waffle-iron serrations on dental instruments; these were claimed to provide adequate friction without irritating the fingers (Atwood & Michalak 1992).

Shock Absorption.   Chronic exposure to power tools or handheld tools with low-frequency vibrating components may thicken vascular tissues and constrict blood flow or injure the digital arteries of the fingers and hand, causing such conditions as vibration white-finger syndrome, hand-arm vibra-

tion syndrome, Raynaud's disease, or carpal tunnel syndrome. Repetitive impact from a hammer also can cause blood vessel spasms, clots, or hypothenar hammer syndrome (National Institute of Occupational Safety and Health [NIOSH] 1989).

Recent research suggests that use of vibrating tools stimulates the tonic vibration reflex in hand and forearm muscles, which stimulates additional muscle contractions during tool use. Researchers also speculate that vibration decreases the worker's tactile sensitivity. Therefore, the worker must grip harder because of the lack of proprioceptive feedback (Armstrong et al. 1987; Radwin et al. 1987). Finally, heavy tools that vibrate may cause the worker to grip the tool more tightly and, consequently, the vibration will resonate to the elbow and shoulder (see Chapter 7).

To decrease the effects of vibration, tool handles should be padded, vibration components dampened, and exposure monitored. Padded gloves may protect hands by absorbing vibration energy, provided the gloves fit properly (Brown 1990). Most tool companies offer kits to decrease vibration effects and specially dampened, custom-made tools. Certain vibration-dampening materials are more effective at certain frequencies. For example, closed-cell foam materials may provide better vibration-dampening qualities above 160 Hz (Hampel 1992; Robinson & Lyon 1994). Hickory wood is recommended as a good material for absorbing shock. Although parameters for vibration do not yet exist, the American National Standards Institute recommends that individuals operate tools for no more than 30 minutes at a time and, cumulatively, for only 4 hours per day (NIOSH 1989).

Tool Weight and Balance

In general, tools should weigh as little as possible. Particularly for precision tasks, a lighter tool will require less force to support than will a heavy tool. In some cases, such as power tools, reducing the weight of a tool will require that more force be exerted to operate the tool, and this will increase shoulder tension. The decision regarding whether to increase or decrease the weight of a tool will depend on how that tool is used.

Guidelines suggest that tools weigh no more than 5 lbs (2.3 kg) if the tool must be supported by the hand and arm or if the tool is being operated away from the body. Tools used in precision work should weigh no more than 1 lb (0.4 kg). Tools that are heavier should be counterbalanced with an overhead sling that is positioned perpendicular to the task. Tools should be well balanced to reduce hand fatigue. The center of gravity of the tool should be located close to the hand grip (Eastman Kodak Company 1983; Armstrong 1990; Robinson & Lyon 1994).

Tool Position

Operating a tool requires a combined effort of supporting and controlling the tool. Often, the body is forced into awkward positions during one of these two acts because of the position of the task or the tool. As stated, the body should be in neutral for the best biomechanical advantage. Shoulders should be positioned at less than 25–30 degrees of abduction, and the wrist should be in neutral. Through use of a vice, the worker can maintain neutral wrist and arm positions and leverage body weight. An assortment of vices, jigs, tilted surfaces, and overhead pulley systems and fixtures can aid the worker in improving the tool position and minimizing the weight needed to support the tool or task itself (Armstrong 1990).

Tool Operation and Activation

A variety of trigger options are available for tool operation. Trigger designs should allow several fingers to activate the trigger and allow both joints of the fingers to depress the mechanism. The proximal joint should activate the trigger initially, thereby using the flexor digitorum superficialis for most of the work.

Many trigger designs require single-finger activation or activation by the distal interphalangeal joint only. With such designs, the potential exists for tenosynovitis or a nodule to develop on the flexor tendon from its repetitive and forceful use (Johnson 1990). In contrast, a strip trigger is approximately 2 in. long and allows two or three fingers to activate the trigger (Robinson & Lyon 1994).

Robinson and Lyon (1994) suggest that trigger forces be determined on the basis of the tool's application. Tools used for high-precision operations or those operated over an extended period of time should require light trigger-force activation, whereas tools used for heavier tasks, such as power tools, may require higher trigger forces.

Work Hours: Shiftwork, Overtime, and Work Breaks

Shiftwork

Continuous production in the industrial arena has made shiftwork (working in the evenings or at night) a reality for nearly 22% of America's work force (Mellor 1986). Shiftwork has become increasingly common in industries requiring around-the-clock attention such as manufacturing, food service, health care, and maintenance. While companies argue that shiftwork is necessary for timely delivery of products and services, many companies fail to consider the effects of shiftwork on workers' quality of life and work.

Shiftwork has the potential to affect many aspects of a worker's life, from health to social relationships. In fact, 20–30% of all shift workers are forced to leave shiftwork within the first 2–3 years because of medical problems (Scott & Ladou 1990).

The effects of shiftwork on individuals result from a disturbance of a worker's own circadian rhythms and a mismatch between the normal activity of shift workers and that of society. The term *shiftwork tolerance* was recently introduced to describe the relationship between circadian rhythms and subjective health effects of shiftwork, such as sleep-wake disturbances, digestion, irritability, and sleepiness (Harma 1993).

The impact of shiftwork on circadian rhythms is as follows. All individuals possess an inherent biological clock called *circadian rhythms*. These rhythms affect bodily functions, work readiness, and an individual's level of general alertness over a 24-hour period. During the day, a person is in the ergotropic (performance) phase, in which body temperature, heart rate, and mental and physical capacities are peaked; at night, a person is in the trophotropic (recuperation) phase, when bodily functions slow down. Within these cycles, circadian rhythms predispose individuals to be tired in the early morning (2:00–7:00 AM) and midafternoon (2:00–5:00 PM). Light-dark cycles are believed to be the major synchronizers of our circadian rhythms. Darkness stimulates the secretion of the hormone melatonin, which stimulates the onset of sleepiness (Colligan & Tepas 1986; Grandjean 1988; Pheasant 1991). When individuals disrupt this rhythm by working at night, health and social relationships are affected.

The most obvious effect of shiftwork on individuals is the interruption of the quantity and quality of sleep. Individuals who work at night and sleep during the day generally do not get adequate deep, restorative sleep, because of daytime noise and general restlessness. Researchers state that, on average, shift workers get 6 hours of sleep per night; informal reports reveal that many workers receive only 3–4 hours of sleep nightly (Smith et al. 1982; Colligan & Tepas 1986; Grandjean 1988).

Although the long-term effects of chronic sleep loss are not well documented, most researchers agree that the immune system of a shift worker is compromised by a long-term sleep deficit. Grandjean (1988) estimates that approximately two-thirds of all shift workers suffer from some type of health problem related to shiftwork because these employees are working out of synch with their natural body cycles.

General Health

Studies suggest that shift workers are at an increased risk for developing sleep-wake disturbances and gastrointestinal and cardiovascular disorders because of a chronic disruption in circadian rhythms (Moore-Ede & Richardson 1985; Scott & Ladou 1990). Gastrointestinal problems are common because of poor eating habits and disrupted digestive cycles; sleep-wake disturbances are typical because of chronic fatigue and the tendency for some workers to use stimulants or sleeping tablets (Grandjean 1988).

Colligan and Tepas (1986) suggest that shiftwork may exacerbate certain health problems and interfere with the efficacy of prescribed medication. Shift workers who take medication at the wrong times during their circadian rhythms may not receive the proper effects of that medication, as the dose-response characteristics of medication cycles are based on a normal daily activity cycle.

Further, workers with chronic musculoskeletal problems such as low-back or neck pain report increased symptoms when they switch to night work, possibly as a result of the overall stress night work places on the body. Many shift workers report problems with maintaining or losing weight, attributing this to difficulty establishing a regular exercise routine and eating properly.

Physical Performance

Most individuals accustomed to working during the day find it difficult to switch shifts and maintain the same quality of work. The effects of shiftwork have been studied on various occupational groups including truck drivers (Hamelin 1987), food-processing workers (Smith et al. 1982), nurses (Minors & Waterhouse 1985), and computer-monitoring operators (Rosa et al. 1989).

Overall, shift workers have been shown to have a higher number of accidents, slower reaction times, and less proficient hand-eye coordination, math calculations, and visual search skills as compared to day workers (Smith et al. 1982; Grandjean 1988; Monk 1989; Rosa et al. 1989). In a study of shift workers who had recently switched to a night and rotating schedule, workers' alertness and performance skills decreased 10% over a 7-month period (Rosa et al. 1989).

Although night workers try to mentally override their body's tendency toward sleep, individuals become vulnerable to accidents or to "falling asleep at the wheel" at low times during their circadian rhythms (Pheasant 1991). Pilots, security guards, and drivers have all reported difficulty staying awake on the job. In a series of confidential interviews reported by Moore-Ede and Richardson (1985), one-third to two-thirds of all shift workers in an industrial plant indicated that they fell asleep at least once per week while on the job.

Decreased alertness would seem to have serious implications for individuals performing continuous monitoring jobs. However, Rosa et al. (1989, p. 31) caution, "It is difficult to speculate on the magnitude of risk associated with the decrements in alertness, or the partial sleep deprivation we have observed." In other words, we cannot translate a certain percentage decrease in performance skills to an estimate of risk for health and safety issues.

Social Adjustment

Our society is based on a 5-day work week and assumes a work-during-the-day-and-sleep-at-night schedule. Workers who rotate shifts often become frustrated and exhausted in trying to coordinate work, family, and social life. Researchers report that shift workers feel dissatisfied with the amount of time spent with family and friends (Tepas & Monk

1987; Sanders 1996). In a survey of 1,490 hourly workers, Tepas and Monk (1987) found a 50% increase in divorces and separations for those on the night shift as compared to those on the day shift. Shift workers report being chronically tired and apathetic about extracurricular activities.

Monk (1989) proposes that successful adjustment to shiftwork depends on a balance between the following three factors: circadian rhythms, sleep, and social and domestic life. Clearly, if workers are not receiving enough sleep, they are prone to absenteeism, irritability, and a poor attitude; if workers are preoccupied with domestic problems, they may be less productive and effective at work.

Monk (1989) associates difficulties in coping with shiftwork with marital problems, working a second job, and excessive responsibilities at home. Female shift workers are particularly susceptible to overwork and fatigue if they do not share child rearing and household responsibilities. Interestingly, up to 33% of all shift workers hold second jobs, which further compromises sleep and social relationships.

Although one would surmise that all shift workers would be dissatisfied with night work, studies on the satisfaction of shift workers yield varying results. Shift workers consistently report fatigue as a major problem. However, a minority of shift workers actually prefer shiftwork, citing as positive factors the slower pace and lack of "hassles" or management supervision at night. Shiftwork provides some individuals with an opportunity to care for children and to participate in hobbies or additional jobs during the day (Colligan & Tepas 1986).

Adaptation to Shiftwork

Workers' abilities to adapt to shiftwork are not as well understood as is the effect of shiftwork on individuals. Studies suggest that it takes individuals anywhere from 1 week to 1 month to adapt to a new sleep and work schedule by reversing circadian rhythms. In most cases, a shift worker's circadian rhythms are never reversed totally if the night worker returns to a normal nightly sleep routine on weekends (Smith et al. 1982; Monk 1989). Current adaptive strategies for night shift are summarized here.

Zeitbergers. Shift workers on a fixed night shift may try to orient their circadian rhythms to night work by using a different set of cues, called *zeit-*

bergers to help set their biological clocks. Examples of *zeitbergers* for night workers may include social interaction at night to increase alertness and a routine of warm milk and a shower in the morning to induce sleep.

Daylight Exposure. Monk (1989) recommends that night-shift workers avoid early-morning commitments after work and wear sunglasses on the way home from work. Those who are least exposed to sunlight before bedtime tend to fall asleep more quickly than those with exposure to daylight and a busy schedule after work.

Light Therapy. Light therapy is being investigated as a means of resetting biological clocks. Most offices use fluorescent lights illuminated at 500 lux. For night-shift workers, this intensity does not simulate natural sunlight (50,000 lux), causing workers to fatigue until approximately 5:00 AM. To determine the relationship between light exposure and individuals' alerting mechanisms, investigators exposed shift workers to bright, full-spectrum light at night during work and maintained darkness during the day. Workers demonstrated increased levels of alertness and cognitive function during work hours and slept an average of 2 hours longer during the day (Czeisler et al. 1990). In the future, bright light may play a role in helping night-shift workers adjust to working at night.

Rotating Shifts. The most difficult schedule for worker adaptation is a rapidly rotating shift from night to day to evening. Workers rarely adjust to a certain shift and are therefore counseled to maintain a body schedule that simulates work during the day and sleep at night. Monk (1989) suggests that rotating shift workers should eat according to a day schedule and seek out light whenever possible.

Personality Types. Research suggests that individuals who adapt better to shiftwork are younger, flexible sleepers, more introverted, and "owl-like"—that is, individuals who enjoy late evening hours. Older workers experience the most difficulty adapting to rotating schedules and night work (Colligan & Tepas 1986).

The literature recommends that, in addition to avoiding early-morning commitments after work and wearing sunglasses on the way home, night-shift workers eat three meals daily, including a "lunch" halfway through the work night (Monk 1989). However, a recent study by Sanders (1996) found that the majority of shift workers needed to devise their own personal strategies and routines to adapt effectively. For example, most shift workers cautioned against trying to sleep immediately after work. Workers usually performed simple chores, watched television, snacked, or exercised as calm-down time after work. Workers explained that a good social life depended on communicating with family members, delegating chores, planning weekend activities, and coordinating schedules (Sanders 1996).

Guidelines for Adapting to Shiftwork.   Health care practitioners can alert companies to the signs and symptoms of chronic fatigue in their workers in an effort to prevent the health and social problems associated with shiftwork. Symptoms of chronic fatigue include weariness even after sleep, depressive moods, and general loss of enthusiasm and motivation to work. Objective signs include loss of appetite, sleep disturbances, ulcers, and digestive problems (Grandjean 1988).

Health care practitioners can offer the following suggestions for shift workers' physical and social adaptation to rotating work hours (compiled from Colligan & Tepas 1986; Monk 1989; Sanders 1996).

Getting to sleep

- Establish a ritual before sleeping, such as relaxation, bathing, stretching, or reading
- Darken and quiet the sleep environment, perhaps using white noise (such as a fan), soundproof curtains, and thick carpets
- Silence doorbells, telephones, and appliances
- Calm down after work
- Exercise regularly
- Sleep and rise at the same time every day
- Try to sleep for one long period of time; use napping as a sleep supplement if needed

Eating healthfully

- Avoid caffeine at night (within 5 hours of sleep)
- Eat low-fat, high-fiber meals
- Eat small meals and frequent healthy snacks
- Bring your own food to work
- Eat at the same time every day

Enjoying home and social life

- Set aside quality time for family
- Communicate schedule to family and friends
- Plan weekend activities
- Delegate chores
- Get extra sleep on weekends

Improving work performance

- Maintain bright lighting at work
- Schedule work breaks to avoid long periods of solitary work
- Socialize with others during work
- Rotate to other jobs
- Walk around when possible
- Concentrate on the job

Work Hours and Overtime

How many hours can a worker work and still be productive? The relationship between work hours and work output has been examined since the 1900s. Various schedules, including five 8-hour days, three 12-hour days, and four 10-hour days, have been examined from all perspectives. The 8-hour workday or 40-hour week consistently bears out as optimal for psychological health and fatigue recovery (Grandjean 1988).

Grandjean (1988) suggests that workers reach and maintain a certain daily output for an 8-hour period. If the workday is shortened, hourly productivity appears to increase; if the workday is lengthened, the productivity appears to fall. Essentially, the length of the day affects workers' paces and their use of spontaneous rest breaks. In a longer workday, workers take more breaks toward the end of the day and slow the work pace.

Psychosocially, a lengthened workday places stress on family members, interrupts leisure and social activities, and may cause workers to feel disconnected from others. Providing an opportunity for a worker's balance of work, rest, and leisure is essential to planning workday hours (Colligan & Tepas 1986).

Overtime presents a further dilemma from economic and medical perspectives. Although overtime pay may be necessary for some employees' financial survival, during periods of prolonged overtime, workers incur increased absences due to illness and risk the potential for poor health and overuse injury. When supervisors attempt to limit overtime hours for workers already injured or at risk for injury, the law suggests that a worker cannot be denied overtime because of an injury if the injury is job-related. The problem becomes a catch-22. Health care consultants agree that overtime increases the risk of overuse injuries to workers involved in repetitive or forceful work.

The advantages and disadvantages of an extended workday (or compressed workweek) have been discussed by industrial planners and ergonomists. The potential advantages of an extended workday (or compressed work week) for the company include decreased daily start-up time and decreased expenses; advantages for the worker include increased blocks of leisure time, an overall reduction in commuting time, fewer workdays, and less night work.

The potential disadvantages of an extended work week seem to outweigh the advantages. Disadvantages for the company include overtime pay, potentially increased worker absenteeism due to illness, and decreased productivity; disadvantages to the worker include increased fatigue and related safety and health problems, increased exposure to toxic hazards, and difficulty scheduling child care and family functions (Colligan & Tepas 1986).

Work Breaks

Work breaks are an essential part of the worker's shift. Work breaks function to restore workers' energy, to alleviate the monotony of routine or vigilant tasks and, importantly, to provide time for socialization. Pheasant (1991) suggests that 45 minutes to 1 hour is the maximum time span for human attention in a wide range of activities, although most people work well beyond this 1-hour span. Work breaks, when designed correctly, may increase overall productivity by deferring fatigue and monotony, which are associated with decreased work output.

The standard for industrial work breaks is 15 minutes in the morning and afternoon and 30 minutes for lunch, but ergonomists recommend a 3- to 5-minute pause every hour, particularly for jobs that are static, repetitive, or paced, or for jobs that require intense alertness such as assembly or com-

puter work (Grandjean 1988; Pheasant 1991). Sjøgaard et al. (1988) suggests that longer breaks may be necessary for complete muscle recovery in heavy work tasks (see Chapters 6 and 7).

Short breaks that involve gentle stretching are more beneficial for increasing blood flow to muscle and increasing one's level of alertness than are breaks that involve only rest (Hansford et al. 1986; Pheasant 1991). Breaks that included some neck motion were found to reduce fatigue and improve concentration among air traffic controllers (Grandjean 1988). Neck, shoulder, arm, and low-back stretches every hour are recommended for computer workers (Pheasant 1991). Neck, shoulder, and finger extension exercises are recommended for dental hygienists between each patient (Atwood & Michalak 1992).

Grandjean (1988) outlines the following types of breaks that have been observed among workers throughout the workday:

- *Spontaneous pauses* are short pauses for rest that workers take on their own.
- *Disguised pauses* are breaks from a worker's routine to perform another, less taxing part of the job (such as emptying the wastepaper basket or consulting a fellow employee).
- *Work-related pauses* are short breaks inherent in the machine pace or work routine (such as waiting for a part or waiting in line).
- *Organizational pauses* are those breaks prescribed by management for certain times of the day.

Observation indicates that the more organizational pauses that are integrated into a worker's schedule for stretches, the less time workers spend in spontaneous breaks (Grandjean 1988).

Although some organizations permit workers to leave early if no breaks are taken, workers should be encouraged to take regular breaks throughout the day to prevent accumulation of stress or fatigue.

Machine Pacing and Worker Control

Machine-paced work is often a major stressor for assembly-line workers. *Machine pacing* refers to work in which the output, rate, and speed of the task is controlled by a machine. Most assembly-line jobs are machine-paced and have the additional problem

Table 8.1. Levels of Illumination from Common Sources

Illumination Source	Lux
Outdoors, noonday sun	160,000
Outdoors, clear day	50,000
Outdoors, overcast day	5,000
Brightly lit office	1,000
Well-lit office	500
Reading light	300
Living room	50
Street lighting	10
Moonlight	0.5

Source: Adapted from S Pheasant (1991). *Ergonomics, Work, and Health*. Gaithersburg, MD: Aspen Publishers.

of being monotonous. Machine pacing has been criticized as incompatible with human variability, as pacing sets a one-way standard against which the worker's performance is measured: The worker can either achieve or fail; there are no gradations. Machine pacing has been related to high stress levels in workers (Arndt 1987; Karasek & Theorell 1990) attributable to the short work cycle and the worker's lack of control over his or her work pace.

Whenever possible, a worker should control his or her own pace. This concept is especially true for overtime work and for critical work tasks (Eastman Kodak Company 1983). Worker rotation to other stations, stretch breaks, and variety on the job (such as inventory, maintenance, or supervisory tasks) can help alleviate the monotony of and intense concentration demanded by machine-paced work.

Lighting in the Workplace

Proper lighting of the workplace is essential to visual comfort and good work performance. Discussion of poor lighting might call to mind an image of a weary watchmaker or jeweler hunched over a high bench with a single light bulb hanging directly overhead. Such an image underscores the strong impact of lighting on posture, eye strain, visual acuity, and overall safety in the work environment.

Most health care professionals are familiar with basic lighting principles from personal experience; most of us have had to deal with computer glare from

backlighting or difficulty reading notes when sunlight is being reflected off a white desk. Health care professionals also realize that the visual demand of the task often determines head and neck postures. However, many are not familiar with the illumination levels appropriate for certain jobs and with common-sense approaches for good lighting. In the following sections, we introduce basic concepts of workplace lighting. Further information is provided by Eastman Kodak 1983; Orandjean 1988; and Pheasant 1991.

Terminology

The terms used to describe and measure lighting are essential to this discussion. *Illumination* is a measure of the quantity of light falling on a surface from a source such as the sun, a lamp, a candle, or a flashlight. Illumination is measured with an illumination meter that is set directly on the surface. Illumination is recorded in lux (1 lux = 1 lumen per square meter). Illumination quantities range from 0.5 lux on a moonlit night to 160,000 lux at noon in summer (Eastman Kodak Company 1983). Table 8.1 identifies some common sources and levels of illumination.

Luminance is the perception of brightness of a surface or the light energy that is reflected back from a surface. Luminance depends on various factors in the surrounding environment, such as color, material, and contrasting articles that reflect different amounts of light energy. Generally, brighter, contrasting colors and shiny surfaces reflect more light and therefore give more luminance to an area. Luminance is measured by a photometer that is placed at a distance from the surface and pointed toward that surface. Luminance is expressed as candela per square meter (cd/m^2) and can be envisioned as a certain number of lighted candles illuminating one square meter (Eastman Kodak Company 1983). Table 8.2 identifies the reflective value of common materials in a room.

To draw a distinction between illumination and luminance, imagine that an office with dark furniture and many windows is illuminated to 300 lux. The luminance in this room will vary from 50 cd/m^2 near the dark-colored desk to 2,500 cd/m^2 near the unshaded window. Although the illumination is the same, the luminance will vary according to the reflective value of the walls (e.g., bright white or mauve), surface of the desk (e.g., dark

Table 8.2. Reflective Values for Common Materials

Material	Reflective Value (%)
Fresh white plaster	95
White paint or white paper	85
Light gray or cream paint	75
Newsprint, concrete	55
Plain light wood	45
Dark gray paint	30
Printer's ink	15
Matte black paper	5

Source: Adapted from S Pheasant (1991). *Ergonomics, Work, and Health*. Gaithersburg, MD: Aspen Publishers.

wood or white panel), paper on the desk, and availability of light (e.g., window blinds open or shaded) (Pheasant 1991).

Most recommended values for lighting are expressed in terms of illumination (Grandjean 1988; Pheasant 1991). However, an understanding of luminance is necessary if one is to determine the best means of decorating and arranging the work environment to provide proper lighting.

Recommended Levels for Workplace Lighting

Recommended levels for workplace lighting have steadily increased throughout history. Pheasant (1991) states that in the 1930s, most offices were lit by incandescent lamps that provided illumination of 100 lux. Today, because of more efficient lighting, a typical office is lit to 500 lux. The generally accepted rule for lighting has been "more is better," but this is not necessarily true. Clearly, more precise work demands better lighting. The extent to which illumination affects performance varies with the accuracy demands of the task, frequency of the task's performance, and safety demands. Pheasant (1991) argues that once a worker has enough light to perform the task optimally, more lighting will not necessarily improve the performance. In fact, Grandjean (1988) found that office workers preferred lower lighting levels (400–850 lux) for office tasks. Further, a high prevalence of office workers complained of eye problems when working at illumination levels greater than 1,000 lux. Although one cannot directly associate bright lighting and eye problems, the reflective glare and contrasting shadows may cause eye strain or blurriness at illumination levels in excess of 1,000 lux.

Luminance affects visibility as well as comfort. For tasks such as reading at a desk, a high contrast between the background and figures (e.g., dark figures on a light background) is beneficial to enhance legibility and ease of reading. However, in the work environment, sharp contrasts in luminance between large surfaces reduces visual comfort and visibility. For example, stark white walls contrasted with dark floor coverings, dark furniture, and dark business machines should be avoided in an office. The recommended luminance or reflective values should be high for ceilings (80–90%) but much lower for business machines, furniture (less than 50%), and flooring (less than 40%) (Grandjean 1988).

Recommendations for lighting vary greatly throughout the world. The U.S. standards are much higher than those in Europe. Regardless of the standards chosen, lighting must meet the minimum lighting level—that is, a level that is sufficient for workers to perform the most critical part of the task. In designing lighting for a workplace, one must remember to consider (1) the reflective value of the surrounding materials, (2) the difference from natural lighting, (3) the age of workers, and (4) the need for artificial lighting during the day. Table 8.3 offers a range of recommendations for lighting for varied work tasks.

Glare

Glare occurs when excessively bright objects interfere with the visual field. This brightness is seen as a reflection of a light source that is superimposed on the visual task. The brightness may interfere with the visual task or may cause discomfort only.

Direct glare occurs when a source of light in the visual field is much brighter than task materials at the workplace. Sources of direct glare for indoor offices or machine shops include light fixtures, bright sky showing through a window, or reflections from brass or polished materials.

Indirect glare is a term used for light that is reflected from materials at the work surface itself. Indirect glare reduces the contrast of materials at the workplace and may reduce task performance (Eastman Kodak Company 1983; Pheasant 1991).

Table 8.3. Recommended Ranges of Illumination for Work Tasks

Type of Work	Examples	Lux
General work, simple visual demands	Work in storerooms	20–200
Moderately precise work, limited visual demands	Rough machining, work in lecture halls, packing, simple assembly, carpentry, locksmith work	200–300
Fine work, normal visual demands	Rough machining, reading, writing, bookkeeping, fine assembly, office and laboratory work	500–700
Very fine to precise work, special visual demands	Hand engraving, technical drawing, color proofing, electrical assembly and testing, watchmaking	1,000–2,000
Prolonged or exacting visual tasks, exceptional visual demands	Microelectronic assembly, surgery	2,000–20,000

Sources: Compiled from E Grandjean (1988). *Fitting the Task to the Man: A Textbook of Occupational Ergonomics* (4th ed). Philadelphia: Taylor & Francis; and S Pheasant (1991). *Ergonomics, Work, and Health*. Gaithersburg, MD: Aspen Publishers.

Direct glare can be reduced by decreasing the illumination level of the light source with shades or by equalizing the luminance of materials near the workstation. The light source should not be in the visual field of the worker. The angle formed between the horizontal surfaces and the light source should be greater than 30 degrees (Eastman Kodak Company 1983; Grandjean 1988).

Direct and Indirect Lighting

Direct and indirect lighting are two types of lighting arrangements. *Direct lighting* is usually from above and directs approximately 90% of light toward the visual surface. Direct light often produces strong contrasts and shadows and may produce glare. However, small lamps may be good for close reading and video-display-terminal work.

Indirect lighting is light that is reflected off the ceiling and walls and back to the room. Indirect light casts no shadows and thus produces no glare. Indirect lighting produces uniformity of lighting but is less efficient because some of the light energy is lost to reflection.

Designers widely recommend a combination of direct and indirect lighting. Such light sources have translucent shades that reflect approximately 40–50% of light to the ceilings and direct the rest downward. This combination of direct and indirect lighting minimizes shadows and permits even illumination. Other designers recommend generally lower levels of office illumination with small lamps directed at the task.

Artificial Light Sources

Daylight is always preferable to artificial light for its aesthetic qualities and for the change of scenery that a window to the outdoors affords. Unfortunately, daylight is not enough to illuminate deep rooms or offices, and thus artificial light is used. Two types of artificial lighting commonly used are electrical filament lamps and fluorescent tubes.

Electrical filament lamps (light bulbs, incandescent lamps) create a subdued, pleasant atmosphere with red and yellow rays. However, filaments are inefficient because they emit heat and usually last less than 1 year.

Fluorescent lighting is created by electricity passed through a gas or mercury vapor that is then converted to light energy. This type of lighting is very efficient; little energy is lost in the conversion from electricity to light. The advantages of fluorescent lighting are that the fluorescent tubes have a high output and long life and the color of the lighting can be controlled by varying the chemical composition of the fluorescent substance lining the inside of the tube. The major disadvantage is a flicker that may not be noticeable in older or defective fluorescent tubes. Normally, fluorescent tubes produce a flicker from alternating current at a much higher frequency than is apparent to the human eye. However, a flicker that is visible can be extremely uncomfortable and annoying because of repetitive overexposure of the retina (Grandjean 1988).

Guidelines for Proper Lighting

The following guidelines should assist in the proper design of workplaces:

Light source

- Direct lighting should be placed at right angles to the work task. Workstations should be at right angles to windows.
- A direct light source should not be in the visual field of the worker.
- For fine work, the light source should be in front of the visual task.
- Avoid fluctuating brightness of light sources or objects, especially when the worker must switch visual fields from one object to another.
- Use more lamps of low power than fewer lamps of high power for equal distribution of light and for diminished glare.
- Avoid glare whenever possible.

Work-space design

- Select colors of similar brightness for large surfaces.
- Choose matte finishes rather than glossy surfaces.
- Avoid reflective color on tabletops, control panels, and machines.

References

Armstrong TJ (1990). Ergonomics and cumulative trauma disorders of the hand and wrist. In JM Hunter, LH Schneider, EJ Mackin, & AD Callahan (Eds). *Rehabilitation of the Hand: Surgery and Therapy.* Toronto: Mosby.

Armstrong TJ, Fine LJ, Radwin RG, & Silverstein BS (1987). Ergonomics and the effects of vibration in hand-intensive work. *Scand J Work Environ Health*, 13,286–289.

Arndt R (1987). Work pace, stress and cumulative trauma disorder. *J Hand Surg [Am]*, 12,866–869.

Atwood M & Michalak C (1992). The occurrence of cumulative trauma disorders in dental hygienists. *Work*, 2(4),1–31.

Brown AP (1990). The effects of anti-vibration gloves on vibration-induced disorders: a case study. *J Hand Ther*, 3(2), 94–100.

Buchholz B, Frederick LJ, & Armstrong TJ (1988). An investigation of human palmar skin friction and effects of materials, pinch force and moisture. *Ergonomics*, 31,317–325.

Bullock MI (Ed) (1990). *Ergonomics: The Physiotherapist in the Workplace*. New York: Churchill Livingstone.

Cochran DJ & Riley MW (1986). The effects of handle shape and size on exerted forces. *Hum Factors*, 28,251–265.

Colligan MJ & Tepas DI (1986). The stress of hours of work. *Am Ind Hyg Assoc J,* 47,686–695.

Czeisler CA, Johnson MP, Duffy JF, Brown EN, Ronda JM, & Kronauer RE (1990). Exposure to bright light and darkness to treat physiologic maladaptation to night work. *N Engl J Med,* 322,1253–1259.

Eastman Kodak Company (1983). *Ergonomic Design for People at Work,* Vols 1 and 2. New York: Van Nostrand Reinhold.

Fraser TM (1989). *The Worker at Work: A Textbook Concerned with Men and Women in the Workplace.* Philadelphia: Taylor & Francis.

Grandjean E (1988). *Fitting the Task to the Man: A Textbook of Occupational Ergonomics* (4th ed). Philadelphia: Taylor & Francis.

Greenberg L & Chaffin DB (1977). *Workers and Their Tools: A Guide to the Ergonomic Design of Hand Tools and Small Presses.* Midland, MI: Pendell.

Hamelin P (1987). Lorry drivers' time habits in work and their involvement in traffic accidents. *Ergonomics,* 30,1323–1333.

Hampel GA (1992). Hand-arm vibration isolation materials: a range of performance evaluation. *Appl Occup Environ Hyg,* 7,441–452.

Hansford T, Blood H, Kent B, & Lutz G (1986). Blood flow changes at the wrist in manual workers after preventive interventions. *J Hand Surg [Am]*, 11,503–508.

Harma M (1993). Individual differences in tolerance to shiftwork: a review. *Ergonomics,* 36,101–109.

Hunter JM, Schneider LH, Mackin EJ, & Callahan AD (Eds) (1990). *Rehabilitation of the Hand: Surgery and Therapy.* Toronto: Mosby.

Jenkins DB (1991). *Hollinshead's Functional Anatomy of the Limbs and Back* (6th ed). Philadelphia: Saunders.

Johnson SL (1990). Ergonomic design of handheld tools to prevent trauma to the hand and upper extremity. *J Hand Ther*, 3(2),86–93.

Karasek R & Theorell T (1990). *Healthy Work: Stress, Productivity and the Reconstruction of Working Life.* New York: Basic Books.

Meagher SW (1987). Tool design for prevention of hand and wrist injuries. *J Hand Surg [Am]*, 12,855–857.

Mellor EF (1986). Shiftwork and flexitime: how prevalent are they? *Monthly Labor Rev*, 109,14–21.

Minors DS & Waterhouse JM (1985). Circadian rhythms in deep body temperature, urinary excretion and alertness in nurses on night work. *Ergonomics,* 28,1523–1530.

Monk T (1989). Human factors implications of shiftwork. *Int Rev Ergon*, 2,111–128.

Moore-Ede MC & Richardson GS (1985). Medical implications of shift-work. *Annu Rev Med*, 36,607–617.

Morse LH & Hinds LJ (1993). Women and ergonomics. *Occup Med*, 8,721–731.

Napier JP (1956). The prehensile movements of the human hand. *J Bone Joint Surg Br*, 38,902–913.

National Institute of Occupational Safety and Health (1989). *Criteria for a Recommended Standard: Occupational Exposure to Hand-Arm Vibration* [DHHS (NIOSH) pub no. 89-106]. Cincinnati: US Department of Health and Human Services.

Pheasant S (1991). *Ergonomics, Work, and Health*. Gaithersburg, MD: Aspen.

Putz-Anderson V (Ed) (1988). *Cumulative Trauma Disorders: A Manual for Musculoskeletal Disease of the Upper Limbs*. London: Taylor & Francis.

Radwin RG, Armstrong TJ, and Chaffin DB (1987). Power hand tool vibration and tool vibration effects on grip exertion. *Ergonomics*, 30,833–855.

Robinson FR & Lyon BK (August 1994). Ergonomic guidelines for hand-held tools. *Prof Safety,* 16–21.

Rodgers SH (1987). Recovery time needs for repetitive work. *Semin Occup Med*, 2(1),19–24.

Rosa RR, Colligan MJ, & Lewis P (1989). Extended workday: effects of 8-hour and 12-hour rotating shift schedules on performance, subjective alertness, sleep patterns and psychosocial variables. *Work Stress,* 3(1),21–32.

Sanders M (April 11, 1996). Circadian rhythms: Implications for shiftwork and occupational therapy. Presented at American Occupational Therapy Association National Convention. Chicago, IL.

Schoenmarklin RW & Marras WS (1989). Effects of handle angle and work orientation on hammering: I. Wrist motion and hammering performance. *Hum Factors*, 31,397–411.

Scott AJ & Ladou J (1990). Shiftwork: effects on sleep and health with recommendations for medical surveillance and screening. *Occup Med*, 5,273–299.

Sjøgaard G, Savard G, & Juel C (1988). Muscle blood flow during isometric activity and its relation to muscle fatigue. *Eur J Appl Physiol*, 57,327–335.

Smith MJ, Colligan MJ, & Tasto DL (1982). Health and safety consequences of shiftwork in the food processing industry. *Ergonomics*, 25,133–144.

Spaulding SJ (1989). The biomechanics of prehension. *Am J Occup Ther*, 43,302–307.

Sunderland RS (1995). Anthropometry. In K Jacobs & CM Bettencourt (Eds). *Ergonomics for Therapists*. Boston: Butterworth-Heinemann.

Tepas D & Monk TH (1987). Work schedules. In G Salvendy (Ed). *Handbook of Human Factors* (pp. 819–843). New York: Wiley.

Tichauer ER (1966). Some aspects of stress on forearm and hand in industry. *J Occup Med*, 8(2),63–71.

Tichauer ER (1978). *The Biomechanical Basis of Ergonomics*. New York: Wiley-Interscience.

Chapter 9

Psychosocial Factors

Dorothy Farrar Edwards

Cumulative trauma disorders (CTDs) are associated with persistent pain, loss of function, and increased work-related disabilities. In spite of comprehensive medical care and substantial attention to the biomechanical and ergonomic factors in the workplace, many persons with CTDs do not improve. Often, psychological factors are implicated in the development of subacute and chronic musculoskeletal pain syndromes (Linton 1995). In some cases, the psychological risk factors in the workplace have been found to be more important than physical work factors as predictors of back injuries (Bigos et al. 1991; Nachemson 1992).

The purpose of this chapter is to examine the effects of psychosocial factors on the etiology and management of work-related musculoskeletal disorders. An understanding of these factors is essential if one is to treat effectively or prevent the devastating consequences of CTDs (Faucett 1994).

Most of our knowledge of the relationship between psychosocial variables and musculoskeletal pain is based on studies of low-back pain (Kelsey & Golden 1988). The applicability of these findings to neck and shoulder pain or carpal tunnel syndrome has not been fully established. However, recent studies suggest that the back pain data may generalize to other musculoskeletal syndromes (Linton 1995). Generally, the psychosocial variables thought to be most highly associated with work-related CTDs are the psychological aspects or emotional tone of the work environment, social support, perceptions of control, coping styles, cognitive responses to stress, and personality traits and states such as anxiety, defensiveness, and depression.

Stress and Work Environments

Seyle's (1936) general adaptation syndrome describes three stages of stress: alarm, resistance, and exhaustion. The last stage, exhaustion, is induced by chronic stress. The term *strain* is used to describe this stage when the worker's psychosocial resources prove inadequate in the face of psychological stressors such as time pressures or conflicts with superiors and coworkers.

The psychosocial characteristics of the work environment are defined as the employee's emotional response to workplace demands and stressors (Feuerstein et al. 1993). Early studies of the industrial implications of stress defined stress as the state induced in an individual when his or her own needs, exertions, and aims are thwarted by the demands and expectations placed on him or her by a superior, work group, or organization. According to Bronner (1965), the employee finds him- or herself in a state of stress when he or she experiences a situation as threatening or frustrating and cannot adopt the behavior needed to reduce the frustration. Bronner associated worker stress in Swedish industrial workers with absenteeism, accidents, and increased emotional problems and psychosomatic disorders.

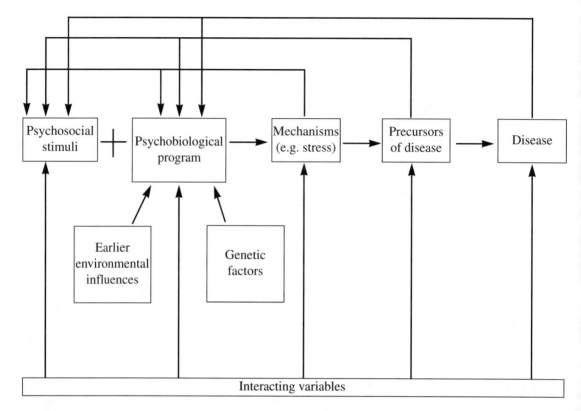

Figure 9.1. Levi's model for psychosocial mediation of disease. The combined effects of each factor may lead to a psychosocially influenced disease or condition such as cumulative trauma disorder. The model shows a system with continuous feedback among the factors. Psychosocial stimuli arise from the social and emotional environments of the person. These stimuli are interpreted based on personal, developmental, and genetic characteristics of the person, which, in turn, may create a stress response. In some cases, the stress response leads to the precursors of the disease or to the disease itself.

Model of Stress and Health

The work of Levi (1972, 1987) expands on the role of psychosocial factors in health and provides the foundation for the current theoretic and empiric models of workplace stress. According to Levi (1972), cognitive, behavioral, emotional, and physiologic reactions influence the development of pathogenic mechanisms that increase the risk of morbidity and decrease perceived health status. Levi (1987) further suggests that linear models of causality are not adequate. Complex, nonlinear systems models are required to account fully for the relationship of these elements to worker health. Levi's model, which was presented first in 1972, still is relevant today (Figure 9.1). The model illustrates the interactions among factors such as social systems, specific physical and psychosocial stimuli,

and the individual's psychobiological program. Levi's model, as well as other related models of worker health, suggest that the stresses present in the workplace may be causally related rather than merely associated or correlated with physical reactions such as cardiovascular disease or musculoskeletal pain.

Objective and Subjective Sources of Occupational Stress

The investigation of occupational or work-related stress was advanced greatly by the passage of the Occupational Health and Safety Act of 1970 through the creation of the National Institute of Occupational Safety and Health (NIOSH) and the Occupational Safety and Health Administration (OSHA). Both

Table 9.1. Subjective and Objective Sources of Job-Related Stress Associated with Musculoskeletal Disorders

Subjective stressors
    Role ambiguity
    Role conflict
    Boredom
    Person-environment fit
    Job insecurity
    Supervisory style
    Job and personal conflicts
    Demand and decision latitude
Objective stressors
    Noise
    Temperature
    Machine-paced tasks
    Electronic monitoring of performance
    Isolation
    Crowding
    Vibration
    Unsafe or hazardous working conditions
    Long hours, overtime

these agencies were charged with the responsibility for conducting the research necessary to support industrial health and safety. NIOSH was directed to include the behavioral, social, and motivational factors associated with workplace safety and health.

The concept of occupational stress is often dismissed because of the difficulty of establishing operational definitions that are acceptable to all the parties involved in the research (Smith 1987). Smith, in his comprehensive review of occupational stress research, suggests that the chief source of confusion is whether to conceive of stress as a situational factor external to the worker or as a reaction experienced by the worker. Most of the work in the field of occupational stress has focused on the aspects of work that have, or threaten to have, negative consequences for the worker. He concluded that the prevalent research paradigm is that stress (independent variable) leads to undesirable consequences such as musculoskeletal pain (dependent variable) under certain conditions (mediating variables). Traditionally, the studies examine either objectively or subjectively defined stress. Different types of stressors are believed to have a differential impact on health and well-being. Objectively defined stressors include the physical aspects of the work environment such as noise, temperature, and exposure to danger, as well as factors such as shiftwork that result in disturbed circadian rhythms and responses to machine-paced manufacturing. Subjectively defined stressors are those defined from the perspective of the worker. Variables such as role ambiguity, boredom, person-environment fit, uncertain job security, and supervisory style have been studied. Table 9.1 presents a list of the most frequently studied objective and subjective occupational stressors. The empiric benefits of separating stress into objective and subjective categories are unclear, as all responses are the result of the psychological reactions of the worker to potentially stressful conditions. Individual differences in perception and response styles ultimately render all responses subjective, regardless of the source of the stressor.

A number of different physical and psychological effects have been used as dependent measures in studies of subjective and objective occupational stressors. The physiologic and clinical aspects of cardiovascular disease in workers have been studied more often than any other stress-related medical condition. Other psychological conditions studied include headaches, peptic ulcers, respiratory diseases, and arthritis. There have been very few studies of cumulative trauma or musculoskeletal disorders. The reported findings follow similar patterns across disease states and health problems. The heart disease studies are considered representative; however, the findings with respect to heart disease are conflicting. According to Chadwick (1980), there is little evidence to support the hypotheses that directly link job-related stress to physiologic indices of heart disease. Chadwick suggests that the "stress causes strain causes heart disease" formula be rejected in favor of the concept of person-environment fit. This concept incorporates the notion that optimal levels of performance and satisfaction are achieved when the worker skills and personal style are matched to the demands of the workplace (Csikszentmihalyi 1993). Within this framework, boredom associated with unchallenging work and a slow pace is as deleterious as work that is too demanding and fast paced. The person-environment fit concept allows investigators to account for individual differences associated with personality traits and coping styles in conjunction with measures of environmental demands.

Methodologic Issues in Workplace Stress Research

Research on the relationship between subjective and objective stressors and health in the workplace is complicated by controversies over design and analytic strategies. There are three major areas of concern. The first focuses on the use of simple and, at times, reductionist models to account for the complex interaction between stress and worker health. Smith (1987) suggests that the traditional research strategy of seeking a linear relationship between an identified stressor and a physical or emotional problem is reductionist and unlikely to produce a clearly identified causal pathway. Correlational models can demonstrate only the associations among variables and should not be interpreted as causal. Because many studies include a number of highly correlated variables, the results can be confounded if the investigator does not use statistical techniques such as analysis of covariance to control for relationships that may mediate the association between stressors and health status. For example, it is generally believed that personality traits influence individual responses to stress. A simple design that does not measure these traits may conclude erroneously that work-site stress causes health problems, without considering the role that personality plays in influencing job choice, response to stress, or comfort in reporting health problems.

The second methodologic concern is associated with the types of scales used to measure both the stressors and the consequences of stress. The majority of studies use paper-and-pencil questionnaires that may not have been appropriately standardized and validated in the population of interest. Also, the tendency to abbreviate or alter existing measures weakens the reliability and validity of a scale even if the scale was robust in its original form (Portnoy & Watkins 1993). A review of the literature reveals that most scales are ordinal. However, many investigators treat these types of scales as continuous measures with normal distributions and use statistical techniques that may obscure the true relationships among the variables or reduce the power of the study to detect significant differences.

The third methodologic problem encountered in research on work-site stress and personality factors in CTDs is the heavy reliance on cross-sectional rather than longitudinal designs. Cross-sectional studies do not allow the investigator to measure the temporal link between stressors and health problems, particularly when chronic problems such as musculoskeletal pain are the focus. Longitudinal surveillance of workers allows the study of changes in health status together with ongoing evaluation of the psychological environment of the workplace. Both types of studies are weakened by the tendency to use very small samples.

In response to these types of methodologic criticisms, a number of investigators have moved beyond the generalized evaluations of occupational stressors to more complex models that examine occupational stress and health outcomes. Many of these studies of worker physical and mental health are based on the models of demand control and autonomy.

Demand Control Models and Worker Health

Karasek and Theorell (1990) have conducted a series of studies examining the impact of occupational stress on mental and physical health outcomes. This model, known as a *demand control model,* posits a relationship between the psychological response to job demands and the worker's sense of control or autonomy. Such models have also been called *job strain models.* According to these models, stress-related illness is the product of the interactive effects of job demands and the worker's perceptions of control.

Demand is defined as work-related feelings such as not having enough time to do one's work, being confronted with conflicting demands on the job, and having to work quickly (Marshall & Barnett 1991). *Control* and *autonomy* are operationalized through two constructs: skill discretion and decision authority. Workers with high levels of skill have control over the specific skills they choose to exercise to accomplish a task. Karasek and Theorell (1990) suggest that the combination of these two constructs results in perceptions of control that influence worker health. The most adverse outcomes are seen in jobs that combine high levels of demand with low levels of control. High-strain jobs include machine-paced manufacturing, computer operations, and service jobs (Repetti 1993). The same job tasks may be defined as low-strain if the worker is allowed to pace him- or herself, contribute information to management, or acquire new job skills. This model has been validated across a variety of work environments and in many different countries. The findings are remarkably consistent across job types and work settings (Evanoff & Rosenstock 1994).

Musculoskeletal diseases have been studied with the demand control model. Most of the research has examined upper-extremity and neck and shoulder pain, although several studies have been directed toward low-back pain. Longitudinal and cross-sectional studies have found that monotonous work and work under time pressures are associated with neck and shoulder pain. In the most elaborate study of musculoskeletal pain using the demand control model (Bigos et al. 1991), jobs classified as having low decision latitude had odds ratios for hospitalization of 1.3–1.9 after adjusting for physical load. Other studies have combined the demand control model with measures of social support, but the findings are less clear (Peate 1994; Nachemson 1992). Social support appears to mediate the effects of high demands and low decision latitude, but the specific mechanisms are highly variable and very sensitive to individual differences.

Demand Control Models and Mental Health

As previously stated, the demand control model has been used to study both mental and physical health outcomes. The combination of job demands and control has been shown to predict general symptoms of psychological distress. A longitudinal study of male power-plant workers found that increased symptoms of psychological distress were associated with the interaction between job demands and decision latitude (Bromet et al. 1988). However, the same study found that decision latitude did not mediate the relationship between job demands and affective disorders. In other words, workers with high job demands and low decision latitude were not found to have higher rates of affective disorders than workers with high job demands and high decision latitude.

Marshall and Barnett (1991) suggest that it is also important to recognize the positive aspects of job challenge and decision authority. They conducted a series of factor-analytic studies and identified six work reward factors (helping others, decision authority, challenge, supervisor support, recognition, and satisfaction with salary) and five work concern factors (overload, dead-end job, hazard exposure, poor supervision, and discrimination). They then estimated separate regression models for well-being and psychological distress as outcome (dependent) measures. This study found that not all work concerns or rewards are equally capable of producing or reducing job-related stress responses. The authors suggest that the narrowing of attention to only two workplace dimensions, such as demand and decision latitude, may be premature. Marshall and Barnett (1991) also found that men and women experience different aspects of work as problematic or rewarding. They concluded that models of workplace stressors and mediators of stress should be broadened to incorporate the growing evidence of gender differences in response.

Immune Responses to Workplace Stress

Evidence from a number of fields points toward a link between neural activity and altered immune responses (Ader et al. 1987). Psychosocial factors such as bereavement, marital separation, depression, and examination stress in students are associated with altered measures of immune reactivity and altered health status. Both animal and human investigations show that the immune and nervous systems communicate through a dynamic process using a variety of hormones and neurotransmitters. This area of research is known as *psychoneuroimmunology*. Stress responses have been proposed as part of the etiology of fibromyalgia and low-back pain. Disturbed autonomic nervous system function has been clearly established in fibromyalgia (Simons 1990). Simons cites several studies that demonstrate that abnormalities in the immune system produce alterations in serotonin pathways, accounting for many of the clinical manifestations. Although still speculative, the association between sleep disturbances, neurohumoral responses, and fibromyalgia may help explain the work-site findings of increased health problems (including musculoskeletal problems) in shift workers. Shiftwork is known to disrupt normal circadian rhythms and to change sleep-wake cycles (see Chapter 8).

One of the first models to emerge in psychoneuroimmunology uses new biomedical techniques to obtain ambulatory recordings of endocrine responses to conditions of daily life. This biopsychosocial model helps to identify stress-inducing environmental conditions and to analyze their influence on health, well-being, and efficiency (Frankenhaeuser & Johansson 1986; Frankenhaeuser 1991). Cognitive appraisal is a key element of this model. When an individual is confronted with an environmental challenge, he or she appraises the nature and strength of the challenge and weighs the importance and severity of the demands against his or her own coping abilities. A stimulus that is perceived as a threat or a situation that creates demands well beyond the perceived resources of the person evokes a complex series of physical and emotional reactions. Threatening stimuli generate the increased secretion of epinephrine and norepinephrine or stress hormones. The pituitary gland also secretes adrenocorticotropic hormone, which is an important element in the body's immune response.

This biopsychosocial model has been used to examine the effects of both chronic and acute stressors in the workplace. Cardiovascular risk factors have been shown to be affected by these neuroendocrine changes, but there is preliminary evidence suggesting that gastrointestinal and musculoskeletal systems are also influenced by the same process (Frankenhaeuser 1991).

Coping, Cognitive Appraisal, and Cumulative Trauma Disorders

Many discussions of the psychosocial attributes of work-related CTDs emphasize the importance of coping styles in dealing with the day-to-day demands of the workplace (Ross 1994). However, most of the research on cognitive appraisal and coping is more relevant to the treatment of CTDs than to understanding the development of musculoskeletal pain syndromes. A significant body of literature has examined the impact of cognitive appraisal and coping mechanisms in persons confronting the consequences of an injury or chronic illness. The findings of these studies are remarkably consistent.

Coping skills are called into action when a person experiences an injury or illness. According to Lazarus and Folkman (1984), coping allows a person to maintain a positive self-image, tolerate negative events, and maintain emotional equilibrium. Coping responses are described as coping styles. Two interrelated factors generally are considered in the investigation of coping styles: The first is appraisal, which involves a person's judgment about what is at stake in a stressful encounter, and the second is coping

process, or the cognitive and behavioral efforts used to manage specific stressful episodes.

Lazarus and Folkman (1984) identified two stages in the appraisal process, *primary appraisal,* or the determination of the challenge, threat, or benefit of an event, and *secondary appraisal,* which reflects the individual's beliefs about the options available to deal with the situation. This appraisal process is believed to mediate an individual's reaction to an event. Measures of appraisal often include questions that tap a person's sense of control. For example, Peacock and Wong (1990) developed a measure—the Stress Appraisal Measure—that assesses both primary and secondary appraisal. They identified three aspects of secondary appraisal in their measure: controllable by self, controllable by others, and uncontrollable.

The type of coping style used depends on the personal characteristics of the individual, environmental factors such as availability of social support and presence of life stressors, and the individual's appraisal of the stressful situation (Parkes 1986). Lazarus and Folkman (1984) identified two primary ways of coping: problem focused and emotion focused. Other investigators have reported similar classifications (Feifel et al. 1987; Carver et al. 1989; Endler & Parker 1990). *Problem-focused coping* is associated with efforts to manage the nature of the problem, whereas *emotion-focused coping* is directed at regulating the feelings that the problem or situation evokes. Coping styles are then classified further into approach strategies and avoidance strategies. *Approach strategies* include trying to identify and solve problems, seeking information, and seeking social and emotional support. *Avoidance strategies* include denial, resigned acceptance, hostility, and passivity.

Pellino and Oberst (1993) used a coping and cognitive appraisal model and found perceptions of situational control and appraisal of illness to be mediators of the outcome of treatment in a group of chronic low-back-pain patients. Those patients who considered the situation beyond their control were more likely to be depressed, reported more negative life events, and experienced more pain.

Personality and Adjustment Factors

The previously described models all note the contributions of personality traits and emotional states to worker response to work-site stress and injury. It is important to remember the differences between personality traits and emotional states that arise in response to the consequences of an injury. The literature in this area often fails to distinguish clearly between the two.

Personality traits are defined as consistent characteristics of a person, including behavior patterns, emotional responses, and emotional predispositions. *Emotional* or *reactive states* are emotional reactions to a particular stimulus or situation. Both are thought to play a role in the etiology and response to treatment of musculoskeletal disorders; however, the empiric evidence in support of this belief is conflicting, despite more than 20 years of interest in the topic.

Personality Traits

Is there a CTD personality? Perhaps the investigations of type A personality and heart disease will shed some light on this problem. Studies of type A personality have identified individuals with high needs for control. This personality type was first investigated in persons with cardiovascular disease, although subsequent research has broadened the construct to include individuals with other diseases. Type A behaviors include competitiveness, aggressiveness, and hostility as coping responses elicited to perceived threats to control (Rhodewalt & Fairfield 1990).

Of particular relevance to CTDs are the studies of type A–personality workers. There is substantial evidence that persons with type A personalities may choose high-pressure occupations. There also are substantial data that report type A workers as having nonsupportive interactions with coworkers, enhanced feelings of time urgency, and decreased levels of perceived environmental control (Bedian et al. 1990). Injury, illness, and treatment resulted in reactive, helpless behaviors and medical noncompliance in a group of injured type A recreational runners with foot injuries when compared to a type B group with similar injuries (Rhodewalt & Strube 1985). The type A runners were more likely to express anger about the injury and to be dissatisfied with their rate of recovery. Smith and Rhodewalt (1986) suggest that type A behavior patterns are elicited by exposure to certain environmental stimuli based on concepts of person-environment fit. It is possible that a similar psychosocial profile increases the risk of work-related musculoskeletal

disorders and that, once injured, these psychosocial states influence response to treatment, recovery, and return to work.

Few longitudinal studies have focused on personality traits and susceptibility to musculoskeletal disorders. In one of the most comprehensive studies, Vikari-Junitura et al. (1991) followed a cohort of Finnish adolescents from 1955 to 1987. One hundred and fifty-four of the original group of 1,084 persons completed a questionnaire about work characteristics and musculoskeletal symptoms and underwent a physical examination. Psychosocial measurements obtained in adolescence showed no consistent association with neck, back, or shoulder symptoms in adulthood. Vikari-Junitura et al. (1991) did find that weak "mental resources for promoting health," such as a poor sense of coherence, were associated consistently with neck and shoulder pain in adulthood.

Leino and Magni (1993) conducted a 10-year prospective study of working conditions, health habits, mental well-being, and physical health in a large cohort of metal workers in Finland. The study was designed to investigate whether distress and depression led to musculoskeletal disorders. They found that depressive and distress symptoms predicted musculoskeletal morbidity of the neck, shoulders, and low back, particularly in men. These investigators did not find the reverse temporal sequence for depression, although the onset of musculoskeletal symptoms was associated with increased distress. Poor adjustment has been associated with chronic musculoskeletal pain. Persons who were anxious, angry, or depressed were found to be at significantly greater risk of a back injury than workers who were not in these states but who held similar jobs and had identical training (Hirschfeld & Banbehan 1963).

Emotional States

A number of cross-sectional studies have compared self-reported measures of personality and adjustment among groups of patients experiencing different types of pain. Early studies classified the pain as either organic or functional. Functional pain was believed to be of psychogenic origin. Measurement of the psychiatric or psychological problems was inconsistent, and the samples were often small. Not surprisingly, the results of these studies are conflicting. Joukamaa (1994) suggests that the use of standardized measures, such

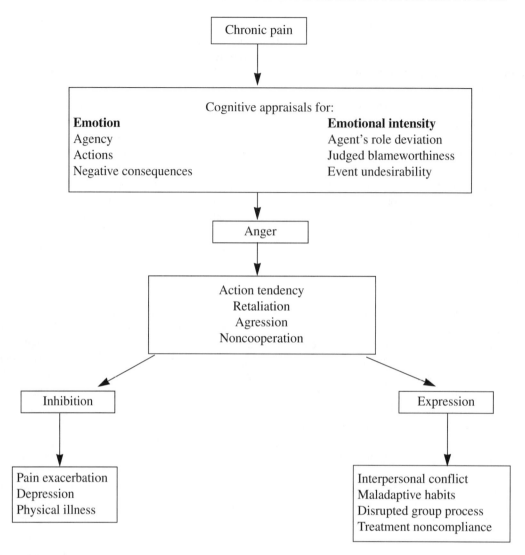

Figure 9.2. Antecedents and consequences of anger associated with chronic pain.

as the Minnesota Multiphasic Personality Inventory or the Millon Behavioral Health Inventory, coupled with large representative samples of musculoskeletal pain patients has increased our understanding of the complex relationship between psychological states and chronic pain. Joukamaa concludes that all pain has psychological consequences, that the relationship between psychopathology and pain is complex, and that depression and anxiety are the most common psychiatric disorders associated with low-back pain. He also proposes an atypical presentation of depression in some low-back-pain patients, in whom the depression is masked by the absence of depressed mood.

Fernandez and Turk (1995) have proposed a similar model. However, they focus on the contribution of anger as opposed to depression as the most salient emotional correlate of pain. Many studies have identified hostility as a common feature of low-back-pain patients (Waddell 1992). Fernandez and Turk believe that anger rather than hostility is the dominant emotion influencing the cognitive appraisals of chronic pain sufferers (Figure 9.2). Most patients inhibit their admission and expression of anger, perhaps because of the perceived social consequences of this emotion. This inhibited anger is believed to be a mediator of depression in persons with chronic pain. Angry, de-

pressed, or hostile persons with painful musculoskeletal disorders are more likely to adopt mal-
adaptive health habits and lifestyles that complicate
treatment and prolong disability.

Impact of Cumulative Trauma Disorders on Quality of Life

CTDs have a major impact on occupational performance. *Occupation* is defined as "the day-to-day en-
gagement in the activities, tasks, and roles that
organize our lives, and meet our needs to maintain
ourselves, to be productive, and to derive enjoyment
and satisfaction within our environments" (Christianson 1991, p. 27). The primary focus of most health
care professionals is on restoring a person's ability to
work. However, it is also important to examine the
emotional impact of CTDs as it relates to decreased
independence in activities of daily living and leisure
activities. The frustration and embarrassment resulting from one's inability to perform simple tasks independently (e.g., buttoning a shirt, tying a shoelace,
combing one's hair, hooking a bra strap, opening a
jar) is thought to increase the anger and depression
experienced by most patients. Anger and frustration
take a toll on families and friends as well, decreasing
the social networks essential for self-esteem and emotional support. As the number of pain-free activities
diminishes, recreational and leisure activities are
abandoned, giving rise to heightened social isolation.
These factors increase the likelihood of sustained
sick-role behaviors, particularly when activities of
daily living provoke pain to some extent.

Unfortunately, the effect of CTDs on quality of
life has not been systematically explored. The
growing emphasis on quality of life and functional
outcomes as determinants of treatment efficacy will
focus attention on the role of self-care, family and
social group responsibilities, and leisure activity
participation in the development of and recovery
from upper-extremity CTDs.

References

Ader R, Cohen N, & Felten DL (1987). Brain, behavior and immunity. *Brain Behav Immun,* 1,1–6.

Bedian AG, Mossholder KW, & Touiliatos J (1990). Type A status and selected work experiences among male and female accountants. In MJ Strube (Ed). *Type A Behavior.* Newbery Park, CA: Sage Publications.

Bigos SJ, Battie MC, Spengler DM, Fisher LD, Fordyce WE, Hansson T, Nachemson AL, & Wortley M (1991). A prospective study of work perceptions and psychosocial factors affecting the report of back injury. *Spine,* 16,1–6.

Bromet EJ, Dew MA, Parkinson DK, & Schulberg HC (1988). Predictive effects of occupational and marital stress on the mental health of a male workforce. *J Organ Behav,* 9,1–13.

Bronner K (1965). Industrial implications of stress. In L Levi (Ed). *Emotional Stress: Physiological and Psychological Reactions, Medical, Industrial and Military Implications* (pp. 225–238). New York: American Elsevier.

Carver CS, Schier MF, & Weintraub JK (1989). Assessing coping strategies. *J Pers Soc Psychol,* 56,267–283.

Chadwick JF (1980). Psychological job stress and coronary heart disease: a current NIOSH project. In RM Schwartz (Ed). *New Developments in Occupational Stress.* Cincinnati: National Institute of Occupational Safety and Health.

Christianson C (1991). Occupational therapy: intervention for life performance. In C Christianson & C Baum (Eds). *Occupational Therapy: Overcoming Human Performance Deficits* (pp. 3–44). Thorofare, NJ: Slack, Inc.

Csikszentmihalyi M (1993). Activity and happiness: towards a science of occupation. *Occup Sci: Aust,* 1,38–42.

Endler NS & Parker JD (1990). A multidimensional assessment of coping: a critical evaluation. *J Pers Soc Psychol,* 58,844–854.

Evanoff B & Rosenstock L (1994). Psychophysiologic stres-
sors and work organization. In L Rosenstock & M Cullen (Eds). *Textbook of Clinical Occupational and Environmental Medicine* (pp. 717–728). Philadelphia: Saunders.

Faucett JA (1994). Depression in painful clinical disorders: the role of pain and conflict about pain. *J Pain Symptom Manage,* 9,520–526.

Feifel H, Strack S, & Nagy VT (1987). Coping strategies and associated features of medically ill patients. *Psychosom Med,* 49,616–625.

Fernandez E & Turk DC (1995). The scope and significance of anger in the experience of chronic pain. *Pain,* 61,165–175.

Feuerstein M, Callan-Harris MS, Dyer D, Armbruster W, & Carosella AM (1993). Multidisciplinary rehabilitation of chronic work-related upper extremity disorders. *J Occup Med,* 35,396–403.

Frankenhaeuser M & Johansson G (1986). Stress at work: psychobiological and psychosocial aspects. *Int Rev Appl Psychol,* 35,287–299.

Frankenhaeuser M (1991). The psychophysiology of sex differences as related to occupational stress. In M Franken-
haeuser, U Lundberg, & M Chesney (Eds). *Women, Work, and Health: Stress and Opportunities* (pp. 39–59). New York: Plenum.

Hirschfeld AH & Banbehan RC (1963). The accident process. *J Am Med Soc,* 186,1939–1945.

Joukamaa M (1994). Depression and back pain. *Acta Psychiatr Scand Suppl,* 377,83–86.

Karasek R & Theorell T (1990). *Healthy Work: Stress, Productivity and the Reconstruction of Working Life*. New York: Basic Books.

Kelsey JL & Golden AL (1988). Occupational and workplace factors associated with low back pain. *State-of-the-Art Rev Occup Med*, 3,7–16.

Lazarus R & Folkman S (1984). *Stress, Appraisal, and Coping*. New York: Springer.

Leino P & Magni G (1993). Depressive and distress symptoms as predictors of low back pain, neck-shoulder pain and other musculoskeletal morbidity: a 10-year follow-up of metal industry employees. *Spine*, 53,89–94.

Levi L (1972). Stress and distress in response to psychosocial stimuli. *Acta Med Scand*, 191,528–538.

Levi L (1987). Definition and the conceptual aspects of health in relation to work. In R Kalimo, MA El Batawi, & CL Cooper (Eds). *Psychosocial Factors at Work* (pp. 5–10). Geneva: World Health Organization.

Linton SJ (1995). Overview of psychosocial and behavioral factors in neck and shoulder pain. *Scand J Rehab Med*, 32,67–77.

Marshall N & Barnett R (1991). Race, class, and multiple role strains and gains among women employed in the service sector. *Women Health*, 17,1–19.

Nachemson AL (1992). Newest knowledge of back pain: a critical look. *Clin Orthop Related Res*, 279,8–20.

Parkes KR (1986). Coping in stressful episodes: the role of individual differences, environmental factors and situational characteristics. *J Pers Soc Psychol*, 51,1277–1292.

Peacock EJ & Wong PT (1990). The Stress Appraisal Measure (SAM): a multidimensional approach to cognitive appraisal. *Stress Med*, 6,227–327.

Peate WF (1994). Occupational musculoskeletal disorders. *Prim Care*, 21,313–327.

Pellino TA & Oberst MT (1993). Perception of control and appraisal of illness in low back pain. *Orthop Nurs*, 11,22–26.

Portnoy LC & Watkins MP (1993). *Foundations of Clinical Research: Applications to Practice*. Norwalk, CT: Appleton & Lange.

Repetti RL (1993). The effects of workload and the social environment at work on health. In L Goldberger & S Brenitz (Eds). *Handbook of Stress: Theoretical and Clinical Aspects* (pp. 368–385). New York: Free Press.

Rhodewalt F & Strube M (1985). A self attribution reactance model of recovery from injury in Type A individuals. *J Appl Soc Psychol*, 15,330–344.

Rhodewalt F & Fairfield M (1990). An alternative approach to Type A behaviour and health: psychological reactance and non-compliance. In M Strube (Ed). *Type A Behavior* (pp. 293–312). Newbery Park, CA: Sage Publications.

Ross P (1994). Ergonomic hazards in the workplace, assessment and prevention. *AAOHN J*, 42,171–176.

Seyle H (1936). A syndrome produced by diverse noxious agents. *Nature*, 138,2–4.

Simons D (1990). Muscular pain syndromes. *Adv Pain Res Ther*, 17,1–41.

Smith M (1987). Occupational stress. In M Salvendy (Ed). *Handbook of Human Factors* (pp. 844–875). New York: Wiley.

Smith TW & Rhodewalt F (1986). On states, traits, and processes: a transactional alternative to the individual differences assumptions in Type A behavior and physiological reactivity. *J Res Pers*, 20,229–251.

Vikari-Junitura E, Vuori J, Silverstein B, Kalimo R, & Videman T (1991). A lifelong prospective study on the role of psychosocial factors in neck-shoulder and low back pain. *Spine*, 16,1056–1061.

Waddell G (1992). Biopsychosocial analysis of low back pain. *Baillieres Clin Rheumatol*, 6,523–557.

PART IV
Work-Site Assessment and Recommendations

Chapter 10

Job Analysis and Work-Site Assessment

Melanie T. Ellexson

In the late 1970s and early 1980s, U.S. industry began to recognize its responsibility for active management and prevention of injury in the workplace. Corporate owners acknowledged that a safer workplace can improve productivity and reduce costly claims. The primary activities for prevention and wellness are education, fitness, and workplace modification. These activities must be based on a functional analysis of work activity.

Government agencies and national law have provided industry with both demands and guidance for regulating workplace safety. In 1990, the Occupational Safety and Health Administration (OSHA) developed guidelines for control of cumulative trauma in the red meat industry. At the heart of these guidelines, which now have been applied to many different industries, is a thorough evaluation of work tasks. The Americans with Disabilities Act, a statement of civil rights for disabled individuals, was signed into law on July 26, 1990. This act, with far-reaching implications for both employment and accessibility, identifies the functional job description as being a key document in determining compliance with the regulations set forth in the law. Knowledge of the tasks workers are required to complete, the effects of these tasks on the human body and mind, and the role of tools, equipment, and the work environment have become mandated and plain good business.

Job Analysis Overview

This chapter discusses the components of job analysis that are necessary for company compliance with laws and regulations and serves as a basis for intervention and prevention programs. The chapter first outlines the steps for job analysis, then discusses the additional steps for assessment of cumulative trauma disorders. The first step in analyzing a job is to determine the essential job functions (see Appendix 10.1).

Essential functions or tasks are the basic job duties that an employee must be able to perform, with or without reasonable accommodation. Each job must be carefully examined to determine which tasks are essential to job performance. The Americans with Disabilities Act provides the following examination guidelines for determining if a task is an essential function (*Federal Register* 1991).

- Whether the reason the position exists is to perform that function
- The number of other employees available to perform the function or among whom the performance of the function can be distributed
- The degree of expertise or skill required to perform the function
- The work experience of present or past employees in the job

195

- The time spent in performing a function
- The consequences of not requiring an employee to perform a function
- The terms of a collective bargaining agreement

Simple examples of essential functions are ringing up sales and making change for the store clerk, answering the phone for the office receptionist, or evaluation of the spine for the physical therapist working in orthopedics.

Work, Worker, and Workplace

An accurate and complete functional job description must include analyses of three major components of work activity: the work, the worker, and the workplace. To make this assessment, one must analyze the task to be completed, the physical and mental requirements of the person doing the work, and the tools, equipment, and work space of the specific company.

The Work

Analysis of the work activity is a systematic study of a specific job in terms of what is done with data, people, and objects. Such analysis requires breaking each essential function down into sequential steps that describe clearly what must be done to accomplish the function. The analysis should organize activity into meaningful units. The following example of this process details a packing position in a food manufacturing operation.

Job title: Packer
Essential function: Packing individual cobbler cups for shipping
Steps:

1. Select a box.
2. Place the box on the conveyor side rack.
3. Pick up one cobbler cup in each hand.
4. Place the cups into the packing box.
5. Repeat steps 3 and 4 until 36 cups are in a box.
6. Place the filled box on the sealing table.
7. Fold down the short flaps of the box top.
8. Fold down the longer flaps of the box top.
9. Tape down the long flaps of the box, using the manual taping machine.
10. Place the sealed box on the pallet.

In an analysis of specific work tasks, the number of repetitions necessary in each core activity must be documented. The foregoing example demonstrates that picking up the cobbler cups to fill each box is repeated 18 times with each hand. It would also be necessary to determine how many boxes are to be filled in a given period and how many hours per day the packing actually takes place. It would be important to determine what the production standards for this task are (e.g., how many boxes are to be packed in a shift; whether pay is based on the number of boxes packed). The weight of the box empty and packed and the height, width, and depth of the box all must be noted. The weight of the filled cobbler cups and the dimensions of each cup must be determined. These measurements, which affect physical function, are the beginning steps in looking at the worker (see Appendix 10.2).

The Worker

In evaluating the workers in a work force, variables such as age, size, and experience must be considered. Studies have shown that younger workers often have a higher rate of injury than do older workers (Brough 1991). Several theories are offered to explain this finding. Frequently, younger, more inexperienced workers are placed in the heavier, higher-risk positions. Younger workers have not yet learned to efficiently use movement patterns. The poultry industry has determined that more experienced workers use fewer motions to debone poultry, thereby reducing their cumulative trauma risk. Knowledge of the work activity and adherence to safety procedures through experience are also believed to play a role in the reduction of injury rates.

It is important to look at the workers as a group to determine the general characteristics of the group. Examples of worker population changes may include shifts in the ethnic population of the work force. This may mean changes in anthropometric measurements and may require changes in worker's tools and equipment. An aging work force could introduce a new group of problems related to older workers. The introduction of women into non-traditional positions may present different problems in a particular worker population.

In evaluating the workers in particular jobs, the therapist uses factors descriptive of activity. These factors are listed in *Selected Characteristics of Occupations Defined in the Dictionary of Occupational Titles,* a supplement to the *Dictionary of Occupational Titles.* These factors include such terms as walking, standing, sitting, stooping, kneeling, crawling, climbing, lifting, reaching, handling, fingering, hearing, and seeing. These factors are correlated with each step of an essential function. For example, the fourth step of the cobbler-packing job requires placing filled cups into the packing box. This function requires *standing* at the conveyor table, *reaching* for the cups, and *handling* the cups to *lift* and place them into the box. Vision would also be an important factor in this step.

Anthropometric measurements can be used to evaluate individual workers or to gather data about a group of workers. The most frequently used measurements are listed here with their relevance to the worker (Pheasant 1986; see Chapter 8 of this book).

- *Stature*: vertical distance from floor to vertex (standing clearance)
- *Shoulder height*: vertical distance from the floor to acromion process (zone of reach)
- *Elbow height*: vertical distance from floor to radius (work surface heights)
- *Hip height*: vertical distance from floor to greater trochanter (functional length of the leg)
- *Knuckle height*: vertical distance from floor to third metacarpal (optional height for heavy lifting)
- *Fingertip height*: vertical distance from floor to tip of middle finger (lowest acceptable level for finger control)
- *Sitting height*: vertical distance from sitting surface to crown of head (clearance required between seat and overhead)
- *Elbow rest height*: vertical distance from sitting to underside of elbow (arm rest and desk-top height, work surface with respect to seat)
- *Thigh clearance*: vertical distance from sitting to top of uncompressed thigh at thickest point (clearance required between seat and underside of work surface)
- *Buttock-to-knee length*: horizontal distance from the back of the uncompressed buttock to the front of the kneecap (clearance between seat back and obstacles in front of the knee)
- *Popliteal height*: vertical distance from floor to popliteal angle (acceptable seat height)
- *Hip breadth*: maximum horizontal distance across the hips in a sitting position (acceptable seat width)
- *Chest depth*: maximum horizontal distance from the vertical plane to the front of the chest (clearance)
- *Abdominal depth*: maximum horizontal distance from the vertical plane to the abdomen (clearance)
- *Elbow-to-fingering length*: distance from back of elbow to tip of middle finger (forearm reach, defining normal working area)
- *Shoulder-to-grip length*: distance from acromion to center of object gripped (zone of convenient reach)
- *Hand breadth*: maximum breadth across the palm of the hand (clearance required for hand access)
- *Hand span*: maximum horizontal distance between the fingertips, both arms stretched sideways (lateral reach)
- *Elbow span*: distance between tips of elbows, both elbows fully flexed, fingertips touching at chest (elbow room)

Anthropometric data must be used judiciously in making assumptions about a group of workers. Averaging worker measurements may provide data that does not fit the worker group if wide disparity in size exists. This could lead to inappropriate and ergonomically incorrect workplace design.

The Workplace

In evaluating the workplace, one must look at space and accessibility, equipment, tools, lighting, temperature, vibration, noise, air quality, the general environment, and aesthetics. One must measure the *space* assigned to various work tasks, clearances between equipment, aisle width, distance from one work area to another, and accessibility to various work areas. *Equipment* evaluation may necessitate measuring the weight to be lifted, the reach, the height of the work surface, seating heights, widths and depths, the height of sighting devices, placement of controls, and force necessary to operate controls. The *tools* used by the worker in the performance of the work should be measured, weighed, and evaluated for the force required in their operation. *Lighting* and visual requirements must be observed and noted for the effect they have on the workplace (see Chapter 8).

Similarly, *temperature* considerations, such as exposure to high heat, humidity, or extreme cold should be documented. Prolonged exposure or intermittent movement between extreme temperatures would be important to note. If a worker was frequently or consistently exposed to direct temperature extremes (e.g., cold running water on the hands and forearms), a measurement of this factor also would be appropriate.

Vibration from tools or equipment or vibrations caused by moving over uneven surfaces must be considered. This measurement is difficult and sometimes expensive to make. The negative effect of any vibration on the worker must be determined. If there is no documented evidence of injury or cumulative trauma attributed to such vibration, one may choose to mention the vibration but not measure this exposure.

Noise can certainly increase stress, create difficulty in communication, and ultimately cause hearing loss in certain frequencies. Audiometric testing may be appropriate if exposure is frequent or over prolonged periods.

Fumes, odors, and general air quality may play a part in worker safety and job satisfaction. Exposure to unpleasant or constant odor must be considered in overall work evaluation.

The general environment, including cleanliness, color, and aesthetic appearance should be noted. Individual perceptions about one's work environment may affect efficiency, attention to detail, and overall satisfaction.

Job analysis can identify those tasks that are of greater risk by identifying forces, postures, and repetitions. It can lead to the development of alternative methods of activity to lower risk of injury and increase productivity.

Ergonomic Assessment: The Basic Plan

Development of technology has led to less physically strenuous jobs. At the same time, psychological stress has increased as the demand for greater proficiency and efficiency has increased. Subse-quently, these developments have created greater risk of repetitive activity and the associated physical degeneration and possibility of injury. Although work environments are often described in terms of technical and physical factors, the psychosocial aspects of the work environment must be considered as part of the broad scope when assessing the workplace (Elmfeldt et al. 1983; Rogers 1988).

Ergonomics, like occupational medicine and rehabilitation, is a multidisciplinary approach encompassing epidemiology, biomechanics, physiology, and psychology. Epidemiology identifies the incidence and distribution of illnesses and injury. OSHA requires most employers to maintain records of work-related injuries and illnesses. Biomechanics concentrates on the physical stresses placed on the musculoskeletal structure of an individual in performing various tasks.

Physiology is concerned with a person's metabolic and cardiovascular responses to various tasks. Research addressing the expenditure of calories and consumption of oxygen during work activity has been well publicized.

A worker's psychological response to physical stress, productivity standards, work environment, and other life stresses has more recently been recognized as a contributing factor to workplace safety. Such response requires assessment and control.

Ergonomic assessment of the work site requires a job analysis that examines the work, the worker, and the work site. A simple seven-step guide will assist the rehabilitation professional in completing an efficient, cost-effective ergonomic work-site assessment.

1. *Job analysis*: Assess the job. Management and employee involvement in this assessment is critical to the accurate documentation of specific job functions.
2. *Problem identification*: Identify the problems and obstacles that require change or adaptation. Again, it is important not to overlook the suggestions of the workers; these are often the most accurate reflections of the work situation.
3. *Problem assessment-solution*: Assess each problem and research solutions. Each problem must be examined, and possible solutions must be developed. Technical and economic factors affecting the implementation of each possible solution must be investigated. Any outside sources of funding should be identified.

4. *Plan development and action*: Devise a plan of action. This plan should describe what measures can realistically be achieved by the team, detail the time frames for the start and completion of each solution, and document the methods by which the plan can be carried out.

5. *Implementation*: Implement the plan. Management and workers must be aware of what is to be changed, why the changes are being made, and what results are anticipated. Worker cooperation and participation are necessary for this step to work smoothly and effectively.

6. *Problem re-evaluation*: Determine what value has been obtained by implementing the plan of action. A decision to continue current activity, to change the activities, or to alter the direction of ergonomic control must be made.

7. *Plan revision*: Take corrective action to alter the plan or to add to the ergonomic management approach in an effort to achieve ongoing utility.

Biomechanical Aspects of Ergonomic Job Analysis

Job analysis requires identification of essential job tasks, describing those tasks, and determining basic physical requirements. Step two of our ergonomic work-site guide requires identification and assessment of problem areas. Biomechanics is one frame of reference that analyzes human activity effectively. The rehabilitation professional then must relate that activity to the work environment and to the cognitive, emotional, and social aspects of function.

Biomechanical analysis can be quite complex and can include concepts of physics, linear motion, gravity, torque, and equilibrium (Brough 1991). The rehabilitation professional must have a working knowledge of biomechanical principles in assessing ergonomic problems. Biomechanical factors include movement, position, weight, force or grip, vibration, and the environment.

Once a problem has been identified, one can begin the assessment by evaluating the factor of movement to find ergonomic solutions. The body requires the right amount of movement to operate efficiently. Too much movement may cause dynamic fatigue; too little movement may cause static fatigue. Each essential task should be analyzed for frequent

repetitive motions or too little motion (Brough 1991; Roberts & Falkenberg 1992). Some tasks can involve both static and dynamic movements. An example is the act of sawing a board (see Chapter 7).

The person holds the board in place with one hand; this is static motion. The hand sawing the board is involved in dynamic movement. In this example, the static motion creates greater fatigue because of the force exerted to hold the board in place and by the extension of the arm away from the body.

Force and distance from the body are two of the components that affect movement. Others are twisting and time spent on the activity. Force is defined as something that causes an object to be moved. Normal forces push surfaces together or pull them apart (Brough 1991). In the preceding example, the upper extremity holding the board pushes the surfaces of the glenohumeral joint together. This compressive force pushes tissue together and causes muscle to shorten and thicken. If the saw were to bind or get caught up in the sawing process, causing the arm in motion to pull against resistance, the anatomic structures would get longer and narrower. This reaction is called *tensile force*. Normally, structures return to their original shape; this ability is called *elasticity*. If elasticity is exceeded, injury may result. Ergonomic assessment requires careful examination of forces acting on the body during movement (Roberts & Falkenberg 1992).

It is important to assess the workers' movement to determine where activity occurs in relation to the body. Generally, activity taking place away from an individual center of gravity creates greater risk. Certain questions must be asked in evaluating movement:

- Is the task necessary?
- Are certain muscle groups overused?
- Can the work be done by calling on larger muscles or groups of muscles?
- Can a variety of motions be introduced into the task?
- Can either the right or left hand be used?
- Can adjustments be made to the work task or work surface to reduce static or dynamic fatigue?
- Is alternating the task or job rotation a possibility?
- Is there a jig or fixture that could add support?
- Is the frequency of the task caused by machine pacing?

- Is the frequency of the task caused by an incentive plan?
- Is overtime involved?
- Are there adequate rest periods between activity?

In the board-sawing example, one ergonomic solution would be to fix the board to the work surface by use of a jig or C-clamp. This would eliminate static movement of the worker's upper extremity (Brough 1991). Generally, a variety of movements within a task or group of tasks creates less fatigue than does the same movement repeated over and over. Proper work-rest cycles are important elements for ergonomic control. Muscles respond better to frequent short breaks than to less-frequent long breaks. Precaution must be taken to ensure that job rotation does not move workers from one task to another with similar motion requirements (Brough 1991).

Positional Posture

Position as an ergonomic factor really must be looked at in two separate ways. First to be examined is the position of a load both before and after it is moved. Critical factors to observe are the angle of the back, extension of the arms, and bending of the legs. For example, picking up and moving a 4-lb object at arm's length places more force on the back than does holding or carrying a 40-lb object at waist level.

Second to be examined is the body position through the task. If the worker maintains one position for long periods, the body will fatigue faster than if it is moving periodically. Soldiers at parade rest often complain of fatigue greater than that experienced in marching. Shoulder position is also important. Stress on the shoulder is reduced when the elbow is kept close to the body. The optimal angle between the upper arm and forearm is dependent on the task to be accomplished. For light and fine motor tasks, the optimal angle is 90 degrees. As the weight of the object being manipulated increases, the angle also increases. Carrying a heavy suitcase is easier with the arms straight down at 180 degrees. Wrist position is also important (Rogers 1988). The wrist in neutral position allows for greatest strength. Wrist flexion to 60 degrees reduces strength by more than 50%. Extension to 60 degrees reduces strength to approximately 60%.

Ulnar and radial deviation also reduce strength of grip (Rogers 1988).

Other questions the health care practitioner may ask include the following:

- Is the position for the task necessary?
- Can the object's shape, size, or placement be changed?
- What keeps the load from being held close to the body?
- Is there room for the feet and legs?
- Is it possible to keep the back straight?
- Is there a mechanical device that could do the job?
- Can the tasks be modified to allow the elbows to be kept close to the body?
- Is there a way to support the arms?
- Can the objects to be manipulated be supported with a counter balance, jig, or brace?
- Can the person use either hand to perform the task?
- Can the work surface be adjusted for better position?
- Can handles be added or changed to improve position?

Position solutions might include designing work stations to provide as much flexibility as possible. Foot- and armrests can be added for support. Periodic stretch breaks allow muscles to move through their entire range of motion. This allowance is particularly important when tasks require static positions or very little movement. Avoiding overhead work by raising the person or lowering the work not only avoids muscle fatigue but reduces strain on the heart, which must pump blood to elevated areas (Brough 1991). The ideal arm position is with the elbows as close to the body as possible. For fine motor activity, the forearms should be kept at approximately 90 degrees to the upper arm. Support should be considered if the arms must be extended for longer periods. Supports must not restrict movement or place stress on the arms or wrist. Whenever possible, workstations should be designed to allow workers to complete tasks at positions of greatest strength.

Force (Weight)

Weight is another factor to be considered in finding ergonomic solutions. Logic tells us that the greater the weight of the object to be manipulated, the higher the risk of injury. Age, weight, height, gender, and physical condition also affect how heavy an object feels to a particular person (Rogers 1992). In the board-sawing example, the saw represents a variable weight. To some it may seem heavy, whereas to others its weight is insignificant.

Questions to consider when examining weight are:

- Is the task necessary?
- Can the object be broken down into smaller components?
- Can the object be handled mechanically?
- Are there people available to assist with the tasks?
- Is employee selection or rotation possible?
- Are there mechanical aids that could be modified or adapted to reduce the physical demands of the lift?

It is important to remember that the force on the body during a lift is a combination of the weight of the upper body, the weight of the object, and the distance of the object from the body (Brough 1991). Simply reducing the weight of an object may not reduce the force on the back to the degree expected. Reducing an object's weight may increase repetitions of task and add to fatigue. In general, the advantage of changing body position will be greater than that of reducing the weight of the object.

Grip Force

Another important ergonomic factor is force as related to grip. The human hand is a nearly perfect processor or end receptor. It can be positioned at desired places, exert force to hold or move objects, provide tactile information about the environment and provide feedback for the control of force and movement. In gripping action, parts of the hand are used in mechanical opposition to each other to exert force on an object and hold it in place. Grip force is discussed in greater detail in Chapter 8.

Gripping actions may be divided into three main categories: (1) A *power* grip requires the fingers to flex around an object and hold it against the palm; (2) a *precision* grip is used to hold an object between the tips or pads of the thumb and fingers; and (3) an *open* grip is used when an object rests on the hands. This grip is used in carrying large objects without handles (Pheasant 1992). The grip used for work activity is dependent on the objects to be manipulated and the demands of a particular task. Some tasks allow for gripping in only one way. An example of this limitation is seen in holding a hammer. This activity requires a power grip. The amount of force necessary to hold the hammer is dependent on hand strength and size, density of the material being hammered, and speed used in the activity. Holding the nail would require a precision grip, and force would be related directly to the size of the nail and the position of the hand in relation to the body. Pounding a nail into a wall above shoulder height generally would require more forceful exertion in gripping the nail. The tendons that connect the fingers to muscle in the forearm pass through the carpal tunnel of the wrist. If the wrist is bent, grip strength is lost.

Gloves also influence the amount of power available. Gloves without seams between the fingers interfere the least with grip force. Thick gloves with seams can reduce grip strength by 40%. If bare-handed grip strength is rated as 100% of available power, wearing rubber gloves reduces strength by 25%, and heat-resistant gloves reduce strength by approximately 40%.

It is important to remember that the greater the force required for a grip, the shorter period of time a grip can be maintained. Recovery time, or the time required for muscles to be able to perform at maximum, also increases with the grip force required for an activity (Rogers 1988).

Certain questions should be asked in evaluating grip force:

- Is the task necessary?
- Are objects as light as possible?
- Can supports be added to reduce the force required?
- Is the body in the best position for the activity?
- Can the activity be performed with the wrist in neutral?
- Are there available tools that would reduce the amount of force required?

The amount of force a person must exert is dependent on body position. Workplaces should be designed to allow for maximum flexibility in moving the body into positions best suited to the individual. Objects to be gripped should be clean and as free of grease or oil as possible. Slippery surfaces require greater force to grip. If gloves are used for work activities, they should fit properly and allow for optimal grip. Tools should fit the hand of the user. Mechanical devices for holding, stabilizing, or assisting with activity will decrease the force required and will reduce fatigue.

Vibration

The body's response to the ergonomic factor of vibration will vary with frequency and duration of time spent on the task. Vibration may cause tissue and nerve damage and cause small blood vessels to close. Vibration causes muscle to contract, thereby adding to fatigue. The use of certain hand tools, machinery, and equipment may cause muscles to tire as they absorb vibration. Tighter grasp is necessary to hold vibrating tools.

Certain questions also must be asked in assessing vibration:

- Is the task necessary?
- Have tools been properly maintained?
- Are new tools designed to reduce shock and vibration?
- Can the tool be mounted in a fixture that will absorb the shock or vibration?
- Can the tool be counterbalanced to help reduce the force required?
- Can the worker assume a position for maximum benefit?
- Can the tool be used (or the activity performed) with the wrist in neutral position and the arms close to the body?
- Can the tool or work area be modified to fit the worker?
- Can the work area be isolated from vibration?

Hand tools are common sources of vibration in the workplace. As new tools are designed to reduce or eliminate vibration, replacements should be considered. Although padded handles and shock-absorbing gloves may reduce vibration, they may also require a person to use greater force in gripping. There is a natural tendency to grip vibrating tools

harder; thus, such hand tools should not be in awkward or end-range positions, as the effects of vibration will increase (see Chapter 8).

Environment

The final ergonomic factor to be considered is the environment. The human body works best within certain temperature ranges—generally 65–75°F (Battie et al. 1989). More specifically, the optimal temperature for mental work is 70°F, with 65°F being the most comfortable for physically active people. Sedentary workers will be most comfortable at approximately 72°F (Pheasant 1992).

Particularly when combined with heavy physical work and high humidity, high temperatures can cause increased fatigue, dehydration, abnormal cardiac function, and even collapse. Perspiration can make the hands slippery, requiring added exertion to maintain grip on tools and equipment. Cold can cause joints to stiffen, because of reduced blood supply. This condition may decrease productivity and can cause hypothermia if workers are inactive. Wearing gloves for protection from cold will increase the force necessary for grip. Extra or bulky clothing may increase fatigue.

Questions to ask in evaluating environmental conditions may include:

- Is the task necessary?
- Can drafts be controlled or eliminated?
- Can cooling fans be added?
- Can warm or cool air be supplied?
- Is heat adequate?
- Can areas be fully or partially enclosed?

Certain materials, such as steel, transfer heat and cold faster than do wood or rubber. Tool handles should be covered or wrapped to prevent exposure (Brough 1991). For the safety of the workers, production schedules may have to be altered during periods of extreme heat or cold. Increased rest periods may offer a measure of safety by reducing fatigue. The effects of the environment may be reduced by work-schedule changes that allow for the most physically demanding work to be done at the most optimal time.

References

Battié MC, Bigos SJ, Fisher LD, Hansson TH, Jones ME, Wortley MD (1989). Isometric lifting strength as a predictor of industrial back pain reports. *Spine,* 14,851–856.

Brough (1991). *Evaluating Your Workplace.* Washington, DC: Brough & Associates.

Elmfeldt G, Wise C, Bergsten H, & Alsson A (1983). *Adapting Work Sites for People with Disabilities: Ideas from Sweden.* Sweden: The Swedish Institute for the Handicapped.

Federal Register (July 26, 1991). Part V: Equal Employment Opportunity Commission 29 CFR part 1630, *Equal Employment Opportunity for Individuals with Disabilities; Final Rule* (p 35736).

Pheasant S (1986). *Body Space: Anthropometrics, Ergonomics and Design* (pp. 71–81). London: Taylor & Francis.

Pheasant S (1992). *Ergonomics, Work and Health.* Rockville, MD: Aspen.

Roberts SL & Falkenberg SA (1992). *Biomechanics: Problem Solving for Functional Activity.* St. Louis: Mosby.

Rogers SH (1988). Matching workers and work site ergonomic principles in work injury—management and prevention. In SJ Isernhagen (Ed). *Work Injury Management* (pp. 65–79). Rockville, MD: Aspen.

Rogers S (1992). A functional job analysis technique in ergonomics. In JS Moore & A Garg (Eds). *State of the Art Review* (Vol 7, no. 4, pp. 679–711). Philadelphia: Hunley and Belfus, Inc.

Appendix 10.1

Sample Job Analysis

Company: Glenstead Sanitary District (GSD)

Position: Laborer

The essential functions of this position are:
1. Course screening
2. Garbage collection
3. Cleaning tank
4. Digging ditches
5. Sampling

The marginal activities are:
1. Indoor cleaning
2. Moving furniture
3. Planting trees
4. Snow removal

An analysis of each essential function was performed on September 23, 1991, at the Southwest GSD and on October 14, 1991, at the West GSD. Results are as follows.

Course Screening

This task is performed by a five-person crew and must be done two times per day. On average, one can is filled at a time. Workers descend metal stairs to enter the lower level of the building. Workers are required to use a pitchfork or shovel to move large bulk waste products from a 23.5 in.–high flat shelf and put it in 3.5 ft–high wheeled metal cans. When 12 cans are filled with waste (on average twice per week), they are emptied by two workers, who push the wheeled cans to a loading area. A large cellar-type door is opened on the upper level, and a motorized hoist is lowered to the cans. The cans are hoisted to the upper level, where a worker, using a vertical chain, pulls each can through the air for 5–10 ft to a large dumpster. While one worker holds the can in place with the chain, the second worker pulls the bottom lever, which is waist- to chest-high. Then they tip the can to empty the contents. The can is lowered by using the hoist and is moved back into place by the workers on the lower level. On average, the process requires 25–40 minutes to fill the 12 cans and 90 minutes to empty them.

Physical Requirements

Standing	To use the pitchforks, pull cans, operate hoist, empty cans
Walking	To pull cans, move about workstation
Climbing	Two flights of stairs
Pulling	To move can to dumpster, to open cellar door
Pushing	To move the cans to the hoist
Lifting	To pick up refuse on shovel or pitchfork
Reaching	With shovel or pitchfork, to move cans on the hoist
Handling	Tools and equipment
Hearing	To coordinate teamwork
Seeing	To position cans, pick up waste
Speaking	To give directions, questions

Measurements

Cellar-type door	40 in. high, 60 lb force to open
Flat shelf	23.5 in. high, 23 in. wide, 12 ft. long
Cans	Pulled 5–10 ft, force required is 60 lb; pushed 25 ft, force required is 80 lb; height 3.5 ft, diameter 26 in.; force to push lever is 10 lb
Pitchfork	Length, 42 in.; weight, 6 lb
Shovel	Length, 42 in.; weight, 6 lb
Waste to be removed	Average 6–8 lb
Stairs	58 stairs
Hoist chain height	36–44 in.

Garbage Collection

Two workers pick up 55-gal drums filled with refuse. Cans are at ground level and are lifted with a two-person lift to a 42 in.–high dumpster. Approximately 15 cans per day are emptied. A five-man team usually takes 45 minutes to complete this task each day.

Physical Requirements

Walking	To get garbage can and to empty it
Lifting	55-gal drums
Carrying	To move cans to dumpster
Handling	Drums
Reaching	To tip drums
Seeing	To handle, lift, and empty drums

Cleaning Tanks

A 40-ft ladder is carried by two people 100 ft, from a storage area to large, open, in-ground tanks. The foot end of the ladder is lowered into the tank. A worker then descends the ladder, carrying two 4- to 6-lb wooden blocks. The blocks are placed under freely moving metal beams so that water can flow under the beams. The worker climbs out of the tank and hooks a 100-ft length of 1.5-in. hose to a hydrant. The hoses are stored outside and must be pulled 100–300 ft to the connection. A nozzle is attached to the hose, and the tanks are hosed out from the top. Then a worker descends into the tank, the hose is lowered to the worker, and the tank floor is hosed down. Two workers clean 5–6 tanks per week. It requires approximately 30 minutes to clean each tank.

Physical Requirements

Standing	To clean tank
Walking	On the ground, in the tank to move hoses and ladder
Carrying	Blocks, ladder
Lifting	Ladder, hoses, blocks, metal beams
Stooping	To attach hose, lace blocks, lift metal beams, maneuver hoses
Pulling	Hose, hydrant valve, ladder (from tank)
Pushing	To place ladder, move metal beams
Handling	Hoses, blocks, ladder, nozzle, hydrant

Measurements

Wooden blocks	6 lb
Metal beams	12 ft × 4 in. × 4 in.; 60 lb
Hose	200 ft long, 60 lb pressure, 20 lb to pull
Tank	35–45 ft deep
Hydrant	12 lb torque to turn faucet on and off

Digging Ditches

A worker uses a shovel to assist a back-hoe operator in digging ditches to access pipe or cable. Typically, ditches are dug to a depth of 9 ft. Excess dirt is hauled away by the back-hoe. A single worker will spend 2–3 days per month digging and refilling ditches for repair of pipe or cable.

Physical Requirements

Standing	To allow back-hoe to work
Stooping	To use shovel
Lifting	Dirt on the shovel
Carrying	Shovels
Climbing	Into, out of ditch
Handling	Shovel
Seeing	Equipment, dirt to be removed

Sampling

A worker positions himself or herself over an in-ground tank. To obtain a sample, the worker dips a 6-ft pole fitted with a 2-cup measure at one end into the sludge in the tank. The worker draws the pole back, removes the cup from the pole, and pours its liquid contents into a gallon jar situated on a 48 in.–high table. When the proper samples are collected, six jars are placed in a wooden carrier and transported to the central lab. Each tank is sampled every 4 hours, 24 hours per day. Each worker samples 12 tanks per hour. There are 40 tanks.

Physical Requirements

Standing	To take samples
Walking	To take samples to the lab, travel between table and tank
Lifting	Sampler stick, wooden carrier
Carrying	Wooden carrier
Reaching	To take sample jars, load and unload samples
Handling	Sample jars, sample cup, carrier, stick

Measurements

Wooden carrier	22 in. × 12 in. × 22 in.; weight empty: 12 lb; weight full: 25–30 lb
Sampler stick	6 ft long, weight: 7 lb
Table	Height, 48 in.
Tank	In-ground, up to 14 ft deep
Distance walked to lab	150–300 ft
Gallon jug	1.5 lb empty, 4–5 lb full

Skill or Specialization Required

A high-school diploma or GED equivalent is required. Within the first 12 months of employment, a worker must successfully complete two 1-week classes in sampling procedures and toxic waste hazards control. This is a nonunion position.

Number of People Available to Perform the Job

There is one 5-person crew. The crew works an 8-hour day from 7 AM to 3 PM. Some tasks are performed by a partial crew.

Psychological Considerations

Workers work in teams and independently. At times, teamwork is important for safety. Work is routine.

Physiologic Considerations

Workers are exposed to chemicals and odors that could affect respiratory function.

Environmental Considerations

Workers are expected to work both inside and outside in all weather. Frequently, noxious odors are present.

Safety equipment includes steel-toed boots, gloves, goggles, and hard hats. Certain tasks require protective clothing, such as disposable coveralls and raincoats.

Cognitive Skill Required

The abilities to read and to follow written protocol for safety are necessary. The ability to follow verbal communication is important.

Appendix 10.2

Job Analysis Worksheet

Essential task: _____

Company: _____

Position: _____

Measurements

Name of item: _____   Name of item: _____

Height: _____   Height: _____

Width: _____   Width: _____

Length: _____   Length: _____

Depth: _____   Depth: _____

Weight: _____   Weight: _____

Reach: _____   Reach: _____

Name of item: _____   Name of item: _____

Height: _____   Height: _____

Width: _____   Width: _____

Length: _____   Length: _____

Depth: _____   Depth: _____

Weight: _____   Weight: _____

Reach: _____   Reach: _____

Name of item: _____   Name of item: _____

Height: _____   Height: _____

Width: _____   Width: _____

Length: _____   Length: _____

Depth: _____   Depth: _____

Weight: _____   Weight: _____

Reach: _____   Reach: _____

Essential task: _____

Company: _____

Position: _____

What Part of the Essential Task Involves

Lifting: _____

Carrying: _____

Pushing, pulling: _____

Standing: _____

Walking: _____

Sitting: _____

Climbing: _____

Balancing: _____

Stooping: _____

Kneeling: _____

Crouching: _____

Crawling: _____

Reaching: _____

Reclining: _____

Handling: _____

Fingering: _____

Feeling: _____

Talking: _____

Hearing: _____

Seeing: _____

Tasting: _____

Smelling: _____

Essential task: _____

Company: _____

Position: _____

Sequential Steps

1. _____
   _____

2. _____
   _____

3. _____
   _____

4. _____
   _____

5. _____
   _____

6. _____
   _____

7. _____
   _____

8. _____
   _____

9. _____
   _____

10. _____
    _____

11. _____
    _____

Job analysis date: _____

Position: _____

Company name: _____

Location: _____

Contact person and phone number: _____

Essential Job Tasks

_____   _____
_____   _____
_____   _____
_____   _____
_____   _____
_____   _____
_____   _____
_____   _____
_____   _____
_____   _____
_____   _____

Marginal Job Tasks

_____   _____
_____   _____
_____   _____
_____   _____
_____   _____

Chapter 11

Reducing Injuries, Claims, and Costs

Donald L. Clark

Determining Whether a Claim Is the Result of a Work-Related Injury

An assembly worker walks hurriedly, unaware of a recent oil leak . . . the slip and fall result in a fractured ankle requiring surgical treatment and immobilization. Another employee comes forward with a chemical burn incurred on the job while mixing solutions. A computer programmer presents with gradual-onset neck pain and numbness in the fingers. The fracture and chemical injury were obvious traumatic incidents that occurred during the course of work; there can be no question in the supervisor's mind that these injuries were job related and compensable. In the case of the worker complaining of finger numbness, the employer is not certain that this problem was caused by work demands.

Many types of musculoskeletal injuries can and do arise during the course of work. Obvious, irrefutable claims include slips and falls, burns, lacerations, objects in the eyes, and the like. Often, it is difficult to verify as work-induced such questionable work-related injuries as insidious-onset muscle aches, tendinitis, numbness, and vague strains. Traumatic, *visible* damage is easy for the employee to prove and the employer to substantiate; the evidence is convincing: discoloration, swelling, bleeding, elevated temperature, disfigurement—classic signs of injury and illness. It is difficult to prove as work-related the *invisible* damage that doesn't produce these basic signs and symptoms; there is only the worker's subjective complaint of pain and inability to function normally.

Work-related cumulative trauma to the neuromuscular and skeletal-ligamentous structures has become a well-recognized phenomenon in highly technological societies. Determination of cause and mechanism of injury may require a comprehensive investigative effort involving the injured worker, medical provider, supervisor, safety official, and workers' compensation insurance specialist. A growing number of such claims have become compensable, with a concomitant increase in attention and research directed to this important modern-day problem.

The Worker's Perception of a Job-Related Injury

An employee who sustains a laceration or burn during the customary course of duty will view such an injury as a simple cause-and-effect incident wherein fault lies solely with the worker, the employer, or some combination of both. For the worker who develops tendinitis or nerve damage over a long period, perceptions of cause and responsibility become more complex among a greater number of involved people (i.e., supervisor, coworkers, medical provider, worker's compensation insurer, and attorney).

To illustrate, we can characterize a typical employee as an *industrial athlete*. Just as a competitive athlete uses physical abilities to undertake a sport, so does the industrial athlete who is being paid to carry out physically demanding job tasks. The very same muscles, tendons, nerves, bones, and ligaments that are called into action to undertake athletic endeavors are used to assemble parts, perform keying operations, lift repetitively, and so on.

Consider the worker who presents with rather nondescript pain and numbness in the upper limbs. Compare this individual to an athletic competitor who severely sprains an ankle. Both were carrying out specified activities under the direction of either a coach or a supervisor. In the case of the athletic competitor, the injury was witnessed by all, thus establishing legitimacy. The victim takes on all the empathy, support, and care deserving of a wounded, highly regarded member of the team. The player rests in confidence that the coach, medical provider, and coplayers will direct extraordinary efforts to encourage and resolve the incident until full restoration to the team is achieved. Throughout the entire course of events, the injured athlete receives the strong message: "I am a valuable and essential part of the team. My absence is a loss, and everyone wants me back on the job (field) as soon as possible."

Contrast this scenario with that of the assembly worker and the telecommunications operator, who claim pain in the neck and shoulders and finger numbness. Because the demands of their jobs require constant sitting and repetitive use of the hands, it is their belief that such symptoms arose because of excessive work stressors. These so-called industrial athletes suffer pain and debility just as real and significant as that of the injured competitive athlete.

Instead of receiving validation, these workers get the clear message from their supervisor and coworkers that their ailments are not real injuries but, rather, that they are either faking it or magnifying their problem to access workers' compensation. In the face of critical suspicion, the suffering employees approach the supervisor (coach) and sense the disbelief and harsh judgment before any evidence is in. As predicted, the supervisor eyes them with suspicion, frowns, and tells them to "quit bellyaching" and go back to work. Humbly, the workers quietly slip back to their assignments. Even they are unsure of themselves; after all, their coworkers don't seem to be having any problem.

This situation may play itself out until symptoms and frustration escalate to the point at which medical intervention becomes necessary. The medical examination is essentially negative: There are no remarkable objective findings, and the doctor dismisses these claims with the usual fare of medications and tells the workers to return to the job and "take it easy." In the workers' eyes, this is a rather cursory response that results in additional erosion of self-worth. Ultimately, the workers have become angry with their supervisor, unsatisfied with medical attention and the prevailing lack of regard for their plight. It is not uncommon for individuals in this state of mind to seek legal counsel in anticipation of an adversarial response to their call for a fair and effective response to their injuries. Enmity has been established between these workers and their employer.

These illustrations readily underscore important considerations of which the employer must be aware in dealing with cumulative trauma disorders (CTDs). Slow-onset musculoskeletal ailments do not reveal obvious, heroic symptoms, as in the case of an injured competitive athlete. It is vitally important for supervisors to become aware of both the physical and the psychosocial impacts of gradual-onset neuromusculoskeletal disorders that usually originate as chronic fatigue and intermittent discomfort.

Impact of Supervisor Attitude and Response to Employee Injury Claim

The foregoing illustration brings to light the significance of injury claims policies and procedures. The injured worker who is not acknowledged properly and respectfully will likely become frustrated in an atmosphere of suspicion and poor injury-management practice. Unlike the competitive athlete whose injury is comparatively heroic, the industrial athlete may suffer alone without the open support and assistance necessary to promote a positive attitude and successful resolution.

Musculoskeletal ailments that arise insidiously over a long period are only recently gaining noteworthy attention from medical researchers, health professionals, the legal community, and public policy makers. That such disorders are work related is often questioned or completely dismissed by many employers. Despite subjective opinions, the incidence, severity, and costs associated with work-related CTDs have escalated pandemically over the past several decades (Jaeger et al. 1991; Franklin et al., 1981; Delgrosso & Boillat 1991; Hebert 1993). Critical, judgmental behavior on the part of managers and supervisors will most assuredly drive many injured workers to their attorneys, creating adversarial relationships that produce excessive workers' compensation costs and damaged lives.

Relationship of Costs to Injury Severity

An on-the-job injury may or may not produce a worker's compensation claim. Principle costs of a claim arise from time out of work, medical expenses, and insurance indemnity payments. Additional costs to the employer include all indirect expenses, such as overtime for other workers to cover the injured employee, cross-training, hiring temporary replacements, and so forth. Expenses increase further when litigation enters the picture. The direct cost of a properly handled claim for a simple nonsurgical elbow tendinitis may be as little as $75–150 for medical treatment, medication, and only several hours of lost time. A mismanaged, adversarial claim for the same diagnosis may result in more than $100,000 of direct and indirect expenses if medical treatment is unsuccessful and significant disability results.

Thus far, we have demonstrated an important link between injury management policies, the worker's perception of injury, the prevailing attitude of the employer, and costs. Those who wish to enlarge their understanding and to uncover cost-saving strategies must give consideration to the foregoing medical, social, and legal influences on costs. Injuries, claims, and costs are separate but related entities. Employers who endeavor to maximize productivity, prevent injuries, and promote good relations must treat each of these segments uniquely to establish successful safety and injury prevention programs.

Emerging Strategies for Ergonomics and Injury Prevention Programs

We can well appreciate the relatively simple cause-and-effect relationship that exists between an obvious sudden injury and its cause. Risk factors for falls or burns, for example, can be reduced or eliminated readily without intensive study and problem solving by a multidisciplinary effort.

By contrast, slow-onset injuries, the so-called CTDs of the neuromusculoskeletal system, often originate from complex and elusive predisposing and precipitating factors (US Department of Health and Human Services 1989; Sandler 1993; Newcombe 1994; Lew & Garfinkel 1983). Problem-solving to avoid this group of disorders often demands input from managers, technicians, supervisors, employees, health professionals, and (possibly) consultants with expertise in ergonomics.

With the rise in the incidence of work-related musculoskeletal injuries (CTDs), increasing attention has been directed to workplace factors that can contribute to or cause such injuries. At the forefront of ergonomic research and problem-solving strategies is the Occupational Safety and Health Administration (OSHA).

Before proceeding, it is useful to develop our perspective and understanding of the terms *ergonomic hazards* and *ergonomic disorders*. The National Institute of Occupational Safety and Health has proposed revised definitions of these terms. Ergonomic hazards relative to work-related musculoskeletal disorders refer to physical stressors and workplace conditions that pose a risk of injury or illness to the musculoskeletal system of the worker. Ergonomic hazards include repetitive and forceful motions, vibration, temperature extremes, and awkward postures that arise from poorly designed workstations, tools and equipment, and improper work methods. The effects of ergonomic hazards may be amplified by extreme environmental conditions. In addition, ergonomic hazards may arise from potentially deleterious job designs and organizational factors, such as excessive work rates, external (versus self-) pacing of work, excessive work durations, shift work, imbalanced work-to-rest ratios, demanding incentive pay or work standards, restriction of operator body movement and confinement of the worker to a workstation without adequate relief periods, electronic monitoring, and lack of task variety. The term *ergonomic disorders* has fallen into disfavor and now is being replaced by the concept embodied in the phrase *work-related musculoskeletal disorders*. Such disorders are those diseases and injuries that affect the musculoskeletal, peripheral nervous, and neurovascular systems and are caused or aggravated by occupational exposure to ergonomic hazards.

In light of the foregoing definitions, consider the implications in the case of a meat cutter who complains of wrist pain and loss of sensation in the fingers. According to the National Institute of Occupational Safety and Health definitions, this worker has sustained a work-related cumulative trauma injury because an ergonomic hazard exists. In this case, the primary hazards are highly repetitive motions, excessive force, and awkward posturing of the upper limb, particularly the wrist and fingers. This model would direct us to an *ergonomic solution*, that is, some type of engineering remedy that reduces or eliminates known hazards. The elements of force and awkward positioning of the upper limb are addressed through redesign of cutting tools that will permit the operator to work with the wrist more in neutral position or midposition. Such tool modification also provides for better leverage of the entire upper limb, thereby reducing average force. This relatively simple sequence, wherein an ergonomic (engineering) fix has resulted in an ergonomic solution, partially fulfills the definition of ergonomics by adjusting work to fit the capabilities of the worker.

Despite such engineering interventions intended to reduce risk factors, workers may still incur progressive stress and fatigue as a result of other factors, such as habitual work style, poor work-to-rest ratios, piecework, and excessive work hours. Commonly, individuals will suffer persistent musculoskeletal ailments due to intrinsic health problems, poor fitness, psychosocial stress, and habitually strenuous posture and body mechanics. The forthcoming discussions stress the importance of ergonomic corrective strategies that complement engineering solutions by attending human performance and psychosocial factors fully.

The OSHA activities that have contributed to our understanding and approach to work-related musculoskeletal injuries include the Occupational Safety and Health Act of 1970, mandating that it is the general duty of all employers to provide a workplace free from recognized serious hazards, including the prevention and control of ergonomic hazards. In January 1989, OSHA published voluntary *General Safety and Health Program Management Guidelines* (1989), which are recommended to all employers as a foundation for their safety and health programs and as a framework for their ergonomics programs. In addition, OSHA has developed *Ergonomic Program Management Guidelines for Meatpacking Plants* (August 1990). These voluntary guidelines mark the beginning of a nationwide effort by OSHA to help reduce or eliminate worker exposure to ergonomic hazards that lead to CTDs and related illnesses and injuries. The suggested program includes a coordinated effort involving enforcement, information, training, cooperative programs, and research.

The essential components of these recommendations are outlined as follows:

I. Management commitment and employee involvement
   A. Top management commitment
      1. Visible, serious commitment to hazard elimination
      2. Same high priority given to safety as production
      3. Delegation of responsibilities among the ranks
      4. Establishing authority and provision of resources
      5. Assigning accountability where appropriate
   B. Employee involvement
      1. Establish employee feedback without reprisal
      2. Reporting procedure (for CTDs)
      3. Inclusion on safety/health committee
      4. Presence on ergonomics team
   C. Written program
   D. Regular program review and evaluation
II. Program elements
   A. Work-site analysis
      1. Medical, safety, and insurance records
      2. Trend analysis by jobs, department, and so forth
   B. Hazard prevention and control
      1. Engineering controls
         a. Work methods
         b. Workstation design
         c. Tool and handle design
         d. Back injury–prevention program
      2. Work practice controls
         a. Proper work techniques
         b. New employee conditioning period
         c. Regular monitoring
         d. Adjustment and modifications
      3. Personal protective equipment
      4. Administrative controls
         a. Decreased production rates, hence decreased repetition
         b. Improving work-to-rest ratios
         c. Provide optimal staffing
         d. Job rotation

e. Job enlargement

f. Maintenance of tools and equipment

g. Housekeeping and workplace organization

C. Medical management

1. Periodic workplace walk-through

2. Symptom survey

  a. Existence and extent of CTDs

  b. Identification, location of CTDs: jobs, departments, etc.

  c. Establishment of baseline disorder rate for trends analysis

3. Establishment of a modified duty program

4. Health surveillance

  a. Baseline health assessment

  b. Assessment following post conditioning period

  c. Periodic health assessment

5. Employee training and education

6. Early reporting of symptoms

7. Appropriate medical care

8. Protocols for health care providers

D. Training and education

1. General, job-specific supervisor and management training

2. Training for maintenance and engineering staff

The OSHA 3123 ergonomic guidelines include detailed policies, procedures, and suggested methods by which employers and employees may study, identify, and solve ergonomics issues that cause or give rise to work-related musculoskeletal disorders.

The OSHA outline conceptualizes and details strategies targeting the elimination of work-related musculoskeletal injuries that typically develop over a long period. This program's bedrock for success lies in the formation of a management commitment with meaningful employee participation. The basic building blocks of this plan are problem identification and analysis (work-site analysis), hazard prevention and control, medical surveillance and treatment, and education directed to management, employees, and other relevant participants. The forthcoming practical workplace recommendations are derived from the OSHA's ergonomic architecture, from this author's practical experience, and from other sources.

Corrective Recommendations in Action

Administrative Controls

The *Random House College Dictionary,* revised edition, defines the word *administer* as "to manage; have executive charge of; to bring into use or operation; to make application." An administrator is "a person or body of persons that administers or manages affairs of any kind." Administrative policies and strategies can be a powerful deterrent to work-related injuries. The following seven categories of intervention represent important administrative domains under which injury-prevention initiatives can be established:

- Sociopolitical atmosphere and employee morale
- New employee conditioning and orientation
- Productivity standards and paced work
- Safety programs
- An ergonomics task force
- Injury reporting and the accident investigation process
- Early return to work and modified duty

Sociopolitical Atmosphere and Employee Morale

Morale and prevailing employee attitudes derive primarily from the human relations policies and the example set by leaders. Managers, supervisors, and others in authority must set a good role model for fair and equitable leadership to promote employee loyalty and enthusiasm. With regard to the management of CTDs, the company's general policy should be based objectively and nonjudgmentally. Workers with early signs and symptoms of slow-onset musculoskeletal ailments should be encouraged to avoid delays in reporting such problems to management. When the prevailing employee perception is that the supervisor will regard such maladies as "griping aches and pains," workers will be reluctant to come forth, thereby prolonging their discomfort until more serious pathology unfolds. In the author's experience, such mismanaged injury claims produced excessive costs to the company and hardship to the injured worker.

In Case 1 (presented on page 221), the employee is diagnosed with left shoulder tendinitis. Early intervention, appropriate first response by the supervisor, and proper management very likely would have yielded a better outcome for both the company and injured party (Lew & Garfinkel 1983). Work-injured persons are more likely to present a bogus or exaggerated claim in the face of contentious attitudes which prolong heated interpersonal issues.

There are practical steps that management can take to establish optimal attitudes among the work force:

- Establish uniform policies and procedures for the management of CTDs. This procedure connotes management's position that such ailments are a real entity deserving of the same attention as the more obvious traumatic injuries exhibiting overt symptoms.
- Educate management-level personnel about work-related CTDs, thereby instilling an appreciation for the broad implications of this significant industrial health and safety issue.
- Educate the employee about CTDs, early signs and symptoms, risk factors (at work and home), individual responsibility for health and safety, and reporting procedures.
- Include employees in problem solving, policy making, and the development of action plans.

These recommendations are only a few of the many initiatives a company can develop to improve morale and the general positive social atmosphere. Management attitude and leadership style are among the most important determinants of a successful injury abatement program.

New-Employee Conditioning and Orientation

In the context of our characterization of the worker as an industrial athlete, employees who engage in physically demanding jobs will be at less risk for injury if allowance is made for adaptation to the task. Just as a competitive athlete must become trained and skilled at a particular sport, so must the new employee, who will benefit from a gradual adjustment to unfamiliar demands physically, procedurally and psychosocially (APTA 1991; Thompson et al. 1951; Wilson & Wilson 1957; Goidi 1964).

It is important to understand that *physically demanding* does not simply apply to such hard labor as heavy manual work. Jobs that demand constant sitting to perform highly focused, repetitive tasks can and do produce significant human effort, fatigue, and injury. It also is true that more physical stress and less economy of motion occur during early adaptation to new tasks. As the worker becomes more proficient, skill increases, as does higher productivity via more economical technique. These factors are important justifications for establishing a new-employee conditioning or break-in period, which should occur over 2 or more weeks. Close monitoring should ensure that acceptable adjustment and performance are being achieved. Even veteran workers who are transferred to another job assignment should be given an appropriate transition period in which to make adjustment.

It is essential to be mindful of the etiology and mechanism of CTDs. They develop insidiously, over an extended time frame. The earliest symptom is fatigue, which is intermittent at first, then constant. Chronic fatigue, especially local tissue fatigue, can give rise to damage sufficient to produce tendinitis, nerve compression, and other CTDs (Lanfear & Clark 1972). Because of the nature and onset of such injuries, workers who are not adapted physically to work demands should not be cast abruptly into job assignments without an adequate break-in period.

Certain tips are recommended. New employees or those with significant changes in work assignments should be given the opportunity to observe, learn, and practice new skills through a progressive adjustment process. The length of this adaptation period should be commensurate with the individual's learning curve and physical tolerance. Also, policies and procedures should exist to evaluate, monitor, and administrate the process by which this transition period is being managed. Further, provision for employee feedback is essential.

Productivity Standards and Paced Work

A worker's level of energy expenditure and physical effort is linked directly to such influences as the work's physical demands, to incentives, and to enforcement policy. A job's physical demands include such factors as repetition, force, and speed. Incentives entail pay rate, bonuses, special recognition, gifts, benefits, and so forth. Enforcement may be executed through performance appraisal, punitive measures, and other administrative controls. Establishing productivity standards and the supportive human output necessary to meet quotas necessitates a thorough understanding of human capacity, physically and psychosocially.

Consider the experience of running at race pace on a treadmill. Speed and rhythm are dictated by a mechanical standard outside human control and choice. If the accelerated pace continues, the runner (industrial athlete) surely will fatigue and eventually will fall off. This scenario is analogous to production workers who must maintain a preset standard for speed and units per hour of production. Not infrequently, workers who must perform highly repetitive tasks under extrinsic controls for speed are subjected to excessive physical demands, increasing risk for cumulative trauma problems.

Case 1.   A 45-year-old highly skilled assembly operator has 15 years of experience as a veteran solder technician. An increase in demand for product necessitates a mandatory change in work schedule, from a 5-day, 40-hour week to a 6-day, 60-hour week.

The essential physical demands of this job (67–100% of the work shift) are constant sitting; constant elevation of one or both upper limbs such that hands and elbows are non-weight-bearing (unsupported) during task; constant highly focused visual attention for viewing small parts and maintaining fixed positions of minute items and hand tools; and occasional walking (1–33% of work shift). Specifically, as part of a group of assembly functions, this position calls for the ability to execute rapid and forceful bilateral pinching, grasping, and highly coordinated manipulatory activity with cables, plugs, and other assorted accessories, machinery, tools, and hardware. Shoulders, forearms, wrists, and hands are frequently (sometimes constantly) postured in extremes of joint position to carry out job tasks. Tools used include small and large cutters, pliers, screwdrivers, hammers, calipers, micrometers, X-Acto knives, solder guns, picking tools, solder holders, and so forth.

A soldering specialist uses both hands in a very precise and highly coordinated fashion to properly position and stabilize multiple small wire leads in readiness for the soldering process. Typically, such workers sit in nonadjustable metal chairs. Foot support consists of metal cross bars under the work table or empty spools that have been appropriated for such use. The work surface is also nonadjustable and provides space for all necessary tools and working materials, including solder vise, tin dip heater, heat gun, and so on.

Several weeks of extraordinary intense work left the solder operator fatigued, complaining of discomfort in the neck, shoulders, and hands. The left shoulder became so painful that this worker took nonprescription medicine to reduce pain so as to tolerate the long workday. Symptoms persisted even off-duty, placing a serious constraint on this individual's ability to engage in normal activities of daily living.

By the end of the fourth week, this worker's left shoulder was so painful that self-medication was ineffective. Because of the imperative for accelerated productivity and the department's prevailing urgency, this operator initially did not approach the supervisor with a complaint; also, this division's particular supervisor was generally regarded as unsympathetic, dictatorial, and insensitive to employee needs. Tentatively, the injured worker finally approached the supervisor, who responded in a suspicious and disbelieving demeanor. Reluctantly, the supervisor directed this worker to fill out a first report of injury, then ushered the operator off to the company nurse. At the first-aid office, this worker received basic medical attention; however, there were no outward, classic signs of injury, such as edema, redness, bruising, only this individual's subjective report of pain and disability. The recommendation was made for this person to be evaluated by the company physician.

The physician issued a diagnosis of severe tendinitis of the left shoulder (rotator cuff), administered an injection, and wrote a prescription for anti-inflammatory and analgesic medicine. The doctor ordered the employee back to work with restricted duty for a 2-week period. Medical work restrictions of the modified duty assignment were: no lifting above shoulder level; no lifting in excess of 5 lbs; no repetitive motion with the hands; no standing or sitting for more than an 8-hour work shift.

On return to work, the impaired worker was hustled off by the harried supervisor to another department, the manager of which tried "to find something for the injured worker to do." The light-duty assignment was to collate and classify reams of files 8 hours per day. This task required constant sitting and handling of files and stacks of paper.

Details of the Environment.   It is revealing to consider in more depth the details of this modified-duty work environment and its physical demands.

The worker is sitting in an old swivel chair with a deep and wide seat pan, nonadjustable armrests with loose forearm supports, and faulty controls for tilt, backrest, and seat height adjustment. It is necessary to sit toward the front edge of this chair to keep from falling backward, and the high armrests prevent positioning close to the table. This inappropriate and defective chair does not allow the individual to use the backrest; therefore, work is being carried out in the presence of excessive loading and tension of the trunk postural muscles. The work table is of the folding conference type, measuring 3 by 6 fcct. On the table are cardboard file boxes filled with thick folders. The task is to remove selected folders and to separate designated paper material for reorganization. Although this worker may opt to stand, the choice is made to remain sitting to carry out this work. An observer readily can note the frequency of forward reaching and fingering, making for awkward retrieval of bulky paper material that is difficult to handle. The shoulders are elevated to eye level much of the time, allowing minimal weight-bearing rest.

Within 8 hours of this so-called light duty, the worker's left shoulder pain intensified. Why did this happen? At this point, it is necessary to consider all the factors that originally caused or contributed to this injury. Furthermore, attention should be directed to additional circumstances that were associated with the modified duty program and further aggravated this employee's shoulder problem:

- Significant increase in daily and weekly work hours
- Increased work pace and intensity, fewer rest intervals
- Lack of task differentiation to use a broader group of working tissues
- Late symptom reporting
- Late medical intervention
- Adversarial relationship between employee and supervisor
- Sustained and prolonged static posturing of trunk and upper limbs
- Minimal upper-limb weight bearing; prolonged, sustained elevation
- Ill-defined modified duty program; poor supervision and duty assignment
- Supervisor and manager uneducated about injury management

- Poor medical definition of appropriate modified duty

This employee was suffering from a severe pathology of the rotator cuff due primarily to the impact of the work's physical demands. As regards the left shoulder, the modified duty work failed to reduce stress to the injured structures significantly (i.e., tendons of the rotator cuff and contents of the suprahumeral space). This person continued to work with the shoulders elevated into the "impingement zone," and stress was intensified by efforts to handle awkward, bulky file folders and papers from a sitting position. Many of the factors that predisposed this operator to injury on regular duty remained in effect during the alternative work assignment. The story does not have a happy ending: This highly productive and valued employee went on to surgery and extensive rehabilitation, unable to return to regular duty for 6 months.

Selected Corrective Workplace Recommendations. The injured solder operator's experience typifies events and shortcomings so common to work-related CTDs. Consider the previously outlined ergonomic program recommendations by OSHA. This framework serves as a focus on the following selected categories under which ergonomic and injury prevention recommendations will be discussed: administrative controls, ergonomic-engineering controls, exposure reduction controls, and education-training for management and employees. The substance of the forthcoming commentary is drawn from this author's field experience as a health professional specializing in workers' compensation technology, rehabilitation, injury prevention, and ergonomics. Additional case histories will serve as illustrations representing broadly diversified types of industry including health care, manufacturing, and service businesses.

Case 2. A typical example of paced work with predetermined external speed is illustrated by two assembly operators positioned facing each other on opposite sides of a conveyor belt. These assemblers are sitting in nonadjustable, high metal chairs without backrests. The hardwood seats are contoured slightly, and brackets connecting the legs serve as foot supports. Each worker is free to sit or stand and face the conveyor line at any angle desired while carrying out the job task. When sitting, space for alternative foot positioning is minimal, owing to barriers below the conveyor unit. In this scenario, 55-year-old operator 1 is sitting directly facing the conveyor belt, whereas 23-year-old operator 2 is sitting at an oblique angle, facing the oncoming belt. Each worker performs identical functions: inserting a 12-space partitioned divider into a pint-sized container made of cardboard; inserting the sales product into each of the 12 spaces; and closing and securing the side flaps and lid of the container with labeled packing tape.

Close observation of the habitual work style of these operators reveals important distinctions that bear significance on work-related injury risks. As noted previously, operator 1 is sitting with the trunk and arms facing the moving assembly line, whereas operator 2 is positioned at an angle of 45 degrees facing the oncoming belt. More detailed scrutiny reveals very telling ergonomic and behavioral details that can broaden our appreciation of many juxtaposed factors that have an impact on worker performance, productivity, and injury risk.

The details of operator 1's work history and behavior are as follows:

- Has been on the job for 15 years
- Sits forward on the front portion of seat with feet supported
- Sits upright and maintains normal spinal curves
- Head and neck remain in midline during course of work
- Minimizes trunk twisting during packaging procedure
- Product supply located 16 inches from worker's right side in forward-tilted box
- Conveyor line set at operator's elbow height when sitting
- Conveyor belt speed provides ample time to complete task without rushing
- Operator patiently waits for all material to arrive in front of torso before assembly
- All motions are rhythmic, coordinated, and synchronized with conveyor
- Good interpersonal relations with supervisor

Operator 2 is working at the same pace; however, significant differences become apparent as follows:

- Has been on the job for 1 year
- Sits leaning forward, with trunk obliquely facing oncoming conveyor

- Holds head forward, with trunk rotated
- Holds slumped posture, with prominent loss of normal spinal curves
- Sustains shoulder-scapular elevation in "hurry-up" posture
- Makes frantic, jerky movements, as if trying to outrun machine pace
- Is impatient, not waiting for product to arrive directly in front of body
- Frequently fumbles, dropping items
- Frequently complains of fatigue
- Criticizes work layout and physical demands
- Has poor interpersonal relations with supervisor

The younger, less experienced operator 2 approaches the supervisor with complaints of pain in the neck, midback, and shoulders. The worker is convinced that this discomfort is caused by the job's physical demands. The older, more experienced operator is not reporting fatigue problems or criticism of work layout.

Questions that now loom before the supervisor or medical provider are the following:

- Is this worker truly incurring excessive stress because of the design and demands of the job?
- Why is only one of many such operators sustaining undue fatigue and discomfort?
- Are *ergonomic hazards* precipitating this worker's *ergonomic injury*?
- Are we dealing exclusively with ergonomic problems that call for ergonomic interventions (purely engineering changes)?
- Was this operator's problem the result of work stressors that obligated this individual to a restrictive, overly laborious work style or, perhaps, was this person exerting excessive, unnecessary effort as a result of habitual, voluntary activity?

This practical work example serves to highlight important considerations applicable to the design of work as it interfaces with human performance and attitudes. The assembly job did have an externally set pace that was satisfactory and acceptable to 99% of the work force. The solution to injury prevention in this illustration lies less with ergonomic intervention and more with appropriate administrative actions (e.g., job-specific training, allowance for a conditioning-adaptation period, and close monitoring and communication with the less experienced operator).

Case 3.   The next illustration demonstrates how financial incentive can be a contributory factor to the genesis of work-related cumulative trauma injury. As a highly experienced, veteran employee of a wire and cable manufacturer, the operator had the arduous task of inserting 10 lead, color-coded wires into small plastic plugs similar to a common telephone jack plug. The physical demands of this job require the capability of constant forceful pinching and finger manipulation, prolonged sitting, and highly focused visual attention for viewing very small parts. Because of exceptional proficiency at this task, this operator consistently produced 50% more units per hour than did coworkers, thereby earning a significantly higher wage because productivity was linked with wages. Over time, this worker began to experience chronic fatigue and increasing discomfort in the arms and wrists. Symptoms advanced to include numbness and decreased ability to maintain high level of output.

This worker was reluctant to report symptoms, knowing that lost work time or a modified duty assignment would result in reduced wages. Also, a negative stigma was associated with claims for "aches and pains" discomfort. This individual persevered until severity of symptoms intensified, resulting in loss of physical ability to participate in regular duty. The long delay and chronicity of symptoms eventually led to severe pathology requiring surgical treatment and extensive rehabilitation. It is evident here that piecework, equating wages with work output, can be a contributing factor to increased risks for CTDs (Lanfear & Clark 1972; Levi 1972; Welch 1972; Arndt 1987).

It is important to distinguish between general, global body energy expenditure and local muscle fatigue in discussing work pacing and rest periods. With reference to our previous illustration, attention is best directed to the work-rest cycle of the upper limbs, particularly the muscles of the forearms and hands. Historically, work-site experience indicates that incidence of upper-limb CTDs is linked most closely to the work-rest cycle of the forearms and hands and less so with overall body energy expenditure (Rohmert 1973; Borg 1982; Arndt 1985; Rodgers 1987; Putz-Anderson 1992). Guidelines are available for estimating rest pauses for repetitive jobs involving various levels of effort, based on maximum voluntary contractions (Roberts 1987; see Chapters 7 and 8).

From an administrative design, deterrents to injury claims associated with work pacing and piecework must address the influence of incentives or penalties associated with job performance and productivity. Helpful administrative strategies to curb work-related injuries include the following:

- Set work pace at a level that meets workers' physical capabilities safely
- Establish appropriate work-rest cycles
- Apply piecework incentives cautiously, with safeguards to minimize injury risk
- Where feasible, create job rotation to diversify physical demands
- Provide incentives for safety and injury prevention and productivity

Safety Programs

The human relations director of a flashlight manufacturer boasted of a superior safety record: "Safety committees do not wholly create a safe workplace." Although this company did not have a formal, management-led safety committee, it did have a laudable track record of success in preventing CTDs in a working environment wherein significant risks were present. How do we account for this success?

A closer view of this company's injury history reveals important administrative initiatives that led the way to such a positive achievement. Although it is true that the recent 3-year period was free from significant injury claims, previously the company was accumulating up to six CTD claims per year. A decisive change in this costly trend occurred through the coordinated efforts of management and previously injured workers. Having recovered from carpal tunnel surgery, two of the workers became a leading force among the employees. Their efforts produced an employee-centered ergonomic safety team that met regularly and had the full support and participation of upper management. This collaborative endeavor resulted in great strides in ergonomic improvements through effective administrative controls and an employee-led safety task force.

The costly rise in work-related CTDs over the past two decades points to increased urgency to define effective safety and injury prevention programs. Safety committees and their policies and procedures should not be just paper-bound; they should be functionally strong. A company's philosophy toward production can be in conflict with its position on safety. If safety is regarded as inferior to manufacturing, priority will be directed to productivity, with a comparatively weaker commitment to the prevention of work injuries. In light of recent exorbitant workers' compensation costs associated with CTDs, industry is appreciating the need to harmonize production needs with preservation of employee health and well-being.

The concept of process safety management is one way of addressing the possible conflict between manufacturing goals and injury prevention. Process safety management is reflective of a company's total plan to integrate safety seamlessly with all operations. As noted previously, safety committees alone, as isolated entities, do not necessarily create the highest possible level of safety. This larger managing process directs attention to more than traditional precautions; it is a comprehensive means of managing process safety by recognizing and understanding the risks of production and by operating in a safe manner, reducing injury risks. In this broader context, the following recommendations are presented for those managers who wish to construct or improve safety committees and programs:

- Give safety the same priority as that given production
- Establish management safety commitment with employee participation
- Provide for all departments to have representation on the safety committee
- Develop comprehensive policies, procedures, methods, incentives, and so forth
- Define a system for collection and analysis of injury data
- Organize appropriate subcommittees (e.g., for plant operations, maintenance, safety education, hazardous materials, accident investigation, ergonomics team)
- Delegate appropriate authority and responsibilities and provide necessary resources
- Provide for necessary education and training of management and staff

As isolated units, safety committees do not ensure safety. Employee well-being and injury prevention is everyone's job. Company injury statistics will improve when safety planning becomes tightly woven into the matrix of a comprehensive plan that blends manufacturing goals with safety necessities.

An Ergonomics Task Force

An ergonomics team may be a subcommittee of the safety committee or a stand-alone task force given the imperative to undertake all issues pertaining to ergonomics and CTDs. Because of the multifaceted nature of ergonomic science, an ergonomics team should be composed of representatives from management, labor, engineering, maintenance, health care, safety personnel, union, and consultants (if necessary). Production workers should play a prominent role in decision making because they are the key players who must live and work with the final outcomes.

The mission of an ergonomics team should be to recognize and solve problems that are predisposing or causing work-related injuries arising from cumulative trauma. Such a task force will become most effective when it becomes educated and skilled in problem analysis, abatement planning, medical management, surveillance, and training. Not infrequently, it becomes necessary for some companies to contract the services of a consultant with expertise in ergonomics to provide the initial start-up team training and organizational layout (Klafs & Arnheim 1973). For additional details and direction on this subject, the reader is referred to Chapter 13.

Injury Reporting and the Accident Investigation Process

Timely reporting of an incident, accompanied by a full explanation of cause, is a critical component of injury prevention and cost-saving strategy. Such obvious traumatic injuries as contusions, lacerations, burns, and the like routinely are reported immediately. The follow-up investigation usually reveals a straightforward cause that can be remedied easily. Uncovering the causes of cumulative trauma–based musculoskeletal injuries is not as exact and becomes subject to diverse opinion.

The term *mechanism of injury* is important in exposing the fundamental cause of insidious cumulative trauma ailments. In the case of a simple laceration, the injured worker will report that the cut resulted from a slip while using a hand knife to open cardboard boxes. The investigation of this incident reveals that the individual was not following proper procedures (i.e., wearing a protective glove on the hand receiving the injury). In this case, the mechanism of injury is straightforward and obvious to all. In another claim, an employee comes forward reporting gradual-onset pain in the left thumb. As a product "picker," this worker continuously holds a standard clipboard in the left hand and a marking pen in the right hand. The clipboard serves a dual purpose: to hold the invoices and as a platform on which multiple small products are carried. On initial reporting of this problem, the supervisor may logically ask when the injury occurred (anticipating a single incident with a date of occurrence). The employee is uncertain of how or when the injury was born but feels the problem is work related. The worker is also seeking the satisfaction of a single, explainable cause that can account for the symptoms. In this case, the mechanism of injury—the exact series of events that contributed to this problem—is unclear to both the investigator and the claimant, because neither of them have the knowledge to ask the types of questions that will yield a reasonable explanation of how this injury developed over time.

By conducting an injury review process (IRP), an investigative group can effectively identify multiple factors giving rise to cumulative wear and tear producing damage to neuromusculoskeletal structures. The IRP becomes most effective when participants include the injured employee, the supervisor, and a health professional knowledgeable in ergonomics and CTDs. In the previously mentioned case of the thumb injury, medical evaluation produced a diagnosis of de Quervain's tendinitis, an affliction of the extensor tendons of the thumb wherein inflammation produces stenosing tenosynovitis. A basic understanding of this diagnosis, its pathology, and the mechanism of injury will be invaluable to the injury review group as it details the events leading to this injury. A careful historical account will acknowledge the importance of such factors as size, weight, and configuration of the clipboard; how the worker must grasp the board; the length of time the board is held without a pause; duration of rest periods; how much weight is placed onto the board; in what position the clipboard is held most of the time; and pressure points against parts of the hand. These factors are some of the important issues that play a contributory role in fatigue and progressive damage. Such an in-depth examination provides the IRP members with the necessary data to establish fundamental cause. The knowledge accumulated by this process generates recommendations for corrective actions and other injury prevention measures.

At first glance, an injured employee may be apprehensive about sitting down with the supervisor, the company health provider, a safety committee designate, and possibly a workers' compensation loss control consultant. The group facilitator should take careful steps to inform the injured worker that the purpose of the IRP is not intended to be punitive or judgmental. The essential function of this meeting is twofold: to uncover the fundamental cause of a reported injury and to implement corrective actions to prevent reoccurrence of such injuries.

Properly administered, the IRP is a powerful problem-solving tool that yields benefits beyond its primary directive. The process of inquiry, interpretation, and resolution is enhanced greatly when multiple contributors provide increased understanding and clarification. It is not uncommon to discover that successful problem solving in one area transfers value to other applications. In the case of the de Quervain's tendinitis, much more attention will be directed to other operations and manual tasks that may pose a risk for injury to wrists and fingers.

Important features and outcomes of the IRP include the following:

- A positive, fact-finding, nonpunitive process. This meeting is not the appropriate occasion for reprimands associated with noncompliance with safety rules.
- An analysis of injury causes and corrective strategies.
- Valuable information and understanding through a formal group process.
- A powerful tool in reducing frequency and severity of injuries, thus lowering workers' compensation costs.
- Establishment of company's commitment to safety and injury prevention.
- Increased companywide safety awareness and participation.
- Strengthened communication throughout the ranks of management and workers.
- Increased accountability for safety and follow-up action.
- Reduced instances of malingering and fraudulent claims.
- A valuable educational and brainstorming opportunity.

Relevant to this discussion is lag time, the time between the onset of injury and notification of the workers' compensation claims representative. Ideally, a *first report of injury* reaches the company personnel office immediately following the incident. This report should be transmitted to the insurance claims representative on the very same day. Such timely communication establishes the best opportunity for obtaining accurate information concerning all circumstances surrounding the incident, for understanding the nature of the injury, and for a resolution satisfactory to both the injured employee and the employer. The longer the lag time, the more cost is incurred by both the employer and insurer. Lag time tends to be much shorter for traumatic types of injuries, whereas many workers tend to put off their complaints of gradually progressing aches and pains.

There are consequences of excessive lag time:

- Increased errors, omissions, and inaccuracy
- Impaired effectiveness of accident investigation process
- Erosion in employee's motivation to return to work or engage in modified duty
- Degeneration of trust and good will between management and worker
- Increased medical costs secondary to late intervention and subsequent reduced effectiveness of treatment
- Increased tendency for fraud and litigation
- Increased potential for additional claims from other workers exposed to similar hazards

It is vitally important that management provide for the early recognition, investigation, and treatment of CTDs. Employees should be encouraged to come forth as soon as significant symptoms first appear. Early intervention is the most powerful primary initiative that can set the stage for the most effective and cost-saving outcomes.

Early Return to Work and Modified Duty

Considering the costly consequences of poor injury claims handling and excessive lag time, it is to everyone's advantage to bring the injured worker back into appropriate employment as soon as possible. Not uncommonly, absence from work of 3 or more weeks significantly reduces the chances that an injured worker will successfully return to the work force. Employers who have committed themselves to a comprehensive injury prevention and management program will discover the value of a strong modified duty opportunity for their injured employees.

The designation *light duty* often carries a negative connotation, as it may stereotype certain workers as lazy and malingering. This connotation has given way to the more objective expressions, *modified* (or *alternative*) *duty*, which does not carry implicit judgmental inference. A well–thought out modified duty program reflects a company's commitment to cost containment and workers' welfare.

A successful modified duty program will fulfill genuine productivity needs of the company, that is, the alternative work is justifiable in everyone's eyes. Such special work assignments fill an important niche that will benefit both the company and injured worker. Ideally, the worker enters alternative duty with the understanding that this duty is essential to the employer; moreover, the employee's continued presence on the job and participation with coworkers is vital to everyone's interest. Managers who hastily fabricate alternative duty assignments with the mindset of *light duty* are likely to set themselves up for resentment and poor morale from the work force.

In summary, a productive program of modified duty will reflect the following guidelines:

- Duty assignments should meet a valid need, not senseless busywork
- Alternative work tasks should be accompanied by written physical demand requirements
- The injured worker's physical limitations and work capacity should be elucidated clearly and fully by proper medical authority
- The designated manager or overseer of the modified duty should be trained fully to observe and monitor a worker's adjustment and tolerance to work tasks
- Policies and procedures and the mission of the alternative duty program should be communicated to all staff, with emphasis directed to positive attitude and conduct toward injured workers on temporary assignment
- The duration of the modified duty should be established via objective criteria that apply uniformly to anyone who should become a candidate
- The employee's progress in this program should be documented carefully via systematic communication between the company, worker, insurer, health provider, and any other relevant parties

The focus of this program is to maintain the employee in a productive capacity while facilitating progressive recovery. The entire process should be directed to restoration of unrestricted work performance that includes return to customary duty.

Ergonomic-Engineering Controls

Ergonomic controls refers to such areas as equipment and tool design, workplace layout, environment, and work processes. In other words, it is often the planner or engineer who directs that segment of design intended to provide optimal assimilation by human operators: fitting the task to the worker.

Consider the broad scope of ergonomics as it has evolved over the last few decades. Recent times have seen increased mechanization, automation, and intensive safety campaigns that have produced increased general safety in the workplace. However, although risk of traumatic injuries is reduced dramatically, cumulative trauma ailments are on the rise. More sophisticated technology has streamlined processes, increased productivity, and economized on human effort. The price tag for this phenomenon—paid by workers—is a new form of physical demand characterized by fixed positions, body stasis, intense concentration, and highly repetitive similar small movements using the same anatomic structures. These physical, mental, and psychological stresses now are well recognized and merit a strategic position in our concept of ergonomics.

For illustration, we may conceptualize an *ergonomics equation* as follows:

Demands of job = Human functional capacity

Ergonomic or engineering controls address the left side of this equation—that is, all factors that will require the full spectrum of human capability (i.e., mental, physical, and psychological). This arena of planning will include such controls as design of machinery, workstations, tools, furniture, products, and so forth. Included are provisions concerned with the reduction of force, repetition, vibration, pressure, and awkward positioning. Assistive devices, hoists, lifts, conveyors, robotics, physical comfort aids, and personal protective equipment are among additional ergonomic considerations. Of final ergonomic importance is the environment: air, noise, temperature, lighting, walking surface, and so forth.

Although it is true that strictly ergonomic interventions (left side of the equation) can remedy existing hazards immediately, it also has been realized that expensive changes in the workplace may not improve injury statistics. The right side of this ergonomics equation presents many opportunities to affect workers' health and well-being. It is in this domain that worker knowledge and behavior can be improved positively, in shorter time frames, and often with comparatively less expense associated with engineering changes. More attention will be directed to specific ergonomic recommendations later. For the moment, consider the following important categories in which employers may enhance safety and worker protection from musculoskeletal problems.

Seating, Standing, and Posture Considerations

Illustrations and practical examples can direct attention to both sides of our ergonomics equation as part of a comprehensive problem-solving process. On many occasions, companies have invested hastily in a highly promoted line of ergonomic chairs only to discover that workers' complaints of fatigue and comfort issues persisted. Not uncommonly, quick ergonomic fixes, whether low-cost or very expensive, will not address adequately the multifaceted problems associated with seated work (e.g., sustained sitting and body stasis with concomitant fatigue, minimal variations of posture, and limb positioning).

The author's observations and worker feedback from diverse industry, including manufacturing, services, and health care, reveal that optimal seating can be achieved best when there is a good match between individual workers' physical characteristics, the task environment, and the specific demands of the job. These considerations are illustrated in the following comparisons of a sewing operator and office telemarketing associate.

Case 4. The sewing operator must sit constantly, allowed only two 10-minute breaks and 30 minutes for lunch. This operator is sitting on an all-metal, nonadjustable chair with a fixed backrest and flat, noncontoured seat. Both the seat and backrest have been cushioned with personally acquired padding. On both sides of this worker are large wheeled laundry bins containing bundles of fabric. The work requires that the operator periodically reach into these bins to grasp a bundle and place it on the flat work surface for accessibility. Some workers choose to remain sitting when they are acquiring their bundles, whereas other operators will get out of their chairs to reach into bins. Those individuals who remain seated while removing fabric bundles are observed to twist, lean, and stretch awkwardly as they extend one hand over the rim of the basket, often groping to grasp and remove the loosely tied material. During the sewing operation, the worker is relatively confined because of the necessity of keeping both feet in fixed positions on controls; also, the right knee is used to activate a lateral switch pad used during the procedure.

A scan of the workplace reveals that other operators carry out similar tasks. However, many individuals are sitting in upholstered swivel chairs from which the wheels have been removed to provide stability. These operators claim more satisfaction and comfort with their modified office chairs, because they have less restricted mobility, a more comfortable seat surface, and a broader back support. Closer scrutiny of workers' sitting postures discloses that most individuals are sitting forward in their chairs, seldom using backrests during actual sewing procedures. Reclining backward only occurs during momentary pauses. The forward-sitting position provides for less total contact with the supporting surface underneath thighs, thus enabling greater freedom of movement of the lower limbs. This positioning also facilitates fewer restrictions to pelvic mobility, making it seemingly easier to pivot or tilt the pelvis while remaining seated to work.

Why do some workers cling tenaciously to the old metal, nonadjustable chairs that have been padded selectively to meet their needs? An explanation for this phenomenon can be derived from an analysis of the foregoing behaviors and choices. It is important to consider how very important are the elements of mobility and positioning choice. Prolonged postural stasis is fatiguing, particularly during focused work, and this is especially applicable during confined sitting wherein minimal opportunity for diversified positioning changes is available. The fixed static posturing of the head and trunk demands sustained tension from all the axial postural maintenance musculature.

Workers committed to such physical demands will discover ways to incorporate as much movement and position choice as possible while maintaining a productivity standard. Sitting far forward in a seat and supplying padding provide one mechanism for operators to exercise more options for body posturing and general mobility while working. Asking such a worker to sit fully back in the seat with the spine pressed upright against the backrest is restrictive and confining.

Still another consideration that has an impact on posturing and movement style is vision or visual access to task. Head positioning is determined by a person's ability to visualize the task adequately. Some workers are observed to work with the eyes only several inches away from the task, whereas other individuals will find it satisfactory to work at a comparatively greater distance from the work object.

Case 5. Consider another type of work: a telemarketing associate whose time is also committed to prolonged sitting, in this case in front of a computer workstation. This job demands constant combined use of the telephone and calculator, writing notes in longhand, and keying while handling data from the video display terminal. Close observation of this worker reveals certain habitual postures and movements that contribute to fatigue and muscular discomfort. This individual already possesses a fully adjustable office task chair and footrest. It should be noted that the chair has armrests and is adjusted too high to position the armrests under the desktop. The operator has adjusted the seat to this height because of other constraints in the workstation. Additional inspection of the work area reveals the presence of numerous personal items, such as pictures, small plants, and decorations placed at arm's reach within the work space.

Observation of this individual executing work tasks provides insight into important factors underlying fatigue and discomfort associated with work demands. For example, this person is holding a telephone between the neck and left shoulder, fingering the calculator with the left hand, and alternately keying and note taking with the right hand, all the while keeping the pencil in readiness in the right fingers. Further, we observe much sustained elevation of the shoulder girdles; the many obstacles in the work space prevent comfortable positioning and weight bearing of the upper limbs. There is highly repetitive reaching over and around the various artifacts throughout the work area. The elements of this scenario explain significant factors that have resulted in this worker's excessive energy demands and subsequent reports of discomfort in the neck, back, and shoulder girdles.

In this context, selection of seating should take into account far more than the singular goal of establishing an artificial concept of good posture (i.e., sitting totally upright, with knees and hips at 90-degree angles and the back in full contact with a backrest). Also, one must assess whether workers' body positions and movements are obligatory, habitual, or some combination of both. *Obligatory* suggests that the worker is mandated to assume a particular position and move in specific patterns to accomplish the job task. *Habitual* implies that the worker has choices and has elected to adopt certain anatomic positions and functional motions for reasons that may be either obvious or obscure. For the individual who habitually sits with pronounced forward head posture and a slumped, kyphotic spine, a new ergonomic chair may not result in desired behavior changes. Most often, ergonomic offerings should be accompanied by appropriate employee education about the justification for the changes and how best to take advantage of such ergonomic improvements.

Examination of some of the finer details peculiar to the sewing operator and telemarketing representative offers a larger appreciation of broad ergonomic factors that play into injury risk. These illustrations highlight certain suggestions that employers will find useful when selecting or adapting seating.

Foot Placement and Lower-Extremity Positioning.   Often, a new chair is unnecessary when it is discovered that provisions for foot placement meet the worker's needs. If footrests are needed, they can be purchased or fabricated. In one company, wooden reels of various sizes were used with much satisfaction. Lack of opportunities for foot placement or obstruction of the lower limbs places increased emphasis on the proper selection of seating.

Mobility.   Do the chairs need to be mobile? Easily moved wheeled chairs can be a great asset when there is need for frequent movement about the immediate work area. The nature of the floor supporting a given chair is important to keep in mind. Not uncommonly, floor surfaces are not level or smooth, a condition resulting in poor stability for the user.

Adjustability.   The ability to adjust a work chair is the most advantageous feature to consider. When complete adjustability becomes a critical factor, the worker should be able to alter the chair's backrest, seat angle, and height quickly without getting out of the chair to perform cumbersome, time-consuming tasks of turning hand cranks or spinning the seat innumerable times to get the right adjustment. Rapid adjustability is particularly advantageous when a given chair will have multiple users.

Position Options.   Sit-stand options are a recent innovation in modern ergonomic furniture. Worthwhile ergonomic choices to consider are increasingly popular workstation designs that provide for sitting, standing, or positioning variations between these limits.

Seat and Backrest.   The shape, contour, size, and covering of the seat and backrest are important details in matching seating to individuals. All too often, flashy, pricey chairs may initially look attractive to the consumer. For example, seat pans may be too large, have excessively deep depressions for the buttocks, or contain incline ramps arising from the rear of the seating surface. This type of design encourages the sitter to move far forward in the chair to gain mobility of the pelvis and lower limbs and thereby minimize tension of the postural muscles.

Armrests.   Armrests can be useful in selected situations, such as in taking a momentary break to lean back and support the elbows. Usually, only the more expensive ergonomic task chairs will have adjustable armrests that will be suitable for upper-limb support during certain work tasks. Standard chairs with fixed armrests tend to be too low, encouraging the body to slide the pelvis forward and slump so as to rest the elbows on the armrests.

Workers who must stand constantly may also incur chronic fatigue, postural stress, and musculoskeletal pain. Important factors to consider include footwear, standing surface, extent of body movement, predominant posture of the neck and trunk, and nature of the work activity. For example, a worker whose job task permits a broad choice of unrestricted lower-extremity movements will very likely become less fatigued than will an individual who must stand with both feet confined to one position, as in the case of foot pedal operation. A hard standing surface (e.g., cement) contributes to joint fatigue because there is minimal shock attenuation.

This factor adds to stresses associated with stasis under compression with minimal joint and tissue mobility. Inappropriate footwear may further contribute to compressive and postural stresses to the feet and knees. Job tasks may demand substantial and prolonged deviations from neutral working alignment through the trunk, neck, and shoulder girdles. Sustained forward bending and reaching, with forward head posture, is a common contribution to painful syndromes in the stressed anatomic regions.

Certain tips can help to reduce fatigue and injury risks associated with prolonged standing:

- Install shock-attenuating pads or mats. If this is not possible, provide workers with access to acceptable footwear or suitable shock-absorbing materials.
- Provide opportunity for changes in foot position, such as a "bar rail."
- Check for barriers in front of the worker's feet. The operator should be able to work as close to a task as possible; even several inches of restriction in front of the toes can result in sustained forward leaning or excessive forward positioning with the upper limbs.
- Consider a "belly rest" or any suitable form of trunk rest against which the operator can take momentary breaks to lean and relax.
- Set work height and task access to permit neutral trunk positioning.
- For individuals with lower-limb circulatory insufficiency, consider pressure gradient leg-length socks to promote venous return.

Physical Comfort Aids. The ergonomics market has seen a proliferation of paraphernalia and gadgets directed at the comfort and safety of the work force. Such items include elasticized back supports, shock-attenuating insoles, vibration-dampening products, wrist and elbow bands, and the like.

It is useful to distinguish a splint from a support. The *International Dictionary of Medicine and Biology* defines *splint* as "a therapeutic device commonly used by the medical community to provide complete restriction of a limb or region of the body." Thus, splinting (or bracing) limits motion (e.g., a wrist splint restricts normal excursions of flexion and extension; likewise, a torso brace will prevent flexion and extension of the lumbosacral spine). According to the same dictionary, a flexible

support "sustains or provides a basis for continued function; a device that maintains or stabilizes something, such as an orthopedic appliance to reinforce the strength of a limb."

It is not uncommon in the workplace to see workers wearing elasticized bands around upper forearms or using garments to restrict wrist motions. Such compression bands and splints are more likely to be seen in work settings that require routine, highly repetitive upper-limb manual tasks. Such products are in response to the rising injury claims for elbow tendinitis and wrist-hand problems, particularly carpal tunnel syndrome.

The definition of splint as a device that limits motion of a joint is important to consider when, for example, a wrist splint is worn by a laborer who must carry out repetitive hand functions that demand a full range of motion with the forearm, wrist, and fingers. When the splint is applied, normal flexibility of the wrist is no longer available; therefore, the individual will direct use of the hand by expanding range of motion from other joints that are not limited. Commonly, the limited wrist motions will demand extra effort from the shoulder, which can create a risk for shoulder strain or tendinitis through repeated elevation and stress in the "impingement zone." Once again, when any device is to be applied or worn on the human body, there are both advantages and consequences to be realized. Just as prescription medicine has indications, contraindications, precautions, and side effects, so do splints, braces, supports, and garments worn by workers. Selection and use of comfort aids necessarily must follow proper study and indications for use of such devices if the anticipated benefits are to be realized.

The use of splints and supports should be judicious. Compressive, elasticized supports can provide comfort and retention of heat in underlying tissues. This is particularly true when a support is constructed from closed-cell material such as neoprene. Caution should be used to ensure proper fit and stability of position. For example, a tennis elbow band should not be so tight as to reduce circulation and not so loose that it slides down the forearm. Precautions should also be taken when any garment is susceptible to being caught in machinery or impeding work performance in any way. Motion-restricting splints may pose a more serious consideration, as noted earlier. In work that demands highly mobile wrist-hand motions, the restrictions imposed by a wrist band, for example, may force accommodation by substituting more forceful finger motions, with concomitant increase in motion and stress to the shoulder. It is necessary to carefully evaluate the need and weight of the benefits and precautions when donning a splint during work. Usually a medical consultation and authorization are indicated before an employee is directed to wear a joint-limiting device; a medical prescription will specify when and how long the user should wear the splint.

Controls to Reduce Force, Repetition, Vibration, and Pressure

The left side of the ergonomics equation (wherein controls address changes that will better adjust the workplace and job tasks to conform to human capacity) provides primary interventions that address force, repetition, vibration, direct pressure, and body posturing. When the design of the work environment and procedures derives from an understanding of human performance and potential, a healthy match can be established between the work and the worker.

The following list of ergonomic controls will serve as a useful reference in problem solving:

- Adjustable workstations
- Workstation design to provide for energy-efficient motions
- Adjustable seating and footrests
- High-density foam seat wedges
- Lumbar supports
- Ergonomic tools: design, counterbalancing
- Assistive aids for lifting, transporting, material handling
- Upper-limb weight bearing
- Upper-limb sling, counterbalance devices
- Antivibration gloves, wraps
- Automation
- Tilting of containers and work surfaces
- Work processes designed to minimize awkward posturing
- Shock-attenuating materials for feet and hands
- Computer document holders, wrist cushions, split keyboards
- Ergonomic writing implements

- Telephone headsets
- Tool maintenance: sharp cutting tools, proper lubrication, calibration

Exposure Reduction Controls

As noted earlier, risks for musculoskeletal disorders are increased with significant exposure to excessive force, repetition, speed, and so forth. In some situations, job demands present a high degree of risk that cannot be controlled readily through ergonomic changes. Costs for such improvements may be prohibitive in a short time frame; therefore, it becomes necessary to explore what opportunities exist to work on the right side of the ergonomics equation discussed earlier. In this area are ways for people to modify their work habits and the intensity with which they carry out the job. Exposure reduction strategies include any method by which such risks can be reduced. Such preventive measures may include sit-stand options, job rotation, adjusting the work-rest cycle, and assistance from coworkers.

Sit-Stand Options

As was discussed earlier, seating and alternative positioning can be a powerful deterrent to fatigue and subsequent musculoskeletal ailments. Wherever possible, job design and procedures should provide for opportunities to increase variety of body positions and economize on motions necessary to accomplish work tasks. The goal is to minimize stasis and prolonged musculoligamentous tension, encouraging blood flow and energy conservation. Office seating and ergonomic supply catalogs now offer a broad variety of specialized furniture to meet contemporary needs. Adjustable sit-stand seating is a welcome alternative to constant sitting.

Job Rotation

Changing job assignments systematically is a proven, highly successful strategy for preserving musculoskeletal health on the job. Added benefit includes additional cross-trained workers who can meet productivity needs more responsively with less costs to the company.

Job rotation becomes a good choice when the level of technical skill is assimilated readily by multiple employees. When rotation of job tasks is called for, the supervisor should ensure that the alternative work requires a significant variation in physical demands (i.e., sufficient variation to relieve a particular group of working tissues). When selected technical ability is too advanced, job rotation becomes less of an option.

Adjusting the Work-Rest Cycle

With increasing physical job demands comes more rapid onset of fatigue. Sustained fatigue results from sustained tension and energy expenditure. Blood flow to working limbs and tissues is restricted under the compressive forces of continuous muscular holding and exertion. Many studies have documented the physiological and cardiopulmonary events occurring during work activity, and the literature abounds with the common theme that there exists an optimal relationship between physical effort and rest. The more strenuous or fatiguing the work activity, the more rest will be required. Rest periods, or cessation from activity, may take the form of periodic minipauses or programmed rest periods of stated frequency and duration.

For further review of this topic, see Chapters 6 and 7.

Getting Assistance

All too often, material handlers are seen working alone when lifting, carrying, pulling, and pushing. Common explanations include time constraint, unavailability of help, absence of physically demanding effort. Once again, safety policies and procedures, and the resources to back them up, must be part of daily working life if effective injury prevention is to be established. When it is recognized that certain job tasks will require more than normal physical demands, company policy should ensure that workers plan for cooperation and assistance where applicable.

Although the concept of assistance readily applies to material handling, its usefulness is also important in any work application. Even in the office setting, much fatigue can accompany exhaustive tasks ranging from keying on the computer to constant phone communications. Such less obvious stressors can be just as incriminating as lifting heavy objects in producing injuries.

On-the-Job Stretching Exercises

There is general agreement in the world of athletics that warm-up and stretching are advisable. It is a commonly held belief that stretching is an injury prevention measure that should be included in every athlete's training program (Hansford et al. 1986; Jacobsen & Sperling 1976; Anderson 1980; Sawyer 1987; Allers 1989). Although evidence is lacking to demonstrate the absolute preventive value of stretching, athletically active persons have more to gain than lose from systematic stretching. In the same vein, employees (industrial athletes), who use their physical abilities to work (game competition), need and deserve the same preventive measures to undergird their well-being and performance.

The theoretic basis for periodic stretching on the job lies with an understanding of the basic physiology of tissue nutrition and pathology of tissue injury. In short, working tissues require oxygen and nutrients if they are to remain healthy. When physical demands or other events result in diminution of blood supply to working structures, fatigue, inflammation, and destructive changes ensue. Some researchers have stated that tendinitis and carpal tunnel syndrome are not so much problems of repetitive motion, or friction wear, as they are a lack of tissue perfusion (Jacobsen & Sperling 1976). In practical terms, is carpal tunnel syndrome derived from high repetition and friction-wear occurring within the carpal tunnel? Does another contribution possibly emanate from restriction of blood flow from more proximal regions, such as the cervicobrachial area, wherein vessels can be restricted by the scalene muscles and other compressive elements in this forest of musculature? This so-called cervicobrachial explanation appears to have merit, particularly when one considers the anatomical positions of tissues and joints when the head is thrust forward, the scapulae are protracted, and the anterior trunk musculature is tight.

In light of these fundamental concepts of physiology, anatomy, and function, we can propose justifiably that position changes of the neck and thorax, with strategies to support increased blood supply and tissue perfusion, warrant preventive stretching on the job. Questions arise, and opinions vary widely on the recommended type and frequency of stretching.

Selection and prescription of on-the-job stretching exercises should take the following considerations into account:

- Exercises should target specific muscles and tendons that incur the most stress and wear during work activity.
- In stretching, consider what tissues are being stretched and the impact on associated joints.
- Proper exercise technique is essential to achieve desired goals.
- Stretching's primary purpose is to increase blood flow and tissue perfusion, not joint flexibility.
- The duration of each stretch should be 5–10 seconds.
- Stretching should not cause pain or pose risk of injury to joints.
- Selected stretching should not be conducted where it is contraindicated medically.
- Instruction in stretching should be conducted by a qualified professional, such as a physical or occupational therapist.
- The frequency of stretching should match intensity of effort. Generally, hard-working tissues should receive a stretch respite at least every hour. If six strategic exercises were selected, they would consume only 1 minute per hour.

Although numerous exercise choices are available, the author supports the following group of stretching movements that target the most needy body areas often implicated in work-related musculoskeletal ailments:

- *Chin tuck*: This is a backward gliding motion of the head with the chin positioned slightly downward. The head remains level as it retracts backward. This movement reduces forward head posture by improving alignment of the cervical vertebrae and re-establishing a better length-tension relationship among the cervical and upper-thoracic musculature.
- *Neck side-bending*: Caution should be taken not to be overly forceful during this movement in which the head is tilted gently laterally while the shoulder girdle remains depressed on the side being stretched.
- *Wrist flexor stretch*: The muscles that flex the wrist originate from the medial epicondyle. Stretching of this group of muscles occurs when the wrist is extended. This can be achieved in

several ways; however, one very effective method is to extend the elbow fully, with the forearm fully supinated. With the other hand, grasp the fingers of the extended arm and gently pull the fingers and palm into hyperextension.
- *Wrist extensor stretch*: The muscles that extend the wrist originate from the lateral epicondyle; therefore, any movement that flexes the wrist will place a stretch on this group of muscles. One of the most effective techniques is referred to as the *Mill's stretch*: To stretch the right wrist extensors, fully extend the elbow, make a tight fist, fully rotate the right shoulder internally, then flex the wrist in this position. The other hand may assist to get more wrist flexion, if this is comfortable.
- *Codman shoulder pendulum exercise:* This seemingly easy movement rarely is performed properly. The purpose of this exercise is to achieve full relaxation of the shoulder mechanism, particularly the glenohumeral joint. This goal is accomplished by bending forward and supporting the upper body with one hand on a knee or some object. The other arm is left to hang totally passively. The passive, dependent arm now can be made to move passively by initiating movement of the trunk while concentrating on dangling the dependent arm with no muscular splinting or guarding from the shoulder girdle. The hanging arm can be made to move back and forth or to circumscribe clockwise and counterclockwise circles.
- *Statue of Liberty stretch*: This author-coined term describes a standing stretch that addresses multiple body areas simultaneously. The individual stands with one foot approximately 18–20 in. in front of the other, measuring from the large toe of the rear foot to the heel of the forward foot. The feet are placed approximately shoulder width apart. The hands are clasped together, reaching fully above the head while gently flexing the forward knee and hip, keeping the rear knee straight. This movement provides a comfortable stretch to the muscles of the upper thorax and the hips as well as providing a lumbar hyperextension stretch to offset prolonged kyphotic posturing of the spine.

These stretches can be a valuable adjunct to the other exposure reduction recommendations outlined earlier. Note that not every exercise stretches muscles and tendons. For example, the Codman pendulum movement functions more as a passive relaxation technique for the shoulder joint. It also provides a rest for frequently compressed and irritated suprahumeral structures (i.e., the supraspinatus portion of the rotator cuff).

Management-Employee Education and Training

The rising incidence of CTDs in the workplace presents one of the greatest challenges for problem solving in U.S. industry. It has become clear that work-related traumatic injuries comprise a group of hazards that are relatively easy to recognize and prevent. By contrast, it is often difficult to diagnose precisely such insidious-onset problems as chronic muscle strain, tendinitis, and spinal ailments and such neurologic compression syndromes as thoracic outlet and carpal tunnel. Determination of root causes and mechanisms of injury is even more difficult.

The complexity of these disorders, some of which may be clearly work related, demands a level of knowledge and problem-solving skills higher than that necessary for the former, more obvious maladies. Abatement strategies, medical management, and prevention programs directed to the elimination of work-related CTDs demand that both management and employees become adequately educated about this subject. Greatest success derives from a collaborative effort between fully informed managers, supervisors, safety personnel, employees, and health care providers.

Because managers have the authority to establish policy and to exercise leadership, it is incumbent on them to become informed and to assign responsibilities, with the appropriate resources, to key players who will implement prevention programs. Suggested objectives for management level training are:

- Develop a practical knowledge of common work-related musculoskeletal injuries and their causes, symptoms, and treatments
- Learn to recognize and distinguish risks associated with job tasks, worker behaviors, and companywide attitudes
- Learn how to analyze and interpret injury data (e.g., OSHA 200 logs, insurance loss runs)

- Develop a methodology of work-site analysis (e.g., study of trends, ergonomic assessment)
- Develop a broad understanding of all issues that contribute to injuries, worker compensation claims, and costs
- Acquire essential knowledge and resources to define, document, and implement fully a comprehensive plan for the prevention of job-related musculoskeletal disorders (i.e., an ergonomics program)
- Learn how to establish, organize, and conduct an *ergonomics team* with supplemental training to address this specialty

Employees have the primary responsibility to follow safety procedures and care for their health. Working individuals should participate in decision making that will have an impact on their performance and well-being on the job. Employee feedback without reprisal is an essential prerequisite to good relations and optimal success. Employees who undertake training directed to the prevention of musculoskeletal problems should achieve the following objectives:

- A fundamental knowledge of common musculoskeletal ailments most frequently encountered in their industry
- Knowledge of how to participate in a total system of health surveillance with procedures for reporting symptoms
- Recognition of inefficient and overly stressful work habits
- Techniques of improving posture and body mechanics, on and off the job
- Strategies to work with more energy conservation and less fatigue
- Procedures for self-management and symptom relief from common, uncomplicated types of soft-tissue discomfort
- Techniques to carry out on-the-job stretching and relaxation exercises

References

Allers V (1989). Work-place preventive programs cut costs of illness and injuries. *Occup Health Saf,* 58,26–29.
Anderson B (1980). *Stretching.* Bolinas, CA: Shelter Publications.
APTA News Release (1991). Physical therapists say most carpal tunnel syndrome injuries preventable through education. *Orthop Pract,* 3(4).

Arndt R (1985). *A Prospective Study of the Psychological and Psychosocial Effects of Machine-Paced Work in the US Postal Service.* Cincinnati: NIOSH (contract 210-79-0072), 1–40.

Arndt R (1987). Work pace, stress and cumulative trauma disorders. *J Hand Surg [Am],* 12,866–869.

Borg GAV (1982). Psychophysical basis of perceived exertion. *Med Sci Sports Exerc,* 14,377–381.

Delgrosso I & Boillat MA (1991). Carpal tunnel syndrome: role of occupation. *Int Arch Occup Environ Health,* 63,267–270.

Franklin GM, Haug J, Heyer N, Checkaway H, & Peck N (1991). Occupational carpal tunnel syndrome in Washington State, 1984–1988. *Am J Public Health,* 81,741–746.

Goidi I (1964). Epicondylitis lateralis humeri: a pathogenic study. *Acta Chir Scand Suppl,* 339,119.

Hansford P, Blood H, Kent B, & Lutz G (1986). Bloodflow changes at the wrist in manual workers after preventive interventions. *J Hand Surg [Am],* 11,503–508

Hebert L (1993). Analytic focus reduces anxiety over cumulative trauma disorder claims. *Occup Health Saf,* 62,56–62.

Jacobsen C & Sperling L (1976). Classification of the hand-grip. A preliminary study. *J Occup Med,* 18,395–398.

Jaeger S, Spitz L, Powell M, & VuTran Z (1992). *The Prevention of Occupational Carpal Tunnel Syndrome.* Cherry Hill, NJ: Occupational Preventive Diagnostics, Inc.

Klafs C & Arnheim D (1973). Scientific basis for conditioning and training. In *Modern Principles of Athletic Training* (p. 65). St Louis: Mosby.

Landau SI (1986). *International Dictionary of Medicine and Biology* (p. 231). New York: Wiley.

Lanfear R & Clark W (1972). The treatment of tenosynovitis in industry. *Physiotherapy,* 58,128–29.

Levi L (1972). Stress and distress in response to psychosocial stimuli. *Acta Med Scand,* 528(Suppl),191.

Lew EA & Garfinkel L (1983). Variation in mortality by weight among 750,000 men and women. *J Chronic Dis,* 32,563–576.

Newcombe G (1994). Cumulative trauma disorders in the workplace. *For The Defense,* p. 2.

Occupational Safety and Health Administration, US Department of Labor (1990). *Ergonomic Program Management Guidelines for Meatpacking Plants.* Washington, DC: US Department of Labor/OSHA 3123.

Putz-Anderson V (1992). *Cumulative Trauma Disorders: A Manual for Musculoskeletal Diseases of the Upper Limbs.* London: Taylor & Francis.

Rodgers SH (1987). Recovery time needs for repetitive work. *Semin Occup Med,* 2(1),19–24.

Rohmert W (1973). Problems in determining rest allowances: part I. *Appl Ergon,* 4(2),91–95.

Sandler H (June 1993). Are we ready to regulate cumulative trauma disorders? *Occup Hazards,* 51–53.

Sawyer K (1987). An on-site exercise program to prevent carpal tunnel syndrome. *Profess Safety,* 5,17–20.

Thompson A, Plewes L, & Shaw E (1951). Peritendinitis crepitans and simple tenosynovitis: a clinical study of 544 cases in industry. *Br J Ind Med,* 8,150–160.

US Department of Health and Human Services (1989). Obesity. In *Surgeon General's Report on Nutrition and Health.* Washington, DC: Public Health Services, Government Printing Office, 017-001-00465-1.

US Department of Labor, Occupational Health and Safety Administration (1989). Voluntary, general safety and health program management guidelines. *Federal Register,* 54,3904–3916.

Welch R (1972). The causes of tenosynovitis in industry. *Indiana Med,* 41,16–18.

Wilson R & Wilson S (1957). Tenosynovitis in industry. *Practitioner,* 178,612–625.

Chapter 12

Employment Examinations

James W. King

Most individuals use their hands to perform the tasks that provide their livelihood. Surgeons, carpenters, butchers, and seamstresses are among many workers whose primary service or product comes directly from the countless simple and complex functions of the hand. Littler (1960) eloquently stated, "With any degree of incapacity of the hand, man's potential is diminished. Function of this unique part is dependent upon its structure, its strength, its critical sensation, and its integration with the mind and the eye" (p. 259). With their concern for the functional ability of humanity, therapists perform many activities to prevent and rehabilitate hand dysfunction.

Gilbreth and Gilbreth (1924) identified specific elements of hand function, such as search, grasp, move, position, reach, and hold, to describe workers' activities. Barnes, as described by Armstrong et al. (1986), modified these elements to include another function: rest, to overcome fatigue. When used repeatedly following the onset of fatigue, the soft tissues of the upper extremities undergo stress. Daily stress may occur when the job exposes a person, either on an intermittent or on a continuous basis, to certain high-risk activities. If the accumulating stress exceeds the body's normal recuperative ability during rest cycles, inflammation of the tissue may follow. Chronic inflammation can lead to the development of cumulative trauma disorders (CTDs). The effect of CTDs can impact the profitability of an industry.

Medical costs, indemnity costs, and the impact on personnel management has become significant and requires intervention. There are several methods of

intervention to reduce this cost: decreasing workers' exposure to environmental risk factors; training workers to manage their working environment and to recognize developing symptoms; minimizing the placement of individuals with existing or developing abnormal conditions in high risk jobs; and initiating early intervention programs for symptomatic workers. This chapter specifically addresses one of these strategies—the development of objective, accurate, valid, and reliable assessments of upper-extremity function to assist in workers' job placement.

Certain individuals may be unsuitable for placement in jobs having one or more environmental risk factors because of their current hand function, which may be influenced by their exposure to risk factors in the past or by their personal risk. Placement in a job with additional risk could lead to the development or exacerbation of the symptoms of a CTD. An objective assessment would assist in three work-related situations.

An initial screening with a standardized, accurate test may identify CTDs in applicants. Consequently, an employee would be matched with an appropriate job. Likewise, when exposed to risk factors, a normal hand may show threshold changes due to increasing inflammation. An ongoing assessment that is sensitive to early changes in hand function could identify an early CTD. Monitoring in this way would clarify the point at which removal of the worker from the high-risk job or referral for medical management would be appropriate. Finally, an objective assessment would identify the point at which previously injured workers have the physical capacity to return to varying levels of hand-intensive work.

This chapter addresses an analysis of the current theories of CTD development in support of medical examinations as one solution to the CTD problem in placing workers in jobs; a history of employment examinations and the typical components of these assessments; the factors to consider in the development and analysis of employment examination accuracy, including the effect of the Americans with Disabilities Act (ADA) on the application-testing-placement process; and a suggested examination, with empiric evidence of its accuracy in both normal and abnormal populations.

Current Theories of Cumulative-Trauma-Disorder Development in Support of Medical Examinations

CTDs of the upper extremities often develop insidiously, then become symptomatic and prevent workers from performing their jobs (Silverstein et al. 1986). Medical examinations that can identify current symptoms or reliably identify a combination of personal and environmental risk and classify an individual accurately will be paramount to long-term management of workers in hand-intensive jobs. Although certainly not all individuals exposed to risk factors in their job will develop CTDs, many risk factors contribute to their development. Risk factors for this disorder in work environments include repetition, abnormal postures of the hand, resistive hand motions, exposure to vibration, and to a lesser degree, exposure to extremes of temperature (see Chapter 7).

CTDs have been identified for many years in the medical literature. Many colorful names—for example, glass arm, telegraphist's cramp, washerwoman's thumb, and gold-beater's palm—have been used to describe them. Increasingly, current medical literature identifies and describes intervention strategies for such CTDs as carpal tunnel syndrome (CTS), epicondylitis, tenosynovitis, and ganglion cysts. Although each disorder has a distinct set of symptoms, common to all is the etiology of inflammation that can occur when excessive stress is placed on the soft tissues of the upper extremity in working (see Chapter 5).

High-risk industries contain work involving one or more hazards. Falck and Aarnio (1983) identified

left-sided CTS in butchers. Workers in electronic assembly (Hymovich & Lindholm 1966; Feldman et al. 1987), investment casting plant workers (Silverstein et al. 1987), and hospital workers (Punnett 1987) are among many at-risk occupations identified in the literature. Other factors can also contribute to the development of CTDs.

By virtue of their gender-related risk factors and their higher percentage of employment in jobs with CTD risk factors, women may be more susceptible to development of the disorders than are men. Hartwell et al. (1964) identified a significant number of women with tenosynovitis in their local industries. In the classical literature presentation of CTS, Phalen (1966) noted that 67% of his 654 subjects with the disease were women.

More than one CTD may occur simultaneously in many workers, and certain tissues are more susceptible than others. Theorists and those who study the incidence of CTDs propose that there is a predisposition in some individuals to these types of disorders. Bleecker (1987) has identified carpal canal size as a risk factor associated with CTS. Castelli et al. (1980) studied the morphology of the median nerve vasculature within the carpal tunnel in cadavers. They identified excessive carpal canal pressure as a factor that could lead to the development of anoxia and secondary destruction of nerve fibers. Differences in individual responses to laboratory-induced pressure in the carpal canal were also identified by Szabo and Gelberman in 1987.

Other theorists believe that work conditions are largely responsible for CTD development, because the soft tissue of the hand and wrist is susceptible, particularly in certain individuals, to the stress of excessive working conditions. Kazarian (1975) has identified a creep effect (viscoelastic deformation of the tissue) related to the duration of loading of musculotendinous units. Chu and Blatz (1972) identified microdamage, leading to the same viscous deformation, from failure on a molecular level of the links between the tissue matrix and filler material in muscle. Additional studies have identified the frequency of these disorders (Hartwell et al. 1964; Hymovich & Lyndholm 1966; Armstrong & Chaffin 1979; Masear et al. 1986). The question still remains as to why some workers develop CTDs and some do not.

For a variety of educational, socioeconomic, ethnic, and familial reasons, workers frequently spend many years in one or more industries where exposure to CTD-associated risk factors is extensive.

Many industries are likely to hire workers who have experience in hand-intensive, production work, yet these are the very individuals who may already have developed CTD symptoms. This set of circumstances has been described as "cumulative trauma roulette" (King 1990). In this scenario, workers who may have developed hand problems during previous work are hired or transferred to high-risk jobs. When a worker with a previously subclinical problem becomes symptomatic, the current employer is liable for the worker's medical care.

Some workers who perform high-risk jobs have successfully avoided CTDs despite exposure to the hazards. The author's clinical observation has been that these individuals often have developed greater than average strength. An assessment that could identify the unique genetic physical characteristics or potential of such workers could lead to future research in predicting workers best suited for high-risk work.

Finally, following medical care, injured workers often return to work with little or no objective measurement of their readiness to perform their jobs. This practice may result in reinjuries, additional lost time, and increased morbidity and antagonism among the injured workers, their employer, and the medical treatment team. One of the best reasons to perform testing is to establish the presence or absence of medical problems or physical limitations in the event that an injury occurs on the job.

History of Employment Examinations

Medical History

Pre-employment examinations have traditionally been used for assessment of the spine. As early as 1947, Stewart described pre-employment examinations of the back. These included x-rays, subsequently refuted and now obsolete as a reasonable predictor of successful job performance. This is an example of how employment tests based on medical history alone have been discriminatory. The correlation between most of the radiographic abnormalities identified on x-rays and the risk of low back pain is weak. In 1973, the American College of Radiology and the American Occupational Medicine Association joined in a conference to evaluate

the effectiveness of such x-rays in comparison with the potential radiation hazards. They concluded that the use of x-rays as the sole criterion for selection of workers was not justified and that more concern was needed to protect workers from unnecessary radiation in such examinations.

Chaffin et al. (1978) found strength testing to be a better indicator of worker performance in heavy-lifting jobs. Medical history has also been identified and used as a factor in screening workers. The literature makes a strong case for the association of certain conditions with the later development of CTDs, and medical screening often includes a review of medical history.

Several authors have presented the incidence of median nerve injuries in fractures of the distal end of the radius, particularly Colles' fractures. Abbott and Saunders (1933) identified a risk of median nerve compression in fractures of the distal radius. Meadoff (1949) noted median nerve injuries in many fractures in the region of the wrist. Cooney et al. (1980) identified median nerve entrapment as one complication of Colles' fractures.

Phalen (1966) described diabetes as a risk factor for CTS. Michaelis (1950) described compression of the median nerve through stenosis of the carpal tunnel and flexor tendon sheath associated with rheumatoid arthritis. In Phalen's study (1966), 49 of the 654 hands studied had rheumatoid arthritis. Forceful gripping and repetitive use of the hand would exacerbate the active synovitis of rheumatoid joints.

Previous surgery for traumatic conditions may inherently impair hand function. Included are limitations from the surgery or trauma itself, the presence of scar tissue, or the residual presence of foreign bodies in the hand (e.g., surgical fixation devices). There is significant literature that correlates development of multiple CTDs. Phalen (1966) reported the following diagnoses occurring with CTS in his subjects: trigger finger or thumb in 34 hands, de Quervain's disease in 10 hands, and the presence of ganglion cysts in several patients.

Although Phalen (1966) reported that surgical carpal tunnel releases are not necessary in most cases, a case severe enough to need surgery may have sustained permanent vascular changes (Gelberman et al. 1981). In the author's experience, there has generally been a small permanent impairment following carpal tunnel release, based on weakness of grip, occasional loss of range of motion, and loss of sensibility.

Analysis of Accuracy in Medical Screening Examinations

In the process of standardization, establishing reliability and validity of an evaluation is a foremost priority. Fess (1986, p. 621) defines reliability as "an instrument's ability to measure consistently and predictably" and validity as "the truthfulness of an assessment tool . . . to measure that which it purports to measure." Chaffin and Andersson (1984) have identified four measures of an instrument's ability to select workers appropriately. They are accuracy, sensitivity, specificity, and predictive value.

Chaffin and Andersson (1984, p. 399) defined accuracy as "a measure of a screening test's ability to provide a true measure of a quantity or quality." The two measures of the accuracy of upper-extremity fitness-for-duty evaluation (UEFFDE) proposed in the research are sensitivity and specificity. Chaffin and Andersson (1984, p. 399) defined sensitivity as "a measure of a test's accuracy in correctly identifying persons with a certain condition. [It is] the fraction or percentage of all persons with a condition who will have a positive test." They used the following equation to describe sensitivity:

$$\frac{\text{True positives}}{\text{True positives} + \text{false negatives}} \times 100$$

Chaffin and Andersson (1984, p. 400) defined specificity as "a measure of a test's accuracy in correctly identifying persons who do not have the condition. It can be expressed as the fraction or percentage of negative tests in persons free of a condition." For this measure, the following equation was proposed:

$$\frac{\text{True negatives}}{\text{True negatives} + \text{false positives}} \times 100$$

Typical Components of Medical Screening

The concept of job-worker matching is well accepted in our society. Industry uses standard qualifications to screen applicants who should be assessed for material-handling or excessively hand-intensive jobs. Assuring the applicant's fitness for duty before he or she enters the workplace is paramount in reducing the number of sudden-onset disorders and CTDs that a company experiences. In addition, thorough physical and functional testing can establish a baseline by which to compare subsequent tests for changes in functional ability or fair impairment ratings in the event of an injury.

Many factors contribute to successful job performance. Strength, flexibility, endurance, and job skill techniques all have been used to establish work readiness. However, the increasing cost of CTDs in industry has brought some urgency (and in many cases, discriminatory methods) into the employment examination picture.

Such general assessments of hand function as grip and pinch-strength testing have the benefit of establishing "normalcy" of the applicant; however, they can be used only individually as a factor to screen out potential workers if the amount of strength required by the job has been established clearly. To establish this criterion, two methods can be used: measuring with sophisticated torque gauges the force needed to perform the job and measuring incumbent worker's strength.

Other, more sophisticated measures of hand function, such as vibrometry, sensibility, and nerve conduction, are being used to establish pass-restrictive criteria (as opposed to pass/fail criteria, which are not appropriate for ADA-acceptable exams) for applicants. The sensitivity of examinations for early CTS was established by Szabo and Gelberman (1987) in the following order: vibrometry, Semmes-Weinstein monofilaments (SWMFs), sensory nerve conduction velocity (NCV), moving two-point discrimination, static two-point discrimination, and motor NCV. Use of these components of hand function must not be used randomly or without thought as to the implications of discrimination when they are used only to eliminate a certain class of potentially disabled individuals.

Constraints on the Use of Employment Examinations: The Americans with Disabilities Act

The ADA of 1990 (Public Law 101-336) mandates equal treatment of individuals with disabling conditions and the rest of the nation's citizens. The act became effective for most employers in July 1992. The ADA mandates accessibility and equality in four primary subtitle areas: Title I, employment; Title II, public services; Title III, public accommodations and services operated by private entities; and Title IV, telecommunications. The directives of Title I affect the use of the employment examinations.

Under the ADA's provisions, applicants to industry can be screened appropriately by the use of standardized medical tests. In such testing, the results are interpreted, and decisions regarding the appropriateness of placement are made, on the basis of pre-established criteria. To be effective in disqualifying, *without discriminating against*, applicants who do not meet physical criteria, such tests must establish appropriate, defensible criteria before examination begins; each applicant for the position must be screened; and interpretation must be made on a pass-fail basis (i.e., the stronger of two applicants—if both meet the criteria established—cannot be chosen on the basis of strength alone).

Employment evaluations can be used to match workers with their jobs but cannot be discriminatory. Examinations can establish the presence of abnormal conditions, but specific portions of the test cannot be interpreted as showing a higher or lower risk for injury. A significant risk—not a nominal risk—of substantial harm must be established. Clearly, workers who are placed in jobs that do not exceed their physical capacity are less likely to become injured. Incumbent workers (those who have been working for the company) also are good candidates for screening once criteria are established. Testing can identify symptomatic and presymptomatic employees, and appropriate intervention can be initiated.

Americans with Disabilities Act Guidelines and the Definition of Discriminatory Testing Methods

The goal of the ADA is to minimize discrimination in the hiring process. Section 102 of the ADA sets forth this standard, providing that:

> No covered entity shall discriminate against a qualified individual with a disability because of the disability of such individual in regard to job application procedures, the hiring, advancement or discharge of employees, employee compensation, job training, and other terms, conditions, and privileges of employment.

The *Texas Employment Law Handbook* defines different types of discrimination. The following are prohibited by the ADA:

- Opportunity status discrimination based on classification

- Participation in a contract or other arrangement or relationship having a discriminatory effect
- Use of standards, criteria, or methods of administration that have the effect of discrimination on the basis of disability or that perpetuate the discrimination of others who are subject to common administrative control
- Discrimination based on a qualified individual's known association or relationship with disabled individual
- Failure to reasonably accommodate, or denial of opportunity due to need to reasonably accommodate
- Use of qualification standards, employment test, or other selection criteria which tend to screen out disabled individuals, unless the criteria are shown to be job-related for the position in question and consistent with business necessity
- Failure to select and administer test concerning employment in the most effective manner to insure that tests measure only necessary skills and aptitude, rather than reflecting the disability

Medical history inquiries are prohibited in the pre-offer stage. With regard to employment physicals (and examination of injured workers who may be covered under ADA), employers may require medical examinations (1) only if they are job related and consistent with business necessity and (2) only after an offer of employment has been made to a job applicant. The physical examination may be given after the conditional job offer and before the commencement of employment duties. An offer of employment, however, may be conditioned on the results of examination only if (1) all employees are subjected to examinations and (2) such information is kept confidential and maintained in separate medical files.

Determining What Constitutes a Disability

To qualify as a disability covered by the ADA, an impairment must limit substantially one or more of the following examples of *major life activities*.

- Walking
- Speaking
- Breathing
- Caring for oneself
- Performing manual tasks
- Sitting
- Standing

- Seeing
- Hearing
- Learning
- Working
- Lifting

It is not necessary to consider if a person is substantially limited in the major life task of 'working' if the person is substantially limited in any other major life activity.

Employers may not make inquiries of a job applicant as to whether the applicant has a disability or as to the nature or severity of the disability. Employers may ask, however, whether the employee can perform job-related functions and then can evaluate the worker for physical capacity to confirm his or her capabilities.

The ADA defines a qualified individual with a disability as a disabled individual who meets the skill, experience, education, and other job-related requirements of a position held or desired, and who, with or without reasonable accommodation, can perform the essential functions of a job. The ADA "requires the employer to evaluate the individual with a disability's qualifications solely on their ability to perform the essential functions of the job, with or without a reasonable accommodation."

When Testing Should Be Done

Examinations may be performed when they are necessitated by business. The ADA's interpretive guidelines state:

> If a test or other selection criterion excludes an individual with a disability *because of* the disability and does not relate to the *essential functions of the job,* it is not consistent with business necessity. [emphasis added]

Testing may also be done when the test is job related. Interpretive guidelines state:

> If a qualification standard, test or other selection criterion operates to screen out an individual with a disability, or a class of such individuals on the basis of disability, it must be a legitimate measure or qualification for the *specific* job it is being used for. [emphasis added]

The key to restricting placement of an individual with a CTD on the basis of the medical examination is to establish the *significant risk of substantial harm.*

Summary: Examinations Allowed Under the Americans with Disabilities Act

Key concepts of the preoffer stage

1. Coordination or agility test related directly to the essential functions of the job
2. Must offer accommodation
3. Disqualification based on inability to meet critical job tasks' requirements with or without accommodation

Key concepts of postoffer stage

1. Medical history and related examinations acceptable
2. Must offer accommodation
3. Disqualification must be based on significant risk of substantial harm when performing essential job function

Testing allowed by ADA

1. Only after an offer of employment has been made
2. Only if all applicants for the position are subject to the examination
3. Only if disqualification is based on job-related and business necessity or placement would pose a significant risk of substantial harm
4. Only if results are kept confidential

Testing prohibited by ADA

1. Use of standard, criteria, or methods of administration that have the effect of discrimination
2. Use of qualification standards . . . unless job related or of business necessity
3. Medical examinations in the preoffer stage
4. Decisions based on physical appearance alone

Suggested Assessment with Empiric Evidence of Its Accuracy in Both Normal and Abnormal Populations

The following assessment arose from the author's frustration with the lack of an objective measure of hand function for use in the purposes previously stated. The UEFFDE and its component evaluations suggest a process to establish other, potentially more accurate groups of assessments.

An initial general description is followed by the specific subsections and their criteria and point values.

General Description

The UEFFDE measures hand function to identify those individuals who have symptoms of CTDs. The physical examination uses clinical signs and observations of actual activity. In the UEFFDE, subjects receive points for failing a subsection of the examination. The higher the total points, the more likely an individual will be placed into the category of *suspect* or *abnormal condition identified*. The subject's hands are scored independently.

In the scheme of the point system, clinical signs based on subjective reports by the patient receive the least points, whereas those objective and clearly observable assessments receive more points. In interpretation of the test results, 0 or 5 points represent a hand within acceptable normal limits, 10 points indicate a suspected condition, and 15 points or more signify an abnormal condition identified.

The UEFFDE includes a stress test that uses certain tools with work-simulation equipment. This specific research used the work simulator manufactured by the Baltimore Therapeutic Equipment (BTE) Company, Baltimore, MD. Stress testing occurs before sensibility testing, nerve conduction testing, and observations for Raynaud's phenomenon, triggering finger or thumb, and the presence of edema. This allows for measuring the influence of resistive and repetitive activity on the hand and would better detect the presence of any dynamic pathologic processes (Braun et al. 1989).

Item Development: Subtests and Their Point Values

The subtests of the UEFFDE are presented in this chapter because of the significant literature citations used to support the rationale and point value for each test as an indicator of the presence of CTDs. Several authors (Hartwell et al. 1964; Hymovich & Lindholm 1966; Kuorinka & Koskinen 1979; American Society for Surgery of the Hand 1983) have described the value of physical examinations

in identifying CTDs. Point values for the subtests of the UEFFDE have been based on three factors.

The first factor was the relative subjectivity of the examination. Deficits noted in objective measurements of hand function receive more points in the UEFFDE than do subjective responses. The second consideration was the strength of support and number of citations in the medical literature for the test as a valid measure of the condition. The third consideration was the results of a survey of certified hand therapists who were members of the American Society of Hand Therapists' Occupational Injuries Prevention and Rehabilitation and Clinical Assessment committees.

The therapists were surveyed regarding their opinion on the relative value of the different examinations in accurately determining the diagnosis of a CTD. What follows are the subtests with definitions, methodology, point values, and literature support.

Intrinsic Atrophy (15 Points)

Phalen (1966) described atrophy of the abductor pollicis brevis muscle as one sign of CTS. Over 17 years, 47% of his patients with CTS had this condition. He stated that often this muscle is the first affected by compression of the median nerve. Loong (1977) found a sensitivity of 53% in CTS patients. Feldman et al. (1987) identified motor weakness of the hand and atrophy of the abductor pollicis brevis muscle in their description of the last stage of CTS. Muscle atrophy involvement has been noted at lower sensitivity by other researchers (Shivde & Fisher 1981; Golding et al. 1986). It has been speculated by MacDermid (1991) that Phalen's group of subjects presented much later for clinical examination than did those of other researchers. This test is based on visible atrophy and is, thus, an objective measure.

Atrophy or weakness of thenar muscles, if not obvious, can be assessed best by comparison with the contralateral side. The abductor pollicis brevis muscle produces the rounded appearance of the thenar muscle group on the radial aspect of the first metacarpal. Flattening or actual depression indicates atrophy (Figure 12.1). This indication can be confirmed by brief muscle testing (the patient points the thumb toward the ceiling while placing the dorsum of the hand and fingers flat against a table surface). For testing of ulnar nerve innervated

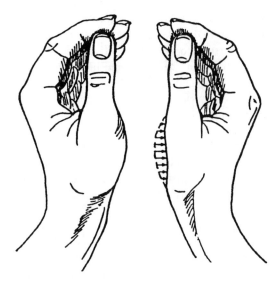

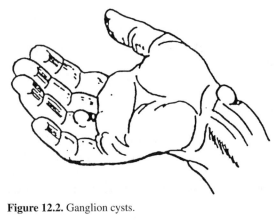

Figure 12.2. Ganglion cysts.

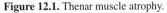

Figure 12.1. Thenar muscle atrophy.

muscles, the dorsum of the hand is observed for atrophy in the interosseous spaces. If atrophy is not obvious, muscle testing of the dorsal and palmer interossei muscles can be performed by resisting abduction and adduction of the fingers.

Ganglion Cysts (15 Points)

Common sites for development of these cysts are the tendon sheaths, the dorsal wrist in the area of the scapholunate joint, and the volar wrist in the region of the flexor carpi radialis insertion (Figure 12.2). Mathews (1973) described the effects of the ganglia on the flexor tendon sheath in the hand. Ganglia that have developed enough to be palpable can become symptomatic and cause pain (American Society for Surgery of the Hand 1983). Phalen (1966) identified a correlation between ganglion cysts and other CTDs. Chaffin and Andersson (1984) have noted ganglia as a risk factor for preventing successful performance in high-risk jobs.

Thus, in the literature it is accepted widely that ganglion cysts can be precipitated and worsened by hand-intensive work. The Texas Worker's Compensation Commission has recognized ganglion cysts as a compensable disorder when the worker has acute trauma or cumulative trauma. Failing to note this as an abnormal condition would not protect employers when a cyst was identified in the preplace-

ment setting. Likewise, failure to identify the cyst as an abnormal condition in a follow-up to baseline testing would prevent workers from making a claim for medical and other appropriate compensation. Palpable ganglia either are present or are not and, thus, represent an objective measure.

Sensibility Loss (10 Points)

Feldman et al. (1987) described paresthesia in the median nerve distribution as early as stage 1 of CTS and identified elevated touch threshold as early as stage 2. Because of its importance in diagnosis of CTS, sensibility testing has received a large share of attention in the literature (MacDermid 1991).

Two common clinical examinations used to measure a subject's sensibility are described frequently in the literature: two-point discrimination (both static and moving) and the SWMFs. The SWMFs have been shown to correlate well with reported sensibility impairment by the patient and sensory nerve conduction tests (Breger 1987). Dellon (1978) reported that significant areas of peripheral nerves and the brain are devoted to discriminative touch of the hand and that the maximum information on nerve function could be obtained with the two-point discrimination test. Gellman et al. (1986) reported 71.4% sensitivity and 80% specificity for sensibility impairment in 67 electrodiagnostic-positive CTS patients compared with 50 normal controls.

Testing vibration-sense threshold changes with commercially available vibrometers has been advocated (Gelberman et al. 1983). However, vibrometry protocols require a subjective response by the individual being tested.

In 1983, Gelberman et al. found a high sensitivity of the SWMFs in identifying CTS. In their research, artificially induced CTS was produced by injecting saline solution into their subjects' carpal canals and was measured with a wick catheter. Their subjects first complained of numbness and tingling leading to loss of vibratory sense. Subjects subsequently experienced loss of perception as measured by the SWMFs, loss of moving two-point discrimination, impairment of sensory nerve conduction, diminished static two-point discrimination, and finally, slowing of motor NCV.

Later, Szabo et al. (1984) compared vibrometry, two-point discrimination, and the SWMFs to evaluate nerve compression. Vibrometry and the SWMFs had a similar sensitivity rate (87 and 83%, respectively) in symptomatic hands. Two-point discrimination had a sensitivity rate of 22%.

For the UEFFDE sensibility test, the SWMFs were used (Figure 12.3). Two-point discrimination and vibrometry were not included in this study because of its time restraints and to limit the number of subjective sensibility tests.

The monofilaments are nylon filaments of descending thickness attached to lucite rods. Their gradation is based on the force required to bend them when they are placed against the skin. The monofilament is applied perpendicular to the finger until it bends. The measure of normal sensory threshold is based on the individual's ability to feel and identify the touched finger.

Bell-Krotoski (1987) has verified the test's repeatability and has provided a standardized format for testing with the SWMFs. The 2.83 monofilament is normal for most individuals. Failure of this section would be a sensibility threshold below perception of the 2.83 monofilament in the median or ulnar distribution of the hand. Even though reliable instruments and methods are used, careful interpretation of the results of this examination is required. Many factors, such as calluses on the subject's fingertips, can influence the examination. Because it requires response from the subject, the test is subjective; however, its interpretation is objective because of the validity of the SWMFs.

Triggering (15 Points)

Triggering can be very painful and can impair hand function significantly (American Society

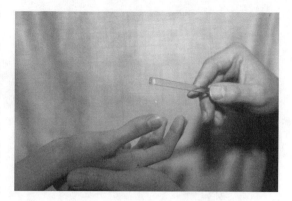

Figure 12.3. Semmes-Weinstein monofilaments.

for Surgery of the Hand 1983). This disorder can be identified by placing the examiner's fingers over the volar, proximal surface of the metacarpophalangeal joints of the fingers and asking the subject to open and close the hand slowly and completely. The thumb is examined in the same manner (Figure 12.4). Snapping or locking of a finger would be a positive response and is measured objectively.

Triggering is one sequela of finger tenosynovitis strongly correlated with repetitive forceful motion, excessive contact, and vibration exposure over the volar surfaces of the metacarpophalangeal joints of the hand (Chaffin & Andersson 1984). Similar to ganglion cysts, triggering has been identified as a compensable disorder in workers who perform high-risk activities. For the same rationale as noted earlier to protect employer and worker, the presence of triggering is identified as an abnormal condition in the UEFFDE. Triggering is an objectively measurable phenomenon.

Raynaud's Phenomenon (10 Points)

If present, Raynaud's phenomenon would be observed most readily following stress testing. It occurs as blanching or coldness in one or more of the fingers (Taylor 1982). For this test, the examiner palpates the fingers to feel for coldness. Each fingernail is pinched to observe capillary refill. In the presence of Raynaud's phenomenon, sensibility may be affected as well. Brown (1990) reported this phenomenon as a significant CTD in industry.

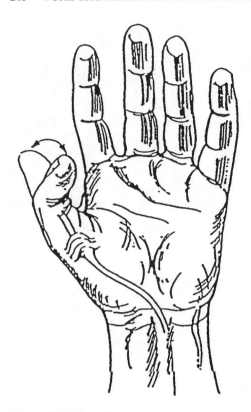

Figure 12.4. Trigger thumb.

Epicondylar Pain (10 Points)

Epicondylar pain is identified as expressed tenderness over the lateral or medial epicondyle and is isolated via palpation of the area during pronation and flexion of the wrist. Lateral epicondylitis is as-

sessed best during the examination for Phalen's test (described later). It is a subjective test.

While the subject is in the position for the Phalen's test, the examiner palpates the region of the lateral and medial epicondyle of the humerus from 1 in. above to 3 in. below the elbow crease. A positive sign is tenderness or wincing by the subject. Epicondylitis also likely would manifest itself as weakness of grip or pinch.

Tinel's Sign (5 Points)

Tinel's sign is recorded as positive when symptoms of tingling occur on tapping over the anatomic distribution of the nerve. As early as 1946, Weddell and Sinclair identified "pins and needles" with mechanical compression of a nerve. In 1966, Phalen described a positive Tinel's sign from percussion of the median nerve at the carpal tunnel in many of his CTS patients (Figure 12.5). A Tinel's sign of the anatomic distribution at the elbow may be present with cubital tunnel syndrome or at the wrist on the ulnar side with Guyon's canal syndrome (American Society for Surgery of the Hand 1983). The test for Tinel's sign requires a subjective response.

A Tinel's sign is not always indicative of a disease process, however, because it may be present in the normal population as well. Although LaBan et al. (1988) reported a sensitivity of 100% in a small population of chronic carpal tunnel patients, in 1990 de Krom et al. (as reported by MacDermid 1991) found 25% sensitivity and 59% specificity in 715 randomly chosen subjects. Gellman et al. (1986) reported 43.9% sensitivity and 94% speci-

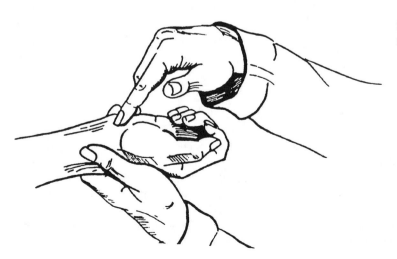

Figure 12.5. Test for Tinel's sign: median nerve at the wrist.

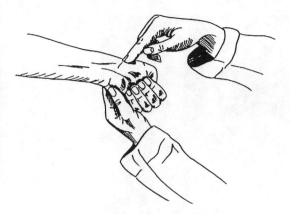

Figure 12.6. Finkelstein's test.

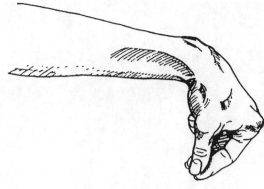

Figure 12.7. Modified Phalen's test.

ficity for Tinel's sign. The relatively low specificity and sensitivity rates given by de Krom et al. and Gellman et al., as well as the level of subjectivity of the response by tested individuals, would favor weighting Tinel's sign lower.

Finkelstein's Test (10 Points)

Finkelstein's test is performed by having the subject grasp the thumb with the fingers (thumb in palm) and ulnarly deviate the wrist (Figure 12.6). This is the recommended method for evaluating de Quervain's disease; if the maneuver reproduces or exacerbates the pain at the base of the thumb, the test is positive (American Society for Surgery of the Hand 1983). Stenosis, or catching of the tendon, in this area is palpable by the examiner. The test requires a subjective response, and no sensitivity or specificity data have been found in the literature.

Phalen's Test (10 Points)

In 1966, Phalen described for CTS a wrist flexion test that is positive when numbness and paresthesia in the median nerve distribution are reported by the subject following holding the wrist in complete flexion for 30–60 seconds. Sensitivity for Phalen's test in CTS patients has been reported as high by LaBan et al. (1988) and moderate by de Krom et al. (1990). It requires a subjective response.

Smith et al. (1977) described a modified Phalen's test (Figure 12.7) wherein the fingers are pinched in addition to flexion of the wrist. The protocol for this test instructs the subject to hold the modified Phalen's

test for 1 minute, with expressed numbness, tingling, or other paresthetic sensory phenomena judged as a positive response. Therapists rated Phalen's test an average of 10.5 points on the survey. This rate is consistent with the test's relatively high reputation for being sensitive to median nerve compression.

Weakness of Grip or Pinch

Ten points are awarded on discovery of more than one standard deviation (but less than two standard deviations) below the norm; 15 points are assigned if more than two standard deviations below the norm are found. Mathiowetz et al. (1984) have shown that grip and pinch strength evaluations performed in standardized positions are reliable and valid. Mathiowetz et al. (1986) presented norms for pinch and grip strength in adults. The instruments used for this portion of the evaluation are the Jamar dynamometer (TEC, Clifton, NJ) and the pinch gauge (Figure 12.8).

Both Feldman et al. (1987) and Phalen (1966) have identified individuals with CTS having decreased grip and pinch strength. Loong (1977) has reported a 53% sensitivity for pinch weakness in CTS patients. Although it requires effort by the subject, grip and pinch testing generally is considered objective.

Abnormal Nerve Conduction Velocity (15 Points)

Feldman et al. (1987) identified slowed motor latency of the median nerve as early as stage 3 CTS. A portable electroneurometer (Figure 12.9) manufactured by Neurotron Medical (Lawrenceville, NJ)

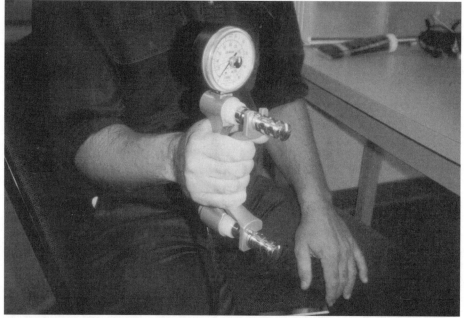

A

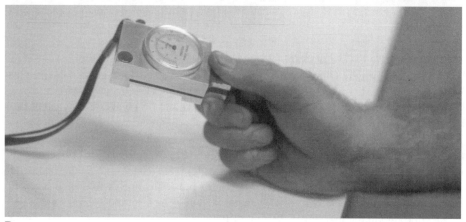

B

Figure 12.8. A. Dynamometer. **B.** Pinch gauge.

was used in the UEFFDE to screen the median nerve motor latency at the wrist.

Rosier and Blair (1984) described the electroneurometer as providing less information than does standard NCV equipment. However, they reported that it served as a diagnostic adjunct for median and ulnar compression neuropathy. Their study supported excellent correlation between diagnoses made with the electroneurometer and standard techniques of nerve conduction. They determined as abnormal NCVs of 4.40 millisec-

onds or greater in the median nerve at the wrist measured with the electroneurometer.

Presence of Edema Following Stress Test (10 Points)

Edema is a symptom of inflammatory disorders. Braun et. al. (1989) stated that provocative testing measures, such as those proposed, would better identify dynamic pathologic conditions of the hand. The presence of edema following exercise similar

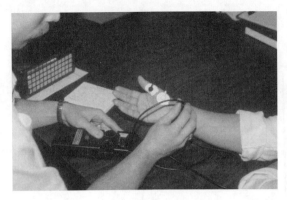

Figure 12.9. Electroneurometer.

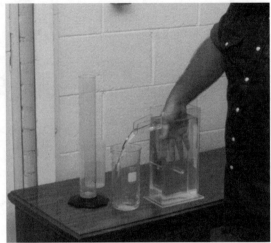

Figure 12.10. Volumeter.

to the subject's work (stressing) can be measured with a commercially available volumeter.

Waylett-Rendall and Sibley (1991) found the volumeter (Figure 12.10) to be accurate within 1%. They recommended consistent placement of the volumeter, careful filling of the tank, and standardized instruction to increase the instrument's accuracy.

In the UEFFDE, the subject undergoes a stress test using tools of the BTE work simulator. Curtis and Engalitcheff (1981) described the work simulator as a way to perform many functional activities in the clinic. The simulator has an adjustable isotonic force-producing mechanism that can be used to alter the amount of resistance to turn a tool in a shaft. Subjects performed at 30% of maximum isometric torque, moving the chosen tool one repetition per second for 90 seconds. Three tools were used. They are the BTE No. 701 (wrist flexion and extension), the No. 302 (wrist ulnar-radial deviation), and the No. 162 (finger flexion and extension; Figure 12.11).

To determine an acceptable percentage of volumetric change, the author reviewed the results of volumetric measurements for 57 uninvolved hands (both male and female) during work tolerance evaluations and 62 pairs of hands in baseline evaluations of workers with no medical history or complaints of symptoms. No subjects in that study were participants in the current research. With the total of 181 hands performing activities similar to those proposed for the UEFFDE, the mean volumetric change at 5–10 minutes postactivity was +1.24% ± one standard deviation of 1.77%. The sum of the mean plus two standard deviations for the population in this study would yield a +4.78% increase in volume.

McGough and Zurwasky (1991) commented on volumetric change following activity. In a pilot study, they reported that the normal increase in volume, measured 5 minutes following similar activities proposed for the stress test, was 3.6% for women and 5.4% for men (mean of total group = 4.5%).

Because the goal was to measure for and identify edema, a 5-minute rest period was taken before the poststress test volumetric measurements were taken. During that time, the subjects participated in the poststress portions of the evaluation. With this stress test and the accurate measure of hand volume before and after, an objective measure indicating 5% change or greater would represent a positive sign and a failing score for that subtest.

Upper-Extremity Fitness-for-Duty Evaluation Accuracy

To measure the sensitivity and specificity of the UEFFDE, two groups of subjects were tested. To measure sensitivity, the first group of data comprised UEFFDE results from 30 male and female workers referred by physicians between January 6 and February 15, 1992, and diagnosed with one of the CTDs for which the UEFFDE screened. Each of these subjects was working or had developed their disorders while performing high-risk activities. Other criteria were that they spoke English and that female subjects were not pregnant.

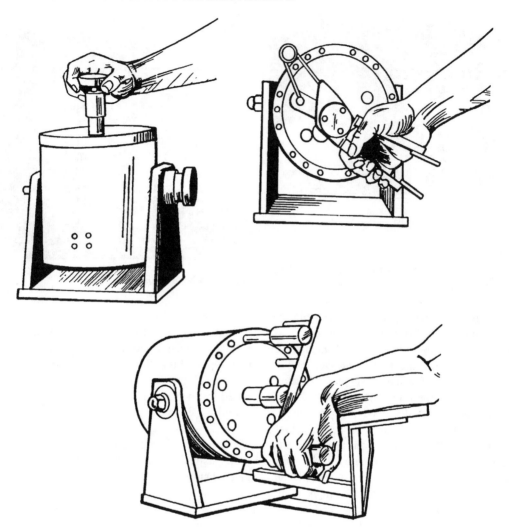

Figure 12.11. Tools in the Baltimore Therapeutic Equipment Work Simulator.

Twenty-two of the subjects in this group performed machine-paced production work or had production incentives. Three workers held clerical jobs wherein they typed or transferred data into a computer for the bulk of the day. Two subjects were mechanics. The remaining three subjects were involved in hand-intensive service industries: a commercial maid, a grocery checker, and a hair dresser.

This group of injured subjects (group A) included 28 women (mean age, 41.3 years) and 2 men (mean age, 43.5 years). Twenty-six were right-hand dominant, and four were left-hand dominant. The 30 subjects had a total of 43 affected hands. The dominant hand was affected in 11 cases, the non-dominant was affected in 6 cases, and 13 subjects had bilateral involvement.

Medical history prior to onset of the current condition was positive in 14 subjects. Five had previous CTDs, two had unrelated hand surgery prior to the onset of the current condition, two had arthritis, and five had had previous surgery for a CTD. The UEFFDE was administered at an average of 36.7 weeks after onset of the presenting condition. This mean was influenced significantly by one subject who was at 6 years postonset. The postonset median and mode for this group were both 12 weeks.

To measure specificity, the second group of data (group B) were UEFFDE results from a convenience sample of eight men (mean age, 36.5 years) and 22 women (mean age, 36.5 years). Subjects had no history of serious upper-extremity trauma or surgery, no congenital defects, and no history of arthritis affecting the upper extremities. No diabetics or pregnant women were included.

A total of 60 hands were measured in this group. Group B subjects included 25 right-hand-dominant and 5 left-hand-dominant subjects. Fifteen were employed in professional occupations, three in service industries, two were homemakers, five were students, and five worked in light (i.e., not typing-intensive) clerical jobs.

Results of Research

The subjects' results were categorized further as (1) false-positive, a normal subject classified as suspect or abnormal; (2) false-negative, a CTD-diagnosed subject classified as within acceptable limits; (3) true-positive, a CTD-diagnosed subject classified as suspect or abnormal; or (4) true-negative, a normal subject classified as within acceptable limits. The equations for sensitivity and specificity were used to determine accuracy for the two groups of data.

The UEFFDE was used to assess 30 injured subjects (group A) with a total of 43 affected hands and a total of 60 hands from 30 normal subjects (group B). Following the evaluation, each of the subjects' hands was scored independently and, on the basis of the score, categorized as *within acceptable limits*, *suspect*, or *abnormal condition identified*. Classification for each hand tested in the two groups and subsequent analysis of accuracy by sensitivity and specificity equations was based on these categorizations.

Hands that were scored 0 or 5 (within acceptable limits) were considered negatives, whereas hands scored 10 (suspect) or 15 or more (abnormal condition identified) were considered positives. Group A subjects could be classified as true-positive or false-negative, and group B could be classified as true-negative or false-positive. The equations for sensitivity and specificity have been used to determine the results of statistical analysis of data from the two groups. Results and subsequent discussion have been based on analysis of sensitivity for the injured hands and of specificity for the normal hands. Results of each subject's test, including

failed subtests and total points for both groups, are presented in Tables 12.1 and 12.2.

Subject Classification

The average score for the hands tested from group A was 33.8 (range, 0–85). The average score for the hands tested from group B was 1.1 (range, 0–10). Group A had 42 true-positives and 1 false-negative. Group B had 55 true-negatives and 5 false-positives.

Statistical analysis of the data reveals results, which are presented in terms of accuracy. Specific analysis of sensitivity and specificity for each group has been accomplished.

Chaffin and Andersson (1984, p. 399) have defined sensitivity as "a measure of a test's accuracy in correctly identifying persons with a certain condition." Statistical analysis indicates the sensitivity of the UEFFDE for group A subjects as 97.67%.

Chaffin and Andersson (1984, p. 400) defined specificity as "a measure of a test's accuracy in correctly identifying persons who do not have the condition." Statistical analysis indicates the specificity of the UEFFDE for group B subjects as 91.97%.

Sensitivity and specificity of the subtests are detailed in Table 12.3.

Analysis of UEFFDE results from the study's subjects indicates a high sensitivity and high specificity rate for abnormal and normal hands tested. The findings support the hypothesis that analysis of accuracy of the UEFFDE would reveal a high percentage of sensitivity in a population of subjects with known CTDs and a high percentage of specificity in a population of normal subjects who have not been exposed to high-risk jobs and have no history of hand disorders. Percentages for both sensitivity and specificity have exceeded the hypothesized percentage of 90%. It is concluded that the UEFFDE, as a clinical assessment, has been an accurate measure for the presence of CTDs in this population.

Subject Classification and Its Implication

The accuracy of the UEFFDE's combined assessment for group A exceeded the sensitivity of most subtests individually. Most subtests individually exceeded the combined specificity for the UEFFDE.

Table 12.1. Group A: Injured Subjects

Subject Number and Hand	Age (yrs)	Gender	Positive Medical History	Diagnosis	Intrinsic Atrophy Present	Ganglion Cyst Present	Sensibility Impaired	Triggering Present	Raynaud's Phenomenon Observed
1R	27	F	Y	DQ					
2R	32	F	Y	TS			X		
3R	51	F	N	CT			X		
3L	51	F	N	CT			X		
4R	60	M	Y	CT	X		X		
4L	60	M	Y	CT					
5R	53	F	Y	CT, TF			X	X	
5L	53	F	Y	CT			X		
6R	67	F	Y	CT	X		X		
7R	56	F	N	CT	X				
7L	56	F	N	CT			X		
8R	36	F	Y	CT					
8L	36	F	Y	CT					
9R	40	F	N	TS					
10R	27	F	N	TS					
10L	27	F	N	TS					
11R	50	F	Y	TF, CT			X	X	
11L	50	F	Y	CT			X		
12R	32	F	N	TS			X		
13R	31	F	Y	TF			X	X	
14R	25	F	N	TS			X		
15R	26	F	Y	TS					
16R	36	F	N	TS			X		
16L	36	F	N	TS					
17R	23	F	N	DQ					
18L	40	F	N	DQ					
19R	42	F	Y	CT			X		
19L	42	F	Y	CT			X		
20L	40	F	Y	EP					
21L	27	M	N	CT			X		
22L	30	F	N	EP					
23R	24	F	N	CT			X		
24R	34	F	N	TS					
25L	38	F	N	DQ					
26R	32	F	Y	TS					
27R	42	F	Y	CT	X				
27L	42	F	Y	CT	X		X		
28R	47	F	N	TS					
28L	47	F	N	DQ					
29R	41	F	N	TS			X		
29L	41	F	N	TS					
30R	47	F	Y	GC, CT		X			
30L	47	F	Y	CT					

DQ = de Quervain's syndrome; TS = tenosynovitis; CT = carpal tunnel syndrome; TF = trigger finger; EP = epicondylitis; GC = ganglion cyst.
Note: Only injured hands were scored.

Epicondylar Pain	Positive Tinel's Sign	Positive Finkelstein's Test	Positive Phalen's Test	Weakness of Grip or Pinch	Abnormal Nerve Conduction Velocity	Edema After Stress Test	Total Score
		X		X			25
X	X			X			35
	X		X	X		X	50
	X		X	X			35
				X	X		50
				X			10
	X		X	X	X		65
			X		X		35
	X			X	X		60
	X				X	X	45
			X				20
	X		X	X			25
			X	X		X	30
	X	X		X			25
			X	X			20
						X	10
	X				X		45
	X			X	X		40
		X					20
		X					35
	X		X	X			35
							0
X	X		X	X			45
X			X				20
		X		X			20
X		X		X		X	40
					X	X	40
							10
X				X			20
	X		X	X		X	45
X		X		X			30
	X			X	X		45
	X	X	X	X			35
		X		X			25
	X		X	X			25
X				X	X		55
	X	X	X	X	X		85
				X		X	25
		X		X		X	35
	X		X	X			35
						X	10
	X		X	X	X		55
	X		X	X	X		40

Table 12.2. Group B: Normal Subjects

Subject Number and Hand	Age (yrs)	Gender	Diagnosis	Intrinsic Atrophy Present	Ganglion Cyst Present	Sensibility Impaired	Triggering Present	Raynaud's Phenomenon Observed
1R	23	F	NA					
1L	23	F	NA					
2R	55	M	NA					
2L	55	M	NA					
3R	39	F	NA					
3L	39	F	NA					
4R	36	M	NA					
4L	36	M	NA					
5R	46	F	NA					
5L	46	F	NA					
6R	36	F	NA					
6L	36	F	NA					
7R	57	F	NA					
7L	57	F	NA					
8R	45	F	NA					
8L	45	F	NA					
9R	44	M	NA					
9L	44	M	NA					
10R	31	F	NA					
10L	31	F	NA					
11R	21	F	NA					
11L	21	F	NA					
12R	44	F	NA					
12L	44	F	NA					
13R	37	F	NA					
13L	37	F	NA					
14R	33	M	NA					
14L	33	M	NA					
15R	22	F	NA					
15L	22	F	NA					
16R	34	F	NA					
16L	34	F	NA					
17R	34	F	NA					
17L	34	F	NA					
18R	54	F	NA					
18L	54	F	NA					
19R	42	F	NA					
19L	42	F	NA					
20R	25	F	NA					
20L	25	F	NA					
21R	43	M	NA					
21L	43	M	NA					
22R	47	F	NA					
22L	47	F	NA					
23R	26	F	NA					
23L	26	F	NA					
24R	35	F	NA					
24L	35	F	NA					
25R	28	M	NA					
25L	28	M	NA					

NA = not available. Note: No patient had a positive medical history. Remainder of 30 subjects exhibited no symptoms.

Epicondylar Pain	Positive Tinel's Sign	Positive Finkelstein's Test	Positive Phalen's Test	Weakness of Grip or Pinch	Abnormal Nerve Conduction Velocity	Edema After Stress Test	Total Score
							0
							0
							0
	X						5
							0
							0
							0
							0
							0
		X					10
							0
X							10
X							10
							0
							0
							0
							0
							0
							0
							0
							0
							0
							0
							0
							0
							0
							0
							0
							0
							0
				X			10
							0
							0
							0
							0
	X						5
							0
							0
							0
							0
							0
							0
			X				10
	X						5

Table 12.3. Sensitivity and Specificity of Subtests

Subtest	Diagnosis	Sensitivity (%)	Specificity (%)
Atrophy	CT	23.8	100
Ganglion	GC	100	100
Sensibility	CT	61.9	100
Triggering	TF	100	100
Raynaud's phenomenon	CT	0	100
Epicondylar pain	EP	100	96.6
Tinel's sign	CT, C	61.9	95
Finkelstein's test	DQ	100	98.3
Phalen's test	CT	52.4	98.3
Weak grip, pinch	All	72.1	98.3
Abnormal nerve conduction velocity	CT	61.9	100
Edema	All	23.8	100

CT = carpal tunnel syndrome; GC = ganglion cyst; TF = trigger finger; EP = epicondylitis; C = cubital tunnel syndrome; DQ = de Quervain's syndrome.

The false-positive and false-negative rates are minimal for both groups of subjects but are worthy of discussion. Increasing the stringency of criteria for a test to be considered positive by removal of subjects classified as suspect decreases the sensitivity for group A to 88.4% but improves the specificity for group B to 100%. Although the groups yielded a small number of subjects classified as suspect, these accounted for all of the false-positive subjects in group B.

The temptation in increasing the accuracy of the instrument would be to eliminate the suspect classification. However, it is felt that by removing this classification, the test becomes less sensitive, and the only benefit would be to increase specificity.

Use of the Upper-Extremity Fitness-for-Duty Evaluation in Industry

It is recognized that, in addition to identifying personal risk factors in applicants in preplacement examinations, the UEFFDE would be useful in establishing a baseline level of function and then following up for threshold changes in workers in high-risk industries. The UEFFDE could also be used to assess individuals with diabetes or other central nervous system problems.

Significant changes in hand function could be indicative of systemic diseases other than CTD. The UEFFDE is a screening test and cannot be substituted for thorough medical examinations. It does have value in its ability to correctly classify individuals who have hand disorders. Within the guidelines of the ADA, the UEFFDE's results are suggestive and useful as a measure of who will need reasonable accommodation.

As a baseline, follow-up examination, routine screening could be used with workers to identify threshold changes and lead either to changing the job or to removing a worker periodically or permanently from such work. Recommended time frames for re-evaluations would be 3 months for newly hired individuals placed in high-risk jobs and 6 months for less hand-intensive work. After that, yearly analysis would be recommended.

Threshold Changes

If threshold changes were noted from baseline function, the worker could be retested within 2 days to confirm the results. Medical treatment or removal from risk factors (depending on the severity of the problem) would be indicated if the follow-up and repeat test indicated a significant change in hand function. A concern is that the UEFFDE may not identify changes until symptoms are present.

Use of the Upper-Extremity Fitness-for-Duty Evaluation as Part of an Overall Prevention Program

Early use of the UEFFDE to follow up on injured workers would assure job-worker matching when such individuals return to work following an injury. As part of an overall program of ergonomic job analysis and changes and of identification of early symptoms to facilitate treatment, the UEFFDE has been shown to be sensitive and specific enough to clearly identify those individuals with problems that should be treated.

Ethical and Legal Rights of Employers and Employees

Prior to employment, identification of any hand impairment would be beneficial to employers in the event that an injury occurred later. For example, if the UEFFDE determined sensibility impairment of 25% to one finger in an applicant, and that worker subsequently had an injury leading to amputation of the finger, the employer would only be liable for 75% of the final impairment.

Another use of UEFFDE information in relation to workers would be to help resolve the question of whether hand-intensive work leads to the development of CTDs. In the past, physicians and therapists have relied on "reasonable medical probability" to make the determination of causation. The incidence and prevalence rates of CTDs in a given population of workers could be established by use of the UEFFDE.

If the prevalence of the disorder in any given group did not exceed that of the average population, any developing disorders would not be compensable under worker's compensation laws. Likewise, the employee would have a claim if the rate exceeded the average population. This arrangement would remove the burden of proof from any one source and would provide a legal definition of financial responsibility.

References

Abbott LC & Saunders JB (1933). Injuries of the median nerve in fractures of the lower end of the radius. *Surg Gynecol Obstet,* 57,507–516.

American Society for Surgery of the Hand (1983). *The Hand Examination and Diagnosis* (2nd ed). New York: Churchill Livingstone.

Americans with Disabilities Act (1990), Public Law 101-336, S. 933.

Armstrong TJ & Chaffin DP (1979). Carpal tunnel syndrome and selected personal attributes. *J Occup Med,* 21,481–486.

Armstrong TJ, Radwin RG, Hansen DJ, & Kennedy KW (1986). Repetitive trauma disorders: job evaluation and design. *Hum Factors,* 28,325–336.

Bell-Krotoski J (1987). The repeatability of testing with the Semmes-Weinstein monofilaments. *J Hand Surg [Am],*12,155–161.

Bleecker ML (1987). Medical surveillance for carpal tunnel syndrome in workers. *J Hand Surg [Am],* 12,845–848.

Braun RM, Davidson K, & Doehr S (1989). Provocative testing in the diagnosis of carpal tunnel syndrome. *J Hand Surg [Am],* 14,195–197.

Breger D (1987). Correlating Semmes-Weinstein monofilament mappings with sensory nerve conduction parameters in Hansen's disease patients: an update. *J Hand Ther,* 1,33–37.

Brown AP (1990). The effects of anti-vibration gloves on vibration-induced disorders: a case study. *J Hand Ther,* 3,94–100.

Castelli WA, Evans FG, Diaz-Perez R, & Armstrong TJ (1980). Intraneural connective tissue proliferation of the median nerve in the carpal tunnel. *Arch Phys Med Rehab,* 61,418–422.

Chaffin DB & Andersson GBJ (1984). *Occupational Biomechanics.* New York: Wiley.

Chaffin DB, Herrin GD, & Keyserling WM (1978). Pre-employment strength testing: an updated position. *J Occup Med,* 20,403–408.

Chu BM & Blatz PJ (1972). Cumulative microdamage model to describe the hysteresis of living tissue. *Ann Biomed Eng,* 1,204–211.

Cooney WP, Dobyns JH, & Linscheid RL (1980). Complications of Colles' fractures. *J Bone Joint Surg Am,* 62,613–619.

Curtis RM & Engalitcheff J (1981). A work simulator for rehabilitating the upper extremity—preliminary report. *J Hand Surg,* 6,499–501.

de Krom MC, Knipchild PG, Kester ADM, & Spaans F (1990). Efficiency of provocative tests for the diagnosis of carpal tunnel syndrome. *Lancet,* 335,393–395.

Dellon AL (1978). The moving two-point discrimination test: clinical evaluation of the quickly adapting fiber/receptor system. *J Hand Surg,* 7,252–259.

Falck B & Aarnio P (1983). Left-sided carpal tunnel syndrome in butchers. *Scand J Work Environ Health,* 9,291–297.

Feldman RG, Travers PH, Chirico-Post J, & Keyserling WM (1987). Risk assessment in electronic assembly workers: carpal tunnel syndrome. *J Hand Surg [Am],* 12,849–855.

Fess EE (1986). The need for reliability and validity in hand assessment instruments. *J Hand Surg,* 5,621–623.

Gelberman RH, Hergenroeder PT, Hargens AR, Lundborg GN, & Akeson WH (1981). The carpal tunnel syndrome: a study of carpal canal pressures. *J Bone Joint Surg Am,* 63,380–383.

Gelberman RH, Szabo RM, Williamson RV, & Dimick MP (1983). Sensibility testing in peripheral nerve compression syndromes. *J Bone Joint Surg Am,* 65,632–638.

Gellman H, Gelberman RH, Tan AM, & Botte MJ (1986). Carpal tunnel syndrome: an evaluation of the provocative diagnostic tests. *J Bone Joint Surg Am,* 68,735–737.

Gilbreth FB & Gilbreth LM (1924). Classifying the elements of work. *Manage Administration,* 8,151.

Golding DN, Rose DM, & Selvarajah K (1986). Clinical tests for carpal tunnel syndrome: an evaluation. *Br J Rheumatol,* 25,388–390.

Hartwell SW, Larson RD, & Posch JL (1964). Tenosynovitis in women in industry. *Cleve Clin Q,* 31,115–118.

Hymovich L & Lyndholm M (1966). Hand, wrist, and forearm injuries—the result of repetitive motions. *J Occup Med,* 8,573–577.

Kazarian LE (1975). Creep characteristics of the human spinal column. *Orthop Clin North Am,* 6,3–18.

King JW (1990). An integration of medicine and industry. *J Hand Ther,* 3,45–50.

Kuorinka I & Koskinen P (1979). Occupational rheumatic diseases and upper-limb strain in manual jobs in a light mechanical industry. *Scand J Work Environ Health*, 5,9–47.

LaBan MM, Friedman NA, & Zemenick GA (1988). "Tethered" median nerve stress test in chronic carpal tunnel syndrome. *Arch Phys Med Rehab*, 67,803–804.

Littler JW (1960). The physiology and dynamic function of the hand. *Surg Clin North Am*, 40,259–266.

Loong SC (1977). The carpal tunnel syndrome: a clinical and electrophysiological study in 250 patients. *Clin Exp Neurol*, 14,51–65.

MacDermid J (1991). Accuracy of clinical tests used in the detection of carpal tunnel syndrome: a literature review. *J Hand Ther*, 4,169–176.

Masear VR, Hayes JM, & Hyden AG (1986). An industrial cause of carpal tunnel syndrome. *J Hand Surg [Am]*, 11,222–227.

Mathews P (1973). Ganglia of the flexor tendon sheaths in the hand. *J Bone Joint Surg Br*, 55,612–617.

Mathiowetz V, Kashman N, Volland G, Weber K, Dowe M, & Rogers S (1986). Grip and pinch strength: normative data for adults. *Arch Phys Med Rehab*, 66,69–74.

Mathiowetz V, Weber K, Volland G, & Kashman N (1984). Reliability and validity of grip and pinch strength evaluations. *J Hand Surg [Am]*, 9,222–226.

McGough CE & Zurwasky ML (1991). Effect of exercise on volumetric and sensory status of the asymptomatic hand. *J Hand Ther*, 4,177–180.

Meadoff N (1949). Median nerve injuries in fractures in the region of the wrist. *Calif Med*, 70,252–256.

Michaelis LS (1950). Stenosis of carpal tunnel: compression of median nerve, and flexor tendon sheaths, combined with rheumatoid arthritis elsewhere. *Proc R Soc Med*, 43,414–417.

Phalen GS (1966). The carpal tunnel syndrome. Seventeen years experience in diagnosis and treatment of 654 hands. *J Bone Joint Surg Am*, 48,211–228.

Punnett L (1987). Upper extremity musculoskeletal disorders in hospital workers. *J Hand Surg [Am]*, 12,858–862.

Rosier RN and Blair WF (1984). Preliminary clinical evaluation of the digital neurometer. *Proceedings of the Twenty-First Annual Rocky Mountain Bioengineering Symposium and Twenty-First International ISA Biomedical Sciences Instrumentation Symposium*, Boulder, CO.

Shivde AJ & Fisher MA (1981). The carpal tunnel syndrome: a clinical-electrodiagnostic analysis. *Electromyogr Clin Neurophysiol*, 21,143–153.

Silverstein BA, Fine LJ, & Armstrong TJ (1986). Hand, wrist cumulative trauma disorders in industry. *Br J Ind Med*, 43,779–784.

Silverstein B, Fine L, & Stetson D (1987). Hand/wrist disorders among investment casting plant workers. *J Hand Surg [Am]*, 12,838–844.

Smith EM, Sonstegard DA, & Anderson WH (1977). Carpal tunnel syndrome: contribution of flexor tendons. *Arch Phys Med Rehab*, 58,379–385.

Stewart SF (1947). Pre-employment examinations of the back. *J Bone Joint Surg*, 29,215–236.

Szabo RM & Gelberman RH (1987). The pathophysiology of nerve entrapment syndromes. *J Hand Surg [Am]*, 12,880–884.

Szabo RM, Gelberman RH, Williamson RV, Dellon AL, Yaru NC, & Dimick MP (1984). Vibratory sensory testing in acute peripheral nerve compression. *J Hand Surg [Am]*, 9,104–109.

Taylor W (1982). Vibration white finger in the workplace. *J Soc Occup Med*, 32,159–166.

Waylett-Rendall J & Sibley DS (1991). A study of the accuracy of a commercially available volumeter. *J Hand Ther*, 4,10–13.

Weddell G & Sinclair DC (1946). Pins and needles: observations on some of the sensations aroused in a limb by the application of pressure. *J Neurol Neurosurg Psychiatr*, 23,26–46.

Suggested Reading

Amadio PC (1987). Carpal tunnel syndrome, pyridoxine, and the workplace. *J Hand Surg [Am]*, 12,875–879.

Armstrong TJ, Fine LJ, Goldstein SA, Lifshitz YR, & Silverstein BA (1987). Ergonomics considerations in hand and wrist tendinitis. *J Hand Surg [Am]*, 12,830–837.

Arndt R (1987). Workpace, stress, and cumulative trauma disorders. *J Hand Surg [Am]*, 12,866–869.

Arons MS (1987). de Quervain's disease in working women: a report of failures, complications, and associated diagnoses. *J Hand Surg [Am]*, 12,540–544.

Barrer SJ (1991). Gaining the upper hand on carpal tunnel syndrome. *Occup Safety Health*, 60,38–43.

Berryhill BH (1990). Returning the worker with an upper extremity injury to industry: a model for the physician and therapist. *J Hand Ther*, 3,56–63.

Bohannon RW (Ed) (1988). *Measurement of Muscle Performance*. Washington, DC: American Physical Therapy Association.

Brain W, Wright A, & Wilkinson M (1947). Spontaneous compression of both median nerves in the carpal tunnel. *Lancet*, 292,277–282.

Fess EE (1984). Documentation: essential elements of an upper extremity assessment battery. In JM Hunter, LH Schneider, EJ Mackin, & AD Callahan (Eds). *Rehabilitation of the Hand* (pp. 49–78). St Louis: Mosby.

Fine LJ, Silverstein BA, Armstrong TJ, Anderson CA, & Sugano DS (1986). Detection of cumulative trauma disorders of the upper extremities in the workplace. *J Occup Med*, 28,674–678.

Gilbert JC & Knowlton RG (1983). Simple method to determine sincerity of effort during a maximal isometric test of grip strength. *Am J Phys Med*, 62,135–144.

Johnson SL (1990). Ergonomic design of handheld tools to prevent trauma to the hand and upper extremity. *J Hand Ther*, 3,86–93.

King JW & Berryhill BH (1988). A comparison of two static

grip testing methods and its clinical applications: a preliminary study. *J Hand Ther,* 1,204–209.

King JW & Berryhill BH (1991). Assessing maximum effort in upper extremity functional testing. *Work,* 1,65–76.

Kurppa K, Pekka W, & Rokkanen P (1979). Paratendinitis and tenosynovitis: a review. *Scand J Work Environ Health,* 5,19–24.

Lundborg G, Gelberman RH, Convely-Minteer M, Lee YF, & Hargress AR (1982). Median nerve compression in the carpal tunnel—functional response to experimentally induced controlled pressure. *J Hand Surg,* 7,252–259.

Louis DS (1987). Cumulative trauma disorders. *J Hand Surg [Am],* 12,823–825.

Matheson, LN (1988). How do you know he tried his best? The reliability crisis in industrial rehabilitation. *Ind Rehab Q,* 1,11.

Meagher SW (1987). Tool design for prevention of hand and wrist injuries. *J Hand Surg [Am],* 12,855–857.

Muffly-Elsey D & Flinn-Wagner S (1987). Proposed screening tool for the detection of cumulative trauma disorders of the upper extremity. *J Hand Surg [Am],* 12,931–935.

Niebuhr BR & Marion R (1986). Detecting sincerity of effort when measuring grip strength. *Am J Phys Med,* 66,16–24.

Occupational Safety and Health Administration (1990). *Ergonomics Program Management Guidelines for Meatpacking Plants.* Washington, DC: US Department of Labor, Occupational Safety and Health Administration.

Pekka W (1979). Epidemiology screening of occupational neck and upper limb disorders: methods and criteria. *Scand J Work Environ Health,* 5,25–38.

Phalen GS (1972). The carpal tunnel syndrome. *Clin Orthop Rel Res,* 1,29–40.

Pinkham J (1988). Carpal tunnel syndrome sufferers find relief with ergonomic designs. *Occup Health Safety,* 8,49–52.

Robbins H (1963). Anatomical study of the median nerve in the carpal tunnel and etiologies of the carpal-tunnel syndrome. *J Bone Joint Surg Am,* 45,953–966.

Schenk RR (1989). Carpal tunnel syndrome: the new industrial epidemic. *J Am Assoc Occup Health Nurse,* 37,226–231.

Smith BL (1987). An inside look: hand injury prevention program. *J Hand Surg [Am],* 12,940–943.

Stokes HM (1983). The seriously uninjured hand—weakness of grip. *J Occup Med,* 25,683—684.

Tanzer R (1959). The carpal tunnel syndrome. *Clin Orthop,* 41A,171–180.

Texas Association of Business (1991). *Texas Employment Law Handbook,* 21-1–21-6.

Chapter 13

Designing a Prevention Program

Michael S. Melnik

Prevention is not a new concept in the field of medicine. Prevention has been applied successfully by the medical and public health communities for years, as demonstrated in the prevention of polio through vaccinations and in the reduced risk of tooth decay through the addition of fluorine to drinking water. Although public health efforts have been successful in preventing disease, the prevention of cumulative trauma disorders (CTDs) and other soft-tissue conditions requires a re-evaluation of our methods for prevention, with a focus on individual commitment, lifestyle changes, and an interdisciplinary approach.

Changes in how the medical community deals with these disorders are also needed to prevent CTDs. Prevention must focus not only on reducing risk factors for CTDs but also on motivating people to make changes and on creating a process that supports these changes. That, in essence, is the focus of this chapter.

Aspects of Cumulative Trauma Disorders

One of the first steps in the prevention process is to define accurately that which you are trying to prevent. The term *cumulative trauma disorder* refers to numerous upper-body conditions, including tendinitis, tenosynovitis, bursitis, carpal tunnel syndrome, cubital tunnel syndrome, de Quervain's disease, Raynaud's syndrome, and trigger finger. These disorders are discussed in Chapter 5. The injury prevention specialist (IPS) first must identify the disorders that are causing problems for the individual or company.

Once the disorders are targeted, the IPS must understand the associated risk factors that can be as varied as the diagnoses. Risk factors include posture or position (Armstrong 1986; Armstrong et al. 1986; Hagberg 1981), force (Armstrong 1986; Astrand 1986), repetition (Armstrong 1986; Armstrong et al. 1986), direct pressure (Eversmann 1983), temperature extremes (Armstrong et al. 1986), vibration (Armstrong et al. 1986), attitude (Bigos et al. 1991; Nathan 1992), stress (Cannon et al. 1981; Arndt 1987; National Safety Council 1993), gender (Cannon et al. 1981), and other disease processes (Bullock 1990). These risk factors are discussed in Chapters 6–9.

Although certain risk factors may respond to a straightforward, engineering approach (Moore et al. 1992; Rice & Rice 1993; The Human Factors Society, Inc. 1988), other risk factors may necessitate a unique combination of approaches. For example, evidence shows that organizational and psychological work conditions are as important in determining the risk for disease in the neck and shoulders as are the physical work conditions (Caplan et al. 1983; Carayon 1993; Simard & Marchand 1994). In addition, a pronounced type A behavior among blue-collar workers has been associated with a higher incidence of musculoskeletal symptoms (Ekberg et al. 1994). Type A personalities are often described as driven, intense, and fast paced. These traits might contribute to a greater risk of CTDs by increasing muscle activity and tension while reducing the amount of time available for tissue recovery. Finally, obesity is considered a possible contributor in some cases (Allen 1993). Given the personal and psychosocial nature of these contributing factors, an isolated engineering change would have limited results in impacting the problem. The IPS must understand the risk factors that necessitate unique, varied approaches.

History of Prevention Efforts

Varied prevention strategies have been discussed in the literature (Joseph 1987; Kilbom 1988; Tadano 1990; National Safety Council 1993; US Department of Labor 1990). These strategies present a core group of activities consisting of ergonomics, training and education, and stretching and warm-up. Benefits and limitations of each are discussed.

Ergonomics

Ergonomics is the science of designing the work to fit the worker. Ergonomics attempts to create an environment in which the most natural way to perform a task is the most efficient and places the fewest demands on the body. In numerous instances, ergonomics processes have been successful at increasing productivity and quality while reducing injuries (MacLeod 1995). However, some ergonomics programs make changes without considering the consequences of these actions (Kroemer 1992; Chong 1993).

For example, how many ergonomics programs consider the personal comfort and familiarity that individuals may have established at their work areas and how they may perceive this change? Many people resist change, regardless of whether the change is beneficial. This resistance can be even greater if people feel that they were not involved directly in precipitating the change. The reaction can present itself in a variety of ways that serve to undermine the ergonomics process.

The author experienced this situation in an industrial setting. It was recommended to management that the company provide antifatigue mats for their employees. The recommendation was approved, and shortly thereafter mats were placed at specific workstations. On returning for a follow-up visit, the author found that nearly all the employees had thrown the new mats away shortly after they arrived. When questioned, they informed the author that they had requested these mats 10 years ago and management had refused, saying that antifatigue mats had no value. Management's change of heart gave the employees the impression that their input had limited value, and the rejection of the new mats was their response. Needless to say, a successful ergonomics program is as much about the perception of change and the level of employee participation in this change as it is about the physical change itself.

Another unanticipated problem can occur when an ergonomic change is made to reduce the demands on a specific body part, without regard to other body parts that may receive an impact from the change. For example, the computer mouse was designed to minimize the amount of keying done on a computer. Excessive keying is considered a risk factor for CTDs, and any reduction minimizes the risk. However, if the mouse is placed at arm's reach, the mouse does not fit a person's hand appropriately, or the person uses too much grip force, excessive demands can be placed on the shoulder, forearm, and hand muscles, creating an entirely different set of CTD risk factors.

Many studies in ergonomics attempt to quantify human capacities and define appropriate work tasks, but those who actually perform the work have difficulty in applying this data to the real world (Buckle et al. 1992). This problem has not gone unnoticed. In an attempt to reconcile such differences, the National Institute of Occupation Safety and Health revised their lifting guidelines specifically to take a more practical approach to the problem of material handling (Waters et al. 1993). It is important for an IPS to recognize that the information coming out of the laboratories may be in conflict with the way in which a company currently runs the business. Many companies do not have the capital (or do not *perceive* that they have the capital) to replace their outdated machinery, purchase material-handling devices, and provide ergonomic training for all their employees. Although this does not mean that ergonomics programs cannot be implemented in these environments until the company managements change their attitude, it does mean that an IPS must take the research coming from the laboratories and "translate" it into a language that is understandable, practical, and useable to industry. Industry management may need some help understanding the relationship between the customary concerns of budgets, cash flow, productivity, quality, and the less familiar topic of ergonomics.

Although the success of ergonomics in preventing CTDs has been cited, implementing an ergonomics process does not ensure that workers will participate. This is due, in part, to the fact that ergonomics is not only about the environment but about the relationship between a worker and the environment. This means that changing the environment is only half of the equation. The other half is employee interaction with this change. As a result of stress, physical condition, motivation, long-standing habits, and many other factors that influence day-to-day choices, workers may continue to make poor decisions in good environments. These choices can be as benign as not adjusting an adjustable chair or as serious as neglecting to use a hoist to lift a heavy or awkward load.

Training and Education

Training and education enable workers to make better choices and to contribute actively to the prevention process. What could be a better source of ideas for making a job safer than the people performing the job? The positive side of training is that if it is done effectively and is reinforced, it empowers employees to take more responsibility for their health, both at work and at home. If done well, training invites ideas, motivates participation, and encourages safe behaviors.

There is some controversy, however, regarding the effectiveness of training as a tool for prevention in the workplace (Tomal 1992). Numerous variables influence the effects of training and educating workers. The most important are the retention capabilities of the audience, the ability of the workers to apply the information to their own work, and the level of motivation they have to use this information. A stressful environment may cause workers to resort to their habitual way of working, regardless of the safety information presented (Tadano 1990). Nearly every job in industry is learned in the process of performing the work. This is the fundamental difference between education and training. For example, education may provide a broad knowledge of the physics of throwing a ball, how baseballs are made, and the history of the game. If a person wants to learn to throw a baseball, there is no amount of classroom education that can compare with picking up a ball and throwing it. Most physical work tasks follow this same principle. Education becomes training when it moves from the classroom to the work environment (Rystrom & Eversmann 1991).

Stretching and Exercise

Stretching and exercise programs in the workplace consist of activities designed to help employees prepare for and compensate for the demands of their work. Typically, these activities include specific stretches designed to help muscles to recover from work activities as well as exercises designed to activate muscles that may not be used otherwise during the workday. In some companies, these activities are performed for several minutes at the beginning of the day; others promote periodic, brief stretching intervals throughout the day, although many programs use a combination of the two.

The efficacy and limitations of stretching and exercise programs have been described in the literature (Sawyer 1987; Clafin 1991; Melnick 1993; Thomas et al. 1993). Although some controversy remains, there is evidence that these types of programs are efficacious, particularly when combined with education, training, and ergonomics. Although most companies are quite capable of developing a stretching program, the real challenges to the IPS include enlisting management approval of this "radical" concept and motivating supervisors to involve skeptical employees. Despite the evidence that demonstrates their success, stretching and warm-up programs are generally resisted by those in industry for reasons unrelated to their potential success. A company's resistance to stretching rarely centers on whether stretching is beneficial. It revolves around management's concern over the time that may be lost while employees are stretching, over supervisor's concerns regarding both the time involved and whether they will have to lead these stretches, and over the employees' concerns over peer pressure, pre-existing injuries, and assorted misconceptions about stretching.

Splints and Braces

Such supports as splints and braces have provided lively discussion with regard to their value as a preventive tool. Ergonomists argue that splinting is an

Table 13.1. Distinctions Between Program and Process

Program	Process
Done to employees	Done with employees
Recognizable beginning and ending	Recognizable beginning and no end
Predetermined course of events	Flexible: able to change and adapt
Considered an "addendum" to productivity	An integral part of day-to-day operations
Energy draining	Energy generating
Short-term benefits	Long-term benefits

attempt to fit the person to the task instead of fitting the environment to the employee. Therapists may argue that although splints may help some workers maintain neutral body postures, the splint may simply shift the problem to another body part that is not splinted and thereby reduce the flexibility and strength of the immobilized area. On the other hand, athletic trainers will prescribe the wearing of splints and braces to protect athletes from environments that are unpredictable and to which it is impossible to adapt.

To determine whether the use of splints or braces is appropriate, the IPS should ask the following questions:

- What is the situation that necessitates supportive splinting or bracing?
- Can the environment be changed to reduce the need for a support?
- Does the employee know why he or she is wearing the support?
- Does the employee know how long and when the support should be worn?
- What problems could occur if workers use the supports incorrectly or wear them too long?
- Do the employees demonstrate increased awareness of proper working techniques when they wear the supports?
- How does the use of splints or braces fit into the larger picture of a comprehensive injury-prevention process?

As the answers to these questions become available, the role of splints and braces as effective preventive tools will be better understood.

In conclusion, it should be recognized that any single approach may be limited in scope because of the comprehensive nature of CTDs. A solution that is undertaken in isolation from other activities may reduce the effectiveness of the overall process. In addition, the roles of motivation and resistance to change are

aspects of an injury-prevention process that may seem less objective than do some of the engineering aspects of ergonomics but can have a dramatic effect on the success of the injury-prevention process. The prevention of CTDs is about ensuring that the right questions are being asked and ensuring that the implemented solutions are appropriate. Injury prevention is not just about making changes in the environment but also about inviting changes in human behavior. Much is known about CTDs and how to prevent them. The challenge to the IPS is to recognize that the reason for the continuing growth of CTD problems is not a lack of information; it remains a problem because of the struggle to deliver this information effectively in a way that makes the prevention process less threatening and more inviting to those we are trying to help.

The Prevention Process

Getting Started

It is important to define the difference between an injury-prevention process and an injury-prevention *program*. Programs generally have a very recognizable beginning and a very recognizable ending. A process, on the other hand, has a recognizable beginning but no foreseeable end. This is a very important differentiation that goes beyond semantics. Many companies have had short-term programs; therefore, gathering support for another program is difficult because the employees are anticipating that the program will be short lived. The IPS must make clear that the process is not temporary.

The fundamental differences between a process and a program are described in Table 13.1.

Identifying the Players

Injury prevention has grown into a field that now involves the services of numerous professionals. The number of experts in the community who provide injury-prevention services has grown dramatically over the last decade (Kohn & Friend 1993) and includes occupational and physical therapists, engineers, occupational health nurses, physicians, chiropractors, exercise physiologists, psychologists, psychiatric social workers, equipment dealers, product distributors, insurance experts, risk managers, and loss-control specialists.

Each of these specialists has a unique set of skills and insights to bring to the work site. To provide the most comprehensive, state-of-the-art services, the IPS should be familiar with the other resources available and how these services complement their role in the prevention process.

There are several benefits of the IPS's familiarity with other professionals in the community:

- Access to more information: The IPS gains access to more information and therefore is able to provide better quality service to the client. For example, a company may want to revamp its medical management system, redesign a job, develop a stretching program, and re-evaluate its worker's compensation carrier. One individual may not be able to provide direct services in all these areas, but the IPS can act as a resource to the client through contacts with experts in other fields.
- Improvement of the success rate: Because numerous risk factors and variables impact the success of a program, the more "eyes and ears" available to help to define the problems and implement solutions, the greater the likelihood for success.
- Increased business opportunities: Establishing relationships with other prevention specialists from different fields can create a referral network. Introducing a competent specialist to an existing client with a need outside the IPS's expertise creates a win-win situation. It provides the client with the best services available and creates a scenario in which other specialists begin to refer the IPS to their clients.

The concept of using more than one expert is not new to business and industry. When companies consider new products, the market research and product development teams first research the need for the product. Engineers then design the product and turn the plans to build the necessary dies over to the tool and die department. The employees manufac-ture the product, the sales department sells the product, and the transportation department delivers it. Each department has a unique set of skills, and each is integral to the overall process.

Similarly, in the prevention of CTDs, the most valuable "experts" are the individuals or departments who are most familiar with the company:

- Management
- Supervisors
- Employees
- Union representatives
- Risk manager or loss-control specialist
- Controller
- Purchasing department
- Medical staff
- Personnel and human resources department
- Tool and die department
- Maintenance department

Each of these departments or individuals plays a role in the injury-prevention process. It is essential that the IPS understand their roles and positions in the company hierarchy so as to solicit the greatest level of involvement and support.

Selecting a Process Leader

To be effective, the injury-prevention process must have a leader. However, one person cannot effectively change attitudes, design workplaces, and foresee all potential obstacles without assistance. IPSs must choose their prevention teams wisely and position themselves strategically to foster a team effort. The most effective IPS knows how to maximize each team member's strengths. If the prevention process already has a leader, the IPS must know how to become a valuable and contributing member of the existing team.

Inviting Change

A successful CTD-prevention process is a series of steps that eventually becomes self-sustaining. Implementation of one idea leads to the development of more ideas; initial participation by a few key individuals leads to the involvement of more. As companies progress through each step, they need to think about the critical ingredients of the process and apply these ingredients along the way. A successful prevention process includes certain basic ingredients.

Flexibility

A company must have in place methods for ongoing evaluation and for subsequent changes to upgrade the prevention process. Many companies begin their program with grandiose plans and lose momentum along the way. Without an alternative plan or the ability to adapt the current program, the company may perceive that, when difficulties arise, the only option is to cancel the program and possibly to abandon its prevention efforts entirely.

Consistency

For effective prevention, a company must maintain consistency throughout the life of the process. It is considered general knowledge that many companies view safety as important only when the company is not busy or after workers have been injured. A good injury-prevention process includes early identification of the methods for enforcing, monitoring, and incorporating injury prevention into the day-to-day operations of the company.

Commitment

Commitment must be demonstrated by management to enlist participation by the workers. Employers who repeatedly start a program, invest energy and funds, and then "pull the plug" generate skepticism about future programs. Ongoing support of the program by management is necessary to promote worker participation.

Communication

The ability to communicate the prevention process effectively to employees and to gather feedback from the participants are two of the most critical and often overlooked variables for process success. Ineffective communication is often identified as a primary reason for program failure. An effective process is more than knowing what to do; it also is knowing how to talk about it.

Accountability

Effective prevention requires that a company determine who is accountable for the various aspects of the prevention process at all levels of the organiza-

tion. Although industry is well versed in defining the specific responsibilities as they relate to productivity and quality, individuals are rarely accountable for safety issues.

The Fatigue Factor

Longevity in a successful prevention process is essential, and its importance needs to be made clear to management. A tool that can affect the process in either a positive or negative way is what the author likes to call the *fatigue factor*. If something is in place long enough, those resisting the change gradually lose the energy to resist it. Once people come to grips with the fact that something is going to be in place for the long haul, they recognize that their resistance is probably fruitless and requires too much energy. It becomes easier to participate in the process than to resist it. This is how the fatigue factor expresses itself in a successful prevention process.

On the other hand, in a struggling prevention process, the fatigue factor is experienced by the few individuals, including the IPS, who are trying to implement it. If the previously outlined essential ingredients are not present and the employees do not think that this process is going to last, those responsible for implementing the process will need to put out an inordinate amount of energy and will fatigue before anything ever takes hold.

Developing the Prevention Process

The methods used by the author are a result of 10 years of direct experience with injury-prevention colleagues, business, and industry as well as exposure to a compilation of approaches used by a variety of published consultants. The prevention strategies used by the author are changing continually. Change and growth are essential components of the injury-prevention process.

Meetings with Management

Management commitment is necessary to get a process started and to keep it going. Critical areas to address in this initial meeting include

- Discussion of goals
- Identification of resources (dollars and manpower)
- Preliminary identification of key team members
- Establishment of preliminary time lines
- Identification of possible obstacles and methods for dealing with them
- Discussion of systems currently in place (including production, quality, maintenance, mandated safety programs, interdepartmental communication, and insurance) and the degree of effectiveness perceived in each system

The background information provided by management can help the IPS to understand what systems or strategies are working for the aforementioned components and what struggles still exist. Those processes that are working well may illuminate the best strategies for implementing the CTD-prevention process. The IPS should use these existing processes to build on those areas in which the company has already succeeded as well as to reinforce the idea that an injury-prevention process need not require drastic changes.

Supervisor Orientation

Participation and ongoing support from supervisors are necessary for the program to realize its potential (Joseph 1987; Minter 1991). In some cases, the supervisors may have been informed by management that the IPS is "in charge" of this process. This places the IPS in an awkward position, because to be successful, the IPS will need the support and insights of the supervisors. The supervisor orientation provides an opportunity to neutralize resentment that may be directed toward the IPS by acknowledging the supervisors' involvement as true on-site experts.

Another purpose of the supervisors' orientation is to introduce them to the process before any activities actually begin. In this first meeting, the IPS describes the process components and each participant is encouraged to ask questions and to express concerns. This initial meeting allows those who will be directly affected by the prevention process to contribute to and adapt the program to their individual needs.

Employee Communication

Supervisors and management can help to identify the most effective methods for communicating the process to the employees and for eliciting feedback. The employees deserve an orientation that informs them of previous actions, coming events, and the role of each prevention team member. The employees will then not be surprised by evaluation of the work site by the IPS or by training sessions that are scheduled without their knowledge. Communication is as important before the process as it is during the process itself. If employee communication is ignored, employees may feel that their concerns are not represented and that the process is management based. Early exclusion of employees may cause resistance to the process and subsequent failure of the process.

Communication strategies include brief tool-box talks (brief meetings usually held at a work site that most often deal with productivity or quality issues), shift meetings conducted by supervisors, or more formal presentations by management representatives. Although a live presentation of this information is preferred, some organizations communicate information through memos or information posted in common areas. The IPS can work with either type of communication to develop the best strategies. It is important that employees be aware of the communication system and who to contact with questions as the process begins.

Establishing a Cumulative Trauma Disorder Task Force

As stated, it is very difficult for one individual to run a prevention process, whereas a task force can perform a variety of important functions (Rystrom & Eversmann 1991). It is important to enlist a variety of in-house players and to have the task force in place before the process begins. This allows representatives from all levels of the company to be involved and to choose their own leader. Once started, the task force should be flexible enough to add motivated individuals (or dismiss unmotivated ones) as the process progresses.

Many companies may have a safety committee already in place. The IPS should learn about the responsibilities and activities of this group. Although safety committees are often responsible for all aspects of safety, CTD prevention may not be their focus. Therefore, it is advisable to assemble an injury prevention task force that is action oriented and focused on one task—CTDs. This group should meet at least once per month and develop an action plan with specific members accountable for implementing these plans.

Task force participants may include the following:

- IPS
- Management representative
- Supervisor representative
- Union representative
- Engineering representative
- Maintenance department representative
- Employee representative(s)
- Medical representative(s)

It is important to keep the task force small enough to manage, yet comprehensive enough to address all the variables. Some of the individuals in the preceding list participate on an as-needed basis as specific issues arise.

Work-Site Evaluation

There are three primary reasons for the IPS to perform a work-site evaluation: (1) evaluating a workplace in preparation for an education and training process, (2) evaluating a workplace as part of an ongoing ergonomics process, and (3) evaluating a specific job as it relates to an individual who is experiencing a specific problem or returning to work following an injury.

Chapter 10 discusses job analysis in more detail. Also, numerous available publications discuss the process (Caplan et al. 1983; Grandjean 1988; Joseph 1989; Johnson 1990; Stankevich 1994). Briefly, at the beginning of a process and before any employee education, the initial work-site evaluation is performed so that the IPS may orient himself or herself to the work environment, become familiar with the layout of the facility, and gain insight into the job demands. It provides the IPS an opportunity to establish dialogue with the employees and to understand their perspectives on the work they perform. The work-site evaluation also provides the IPS with an increased level of credibility that can transfer to the educational sessions.

The initial objective of a work-site evaluation is to ask pertinent questions and to define problems—not to find solutions. Finding a solution is the end product. Asking questions and getting the opinions of veteran workers not only provide valuable insight but help the IPS to increase the level of employee involvement.

Another objective of the work-site evaluation is to identify other, "invisible" factors that may contribute to the breakdown of an injury-prevention process. Although these factors may not be observed readily during this visit to a facility, their presence can have a dramatic impact on the success or failure of an injury-prevention process. An abridged list of these factors includes:

- Anticipated layoffs
- Anticipated plant shutdown
- Labor negotiations
- Personnel changes
- Changes in production or quality standards
- Changes in company ownership
- Beginning or ending of an existing program (safety or non-safety related)

These factors tend to influence people's perceptions about the injury-prevention process. In one situation, the author was invited to provide education sessions during a time at which layoffs were occurring. One of the employees in the class asked the author how many employees had to be laid off to pay for these classes. Although the author's presence and the impending layoffs were not related, it is the perception of the timing of these events that must be dealt with effectively. Had the author been aware of the layoffs beforehand, a discussion with management to determine the appropriateness of training at this time could have taken place. Of course, education and training can be conducted during stressful times but, as an IPS, the author is responsible for informing clients of all the variables that will effect the service they are purchasing. Working with a client to deal effectively with some of the invisible issues will increase the likelihood that the services will have the desired results.

In some instances, a certain event may change the time lines of the process or the method in which it is presented to the employee population. In any case, recognition of these events can add to the credibility of the IPS. Finally, the IPS should increase personal awareness of the following critical workplace issues:

- *Stress:* Includes both work and home issues.
- *Lack of job control:* Can range from having little say about quality and productivity issues to concerns over potential layoffs or salary cuts.
- *Poor communication at the job site:* For a prevention process to work, it is essential that management effectively communicate its goals to supervisors and that the supervisors communicate safety to the employees. Although productivity and quality are languages that most successful companies communicate well, often safety is an unfamiliar language, and it should not be assumed that companies will make the transition into safety communication without a struggle.
- *Power struggles:* These struggles may take place between supervisors and employees and can have an impact on the prevention process, particularly if the IPS is attempting to increase the supervisor's role and is encouraging the employees to communicate more with their supervisors.
- *Hidden agendas:* They are a lot harder to detect but can be deadly to a prevention process. These agendas can be the result of a supervisor who speaks highly of the process but knows that the department is being evaluated only on the basis of production. They can be the result of a safety person who would rather be in another department or of a management team that has been told by its insurer that prevention is something it needs to do and in the midst of the process begins looking for an insurer whose expectations are not as high. Regardless of the agenda and its origin, the IPS needs to keep a sharp eye out for behaviors that seem inconsistent with the goals of the process.

The IPS should be cautious about drawing conclusions on the basis of personal perceptions or conflicting reports from management and workers. Many of the foregoing factors exist at least to some degree in all companies, and this should be taken into consideration as the process evolves.

The following considerations should be included in a work-site evaluation:

- *Be prepared:* Bring your own hard hat, safety shoes, safety glasses, work gloves, and hearing protection. Although nearly all companies will make these items available to their consultants, you will be viewed as more competent if you come prepared. Obviously, a pad of paper and a pen or pencil and some sort of photographic medium are necessary for recording observations.
- *Be a good listener:* Ask the employees to describe their jobs. Most people are proud to talk about what they do in great detail. There is a tendency for the IPS to be viewed as the expert when going into industry; however, the experts are the ones that have worked in this environment for years. The IPS should discover the best ways to tap into workers' expertise.
- *Communicate with employees:* Ask a lot of questions. Good questions can help the IPS to get a good feel for the environment:

1. Is this a typical day (with regard to workload, pace, noise, temperature, etc.)?
2. Who else works at this workstation?
3. What happens when this machine goes down?
4. Does everyone perform this job the same way?
5. What are the easiest and hardest parts of the job?
6. Where (if anywhere) do you feel the physical effects of your job at the end of the day?
7. What do people do (where do they go) on breaks?

- *Do not make assumptions:* It is very natural to want to come up with "the" solution that makes the IPS a hero. Keep in mind that the greatest value of an IPS is to help a company to identify problems thoroughly. Before any attempts are made to change a work area, specific variables need to be taken into consideration, including the following:

1. What has been tried previously to improve this area, and what worked or did not work?
2. How many people work at this work area and will it affect each person the same way?
3. Have any of the employees who work at this job made recommendations for improvement? If so, how did management respond?
4. How will a change affect production, quality, and overall safety? Does the change make it easier on a specific body part but pass the demands on to a different area?

5. What people, either in house or in the community, have the most expertise in this area? Is it feasible to enlist their support?

• *Remember that the IPS is a guest:* The IPS is a visitor in someone else's "home." The initial work-site evaluation is a time of first impressions; it is important that they be good. Before observing a workstation, introduce yourself to the employee and explain why you are there. Ask employees for permission before taking a picture. If you want to "catch them in the act," ask employees if they will repeat the activity.

• *Perform the jobs you are evaluating:* Performing the job allows the IPS to "feel" the skills needed to perform the job. It helps to identify the job demands more accurately and puts the IPS in a position to acknowledge the skills required by the employee to perform this job. Be sure to ask the company beforehand if it is all right to perform the job. Some companies may refuse, due to liability issues.

Employee Education

It is important to recognize that most companies do not provide training. A recent survey revealed that 90% of the companies contacted do not train their employees formally (LaBar 1991). In the author's experience, the effects of education and training have been overestimated regarding what can be accomplished in a single training session. A single training class constitutes neither education nor training. Education and training take place over time and are impacted by repetition and reinforcement (Tadano 1990; Rystrom & Eversmann 1991). For years, consultants have provided classes to workers with the expectation that workers will change as a result of exposure to new information. There are some *assumptions* that underlie our belief that education will create change. One is that the audience is interested in the information presented. Many participants will ask, "What's in this for me?" Relative to other concerns of the employee (finances, family, illness, etc.), keeping the wrist in a neutral position may seem superfluous or unimportant.

Another assumption is that the audience will retain the information presented. If the information presented is not reinforced in the work environment, the information will not be retained for long (Carlton 1987). Most employees do not bring notepads and pencils to education sessions and do not go home to study what was presented. Many employees believe that if the company thinks that this information is important, they will certainly hear it again.

Yet another assumption is that the audience can use the presented information effectively. Everyone has long-standing habits, both in thought and in movement. Many worker movements are not the result of conscious thought but rather of movement habits. Teaching individuals to hold their tools differently or to use different motor patterns is akin to telling a person to kick a field goal or hit a baseball with no previous experience. The ability or opportunity to practice needs to be built into the injury-prevention process.

As an exercise in demonstrating the difficulty of changing movement patterns, ask all the participants in an educational session to cross their arms. Then ask them to uncross and recross their arms quickly the opposite way. Many struggle to accomplish this task and admit that it feels awkward to change.

Everyone has movement patterns that feel normal. No matter how much the author lectures on better ways to work, the only thing that will allow different movement patterns to feel normal is *practice*. This exercise allows the author to demonstrate recognition of the difficulty in change and the need for practice to make the change feel more comfortable.

Management must support your strategies and be willing to make changes when necessary. Many environments do not physically permit or support the changes in work methods advocated by prevention processes. If you teach a person in a class to minimize certain movements but the job still requires these movements, workers must choose between what they have been asked to do and what they are required to do.

An additional assumption is that the information is presented in a way that makes sense to the audience. The educational program is, in part, entertainment. An initial education session cannot be expected to create change, but it should be expected to generate interest. The IPS should evaluate the content of the class critically and ask if the information presented is something audiences need or want to know, if the information is presented as something they can use, and if the information is presented as something they will hear again.

Excessive information can overload the participants and bury the most valuable points made during your presentation. Initially, the purpose of education is to expose the employees to information that will help them participate in the process. For this reason, the author likes to call the initial classes *employee orientations*, not education. The education will come as the IPS makes a few major points that employees will hear, practice, or experience over and over again.

Although the role of training in changing behaviors may have been overemphasized, what has not been emphasized enough is the effect that education sessions have on the attitudes and perceptions of the audience. Although a single class may not get a person to choose different work postures or to perform stretches throughout the day, the way in which the class is presented and how well it is received will have a major impact on future activities.

Recognizing the Audience's Reality

In an education session, as in a process, it is important to establish a baseline on which to build. It is important that the IPS avoid making the assumption that everyone who attends an educational session in industry is willing and eager to learn. The author initiates the educational program by acknowledging the certain realities in this type of learning situation:

- Change is not expected as a result of one talk on prevention.
- This subject may not be the most important event in lives of the attendees.
- Prevention does not begin until the class is over; prevention involves all levels of workers and management.
- We do not yet know everything about CTDs, but we know enough to take action.
- The audience will hear this information again.
- The audience will need to think about the following questions:

  1. What information made the most sense?
  2. What information would help them the most if it were repeated?
  3. How often would they like to hear it?
  4. What would be the best methods for delivering this information?

The main points presented by the author in an educational session for employees include:

- *The cumulative nature of CTDs*: It is important that employees not look for the *one thing* that causes the problem. Numerous activities, positions, and other factors contribute, and the goal is to minimize the impact of each.
- *Basic anatomy and mechanics of the upper body*: The employees need to know enough about how they are designed to be able to understand the concept of better or more efficient work positions. The author uses the term *neutral* to describe the most efficient and least demanding positions for the upper body. Using the employees' actual work tools can emphasize these points (e.g., have the employees attempt to grasp a tool with a straight wrist, then with a bent wrist).
- *General principles of prevention*: This portion provides practical solutions for minimizing the demands of work, recreational, and home activities.
- *Compensating for demanding positions:* This topic places a great deal of the responsibility for prevention on the employees. Employees can learn to minimize the demands on their bodies by understanding compensation techniques. These include specific stretches, position changes, and awareness of inefficient work methods.

Providing Effective Presentations

To create a good impression and an effective presentation, the IPS should attempt to troubleshoot in preparation for the presentation. Consider the following issues:

- How will the IPS handle a difficult question?
- Can the IPS present in a variety of environments?
- Does the IPS have flexibility if there are time constraints?
- What will the IPS do if the projector breaks or a slide gets stuck?
- How will the IPS handle a difficult audience or employee?
- Can the IPS effectively bring humor into the session?

Preparing to deal with these types of situations is essential in being an effective presenter in an industrial setting. Presenting information effectively is no different from providing effective treatment. The same preparation needs to be made to ensure that the desired results are achieved.

Supervisor Educational Session

A recent article reported that more than 20% of supervisors surveyed receive no ongoing training regarding safety matters (Krout 1994). In 1967, the National Safety Council determined that supervisor participation is the most important ingredient in an effective safety program (Krout 1994).

The goal of supervisor education is to assist the supervisors with providing cursory work-site evaluations and eliciting change in their departments and with developing methods for communicating safety in those departments on an ongoing basis. Ideally, this session identifies the role of the supervisors in more detail, improves communication between the supervisors and the IPS, and allows supervisors to ask questions or voice concerns generated from the initial employee sessions. In an effective process, supervisors are held accountable for safety in their departments. By providing supervisor education, the company reassures the supervisors that, if more is going to be asked of them, the company will provide them with the necessary tools to be successful.

Ongoing Activities (Program Maintenance)

Ideally, by this point, management has demonstrated commitment to the process. The task force is in place, the employees have been oriented, and the supervisors have acquired skills to help support the process. At this point, the process actually begins. To be successful, *repetition* should be built into every aspect of the CTD-prevention process (Topf & Preston 1991). The maintenance of an effective injury-prevention process must be a normal part of the workday. It should not be looked on as being a burden or time consuming. Certain maintenance activities are essential for success of the program.

Ongoing Task Force Meetings

The task force meets on a regular basis. It continuously evaluates the progress of the process, gathers feedback from the participants, and makes plans for the future.

Developing and Maintaining an Ergonomic Process

Developing an effective ergonomics process follows the same steps as those found in the global CTD-prevention process. In a survey of supervisors in an industrial environment, ergonomics was rated the least effective of all their programs. Only 54% of the supervisors believe they even need an ergonomics program, and as few as 33% report being trained in ergonomics (Arndt 1987).

An ergonomics process involves more than the development of a task force, educational programs, and ongoing work-site evaluations. The successful ergonomics process will include a system for modifying workstations and a prioritization system to identify the most critical issues. This system demonstrates to the employees that there is a method for determining the order and timing of work-site changes on an equitable basis. In many companies, the prioritization system is based on determining which projects are the least expensive or require the fewest hours to complete, which work area has the greatest exposures, and which project will demonstrate the greatest return on investment.

By answering these questions, a company can create a ranking system that continuously moves projects through the process. Articles that discuss the implementation of an ergonomics process can be found in numerous publications (Kilbom 1988; The Human Factor Society 1988; Rice & Rice 1993; Sehnal & Christopher 1993). The OSHA is working on identifying the traits of those processes that have the greatest impact on the problem (Smith 1993).

Stretching and Warm-Up

Developing a stretching and warm-up program follows the same "process" procedures. Numerous articles report success when such activities are incorporated as part of a comprehensive, ongoing process (Sawyer 1987; ErgoTech, Inc 1991; Wilson 1992; Thomas et al. 1993). Although controversy still exists about whether stretching is effective, the biggest obstacle remains the reasons for not wanting to participate, reasons such as:

- *It is embarrassing*: Many employees are self-conscious about stretching in front of their peers.
- *It is too difficult or physically demanding*: Many employees perceive this to be a fitness or exercise program.
- *This takes too much time away from production*: Many employees are concerned that they will lose money or that management or supervisors will not appreciate their participation.
- *I have a pre-existing injury*: Many employees are concerned about reinjury or aggravation of an existing or previous injury.

These are valid concerns, and each should be addressed by the IPS as part of the introduction to a stretching program. There are some sound physiologic reasons for encouraging people to stretch. For example, it has been demonstrated that as little as a 15% maximum voluntary contraction held for an extended period can lead to fatigue (Headley 1992). The appropriate stretches can offset this fatigue and speed up muscle recovery. However, an effective stretching program will recognize that the majority of employee resistance does not occur because employees do not think stretching will help but rather because of the foregoing concerns.

New Program Ideas

It is important that the process continue to absorb and integrate new information into the programs. For example, there is a relatively new body of evidence that implicates the muscles of the neck and shoulders as contributors to a variety of upper-body disorders (Pronsati 1992; Headley 1994). A pattern of fatigue and resulting dysfunction has been identified in the muscles of the neck and shoulders, muscles that are under increased demands during extended periods of sitting, keying, or light assembly work. The Controlling Symptoms at Work, or C-Saw, program (Headley 1993) involves a series of stretches that address the specific pattern of fatigue

and muscle shut-down. This program identifies prevention of symptoms at their earliest stages, rather than waiting until symptoms have reached a level at which continued work is no longer possible and a physician visit and lost time are inevitable. A company can incorporate this type of information into a program if a prevention process is already in place.

Toolbox Talks and Shift Meetings

These periodic, brief, department meetings allow the IPS more frequent contact with the supervisors and employees so as to discuss the highlights of the process, address questions, and provide any new information on the topic of CTD prevention. These meetings can be conducted by the IPS or department supervisor, with input from the IPS on materials related to the prevention of CTDs.

Informal Discussions

These discussions can be initiated by either the IPS or the supervisors. Ideally, the supervisors will gradually become more comfortable in delivering safety messages to the employees on an ongoing basis. These messages include statements consistent with the information that was presented in the employee education sessions. Messages can include queries about whether they are able to use what was presented in the CTD class, whether there are any simple changes that can be made now with regard to CTD information presented, and whether they have made any changes since the class. Such a message also might remind workers to change positions frequently.

These statements are not formal. However, they support the process with content of the message, repetition, and consistency. These frequent messages keep the employees aware, help them to retain the information presented in the initial sessions, and encourage injury prevention to become an integral part of the workday.

Posters, Check Stuffers, and Bulletin Boards

There are limits as to the value of certain items—posters, check stuffers, and bulletin boards—as stand-alone programs. Posters do not create change; however, if their messages are related to topics covered at shift meetings and informal discussions, they can reinforce the desired changes and demonstrate a consistency to the participants.

Medical Management

By definition, injury prevention applies to people who are asymptomatic as well as to those who are experiencing symptoms. The IPS should identify community health professionals who understand state-of-the-art CTD treatment, the operating procedures of industry, and the psychological impact of involvement in the worker's compensation system. Once a relationship is established between the industry and the clinic, the chances for early return to work are greater. IPSs can benefit their clients by working closely with the medical providers and "translating" the clinical terminology from the clinic to the work environment.

During the return-to-work process, the IPS can work with industry to ensure a smooth transition back into the workplace via many aspects of the prevention process. These aspects include the *ergonomics* process to ensure effective job modification, the *stretching* process to ensure that the employee knows the proper stretches, and the *maintenance* process to reinforce education and training.

Identifying Potential Problems: Surveying

Identifiable stages of CTDs have been described in the literature, and methods of detecting the presence of CTDs in the earlier stages are being pursued (Fine et al. 1986; Katz et al. 1991; Berg & Ackerman 1992; National Safety Council 1993). The literature supports the idea that the earlier a CTD is diagnosed and treated, the easier it is to treat (Headley 1993, 1994). Chapter 12 discusses medical surveillance methods and current tests to identify early CTD involvement in more detail.

To help to reduce the extent of injury (and related costs to the company), management and supervisors should be encouraged to pay attention to the early complaints of workers, particularly those of neck and shoulder symptoms. These symptoms generally go untreated until the more advanced symptoms appear in the arms and hands, the level at which treatment usually begins. Teaching supervisors to recognize early symptoms (e.g., employees rubbing their necks or hands and arms) and developing strategies for dealing with mild symptoms before at-risk employees ever have to leave the work environment can, in many instances, interrupt the onset of more serious problems (Moore et al. 1992).

Marketing the Process

One of the easiest ways to market services is by tapping into an existing patient population through a medical facility. When a number of CTD patients from a specific company are being seen, that company may appreciate a phone call letting them know what can be done to reduce these numbers.

When a client has completed treatment, a return-to-work consultation, involving a visit to the workplace by the treating health care provider, ensures a safe transition to the workplace. It also helps to familiarize the company with the capabilities of the IPS in a non–direct marketing way.

Other marketing opportunities include sponsoring local seminars, speaking at local events, and becoming a resource for local businesses by sending them updates of information that may be of interest.

Selling Your Services

Marketing is making people aware of your services. Selling is getting them to buy your services. In the business of injury prevention, it is important to be able to separate oneself from the competition. One effective method is to create a niche or specialty. Some IPSs have a reputation for being great motivational speakers enjoyed by the employees, whereas others are recognized for their ability in problem-solving effectively in a work-site situation. Still others are seen by businesses in the community as being effective at orchestrating a variety of professionals in the prevention process. Whatever your own strengths may be, play on these and be secure in the presentation of your services. As mentioned earlier, establishing alliances with community professionals who provide services that differ from yours can create a valuable referral network.

Cost

In the author's experience, the number one factor that keeps a company from implementing a prevention process is *money*. Many companies will verbalize that injury prevention costs too much. The IPS can offset some of their financial concerns by providing information on cost savings and program effectiveness (MacLeod 1993, 1995). The IPS can also relate that injury prevention not only has a positive effect on recordable injuries and worker's compensation but that it can also improve productivity and quality control. Listen carefully to managers when you try to sell them a process. They will guide you to the areas that most concern them and the areas of greatest resistance. For example, prevention can be sold effectively in one of three (or all three) ways: injury prevention as a *productivity* issue, injury prevention as a *quality* issue, and injury prevention as a *safety* issue. By being able to incorporate discussions about increases in productivity or quality, the IPS is able to speak in a language that is often more familiar to the client.

Putting Together a Proposal

In reviewing a proposal prepared by the author, many potential clients will notice that there is no specific end point. This prompts them to ask the question, "When is this process over?" The author's response is, "When injury prevention no longer is important to this organization." In the author's opinion, finding a new client is a lot harder than maintaining an existing one. The key to the success of both the IPS and the process itself is maintenance. It provides ongoing income for the IPS and dramatically improves the odds for success of the prevention process.

In preparing a proposal, meet with the client to learn more about the company. From this discussion, a series of proposed activities are assembled. Then these activities are discussed with the client. The necessary changes or additions are made in the proposed activities; then they are resubmitted to the client as a proposal. Because discussion has preceded the proposal, further discussion is rarely needed before getting the process started. This final proposal is amenable to change based on input from the supervisors in the supervisor orientation. As the process progresses, it may be necessary to change the order or schedule, or to deal with the numerous variables that can affect a business. Although this factor may alter the look of the proposal, the underlying commitment to process success must be unwavering. An effective process is pliable. The strength comes from the commitment to the process and the ability to adapt.

In some instances, it may be appropriate to be on retainer with a client. A retainer is an agreement for a specific level of activity, generally measured in hours per month. For example, at the time of this writing, the author is working under a retainer from a power company for a specific number of hours per month. In this arrangement, each of the numerous locations can schedule activities without needing prior authorization from the purchasing department; the author knows how much time to allot each month for client activities, and the employees see a commitment from management to keep the process alive. It is much easier to get on a retainer with a process than with a program, because process success is based on an ongoing presence and reinforced messages.

Fees need to be set relative to acceptable rates in the community. The author does not recommend that an IPS promise results. Simply by limiting support or undermining activities, a company can take a process with the best of intentions and drive it into the ground. Inform the company that when the process is in place and support is gathered, the company might expect certain results. Remember that many companies are not experienced in implementing an effective injury-prevention process. Part of the IPS's responsibility is to educate industry as to what is and is not working. The IPS can educate in a way that does not make owners feel as though they have been doing everything wrong but that there are new information and techniques that can be used.

In the author's experience, for any process that was to be implemented, money was a perceived (though often not a real) problem. A process does not fail because of a lack of money. It fails because of a lack of flexibility, accountability, commitment, and consistency. An IPS cannot forget how long it has taken people to develop the attitudes they hold. It is naive to assume that an event, whether it be ergonomics, education, or stretching can impact on a problem with so many risk factors. Therefore, the purpose of the process is to ensure that we are keeping our eyes open, enlisting support, asking the right questions, making appropriate changes, and looking to the future for new and innovative ways of reducing everyone's risk of experiencing CTDs.

Case Study

In one warehouse operation with approximately 30 employees, a task force was developed to explore the idea of stretching. The process started with an orientation to the employees on stretching and a series of meetings with the task force to address specific issues. This was followed by a work-site evaluation to determine the most appropriate stretches. The employees were then instructed in the stretches, and the author returned to the workplace weekly for the first few weeks to answer any questions and to ensure that the stretches were being performed correctly.

An ongoing series of educational seminars was scheduled throughout the year, with topics determined by the employees. This was a voluntary program that enjoyed full participation. Three years into the program, the company still has full participation and has experienced no recordable injuries since implementing the program, a safety record for this department. The key was not that the stretches were somehow special; it was the fact that a process put into place could continuously evaluate effectiveness, make changes and updates, and keep the concept of health in wellness in front of the employees on a daily basis.

References

Allen CW (1993). Weight of evidence links obesity, fitness to carpal tunnel syndrome. *Occup Health Saf,* 64(11),51–52.

Armstrong TJ, Ardwin R, Hansen DJ, Kennedy KW (1986). Repetitive trauma disorders: job evaluation and design. *Hum Factors,* 28,325–336.

Armstrong TJ (1986). Ergonomics and cumulative trauma disorders. *Hand Clin,* 2,553.

Arndt R (1987). Work pace, stress, and cumulative trauma disorders. *J Hand Surg [Am],* 12,866–869.

Astrand I (1986). *Textbook of Work Physiology* (3rd ed). New York: McGraw-Hill.

Berg DR & Ackerman E (1992). Use of vibrometry in conjunction with ergonomic evaluation and conservative medical management as an ongoing surveillance program for median nerve function. *Work Injury Manage,* 1(5),7.

Bigos SJ, Battie MC, & Fisher LD (1991). Methodology for evaluating predictive factors for the report of back injury. *Spine,* 16,669.

Buckle PW, Stubbs DA, Randle IPM, & Nicholson AS (1992). Limitations in the application of materials handling guidelines. *Ergonomics,* 35,955–964.

Bullock MI (Ed) (1990). *Ergonomics: The Physiotherapist in the Workplace.* London: Churchill Livingstone.

Cannon LJ, Bernacki E, & Walter S (1981). Personal and occupational factors associated with carpal tunnel syndrome. *J Occup Med,* 23,255–258.

Caplan SH, Champney PC, Corl K, Crist B, Cushman W, Davis H, Faulkner T, Little R, Lucas R, Murphy T, Nielsen W, Pugsley R, Rodgers S, & Stevens J (1983). *Ergonomic Design for People at Work.* New York: Van Nostrand Reinhold.

Carayon P (1993). Job design and job stress in office workers. *Ergonomics,* 36,463–477.

Carlton RS (1987). The effects of body mechanics instruction on work performance. *Am J Occup Ther,* 41,16–20.

Chong I (1993). Prioritize office workstation goals and watch out for "voodoo ergonomics." *Occup Health Saf,* 62(10),55–60.

Clafin T (1991). Woodmill stretching program works for fitness, morale, lower costs. *Occup Health Saf,* 60(11),34.

Ekberg K, Bjorkqvist B, Malm P, Bjerre-Kiely B, Karlsson M, & Axelson O (1994). Case-control study of risk factors for disease in the neck and shoulder area. *Occup Environ Med,* 51,262–266.

ErgoTech Inc. (1991). *Setting up an Ergonomics Program.* Minneapolis: ErgoTech, Inc.

Eversmann WW (1983). Compression and entrapment neuropathies of the upper extremity. *J Hand Surg,* 8,759–766.

Fine LJ, Silverstein BA, Armstrong TJ, Anderson CA, & Sugano DS (1986). Detection of cumulative trauma disorders of upper extremities in the workplace. *J Occup Med,* 28,674.

Grandjean E (1988). *Fitting the Task to the Man* (4th ed). New York: Taylor & Francis.

Hagberg M (1981). Electromyographic signs of shoulder muscular fatigue in two elevated arm positions. *Am J Phys Med,* 60(3),111–121.

Headley BJ (October 7, 1992). EMG analysis: examining muscle activity in the workplace. *Occup Ther Forum,* 4–5.

Headley B (1993). C-Saw. *Preventing Injury,* 2(1),2.

Headley B (1994). Strategies for management of CTD symptoms at the work site. *Work Injury Manage,* 3(3),1–5.

Headley BJ (July 1994). Carpal tunnel syndrome: finding its beginning. *CTS: Advance Dir Newsletter,* 19–23.

Johnson SL (1990). Ergonomic design of handheld tools to prevent trauma to the hand and upper extremity. *J Hand Ther,* 3(2),86.

Joseph BS (1987). Analysis of a program for control of cumulative trauma disorders in the auto industry. *Ergonom Interventions,* 133–149.

Joseph BS (1989). Ergonomic considerations and job design in upper-extremity disorders. Occupational hand injuries. *Occup Med,* 4,547.

Katz JN, Larson MG, Fossel AH, & Liang MH (1991). Validation of a surveillance case definition of carpal tunnel syndrome. *Am J Public Health,* 81(2),189–193.

Kilbom A (1988). Intervention programmes for work-related neck and upper-limb disorders: strategies and evaluation. *Ergonomics,* 31,735–747.

Kohn JP & Friend MA (1993). Quality and ergonomics: the team approach to the occupational people factor. *Profess Safety,* 38(5),39–42.

Kroemer KHE (1992). Personnel training for safer material handling. *Ergonomics,* 35,1119–1134.

Krout K (1994). Study of supervisors reveals need for more extensive training efforts. *Occup Health Saf,* 63(2),54–60.

LaBar G (August 1991). Worker training: an investment in safety. *Occup Hazards,* 23–26.

MacLeod D (1993). Competitive edge: good ergonomics is good economics. *Prevent Injury,* 2(3),14.

MacLeod D (1995). *The Ergonomics Edge.* New York: Van Nostrand Reinhold.

Melnik MS (1993). Implementing a stretching-warm-up program in industry. *Prevent Injury,* 2(1),8.

Minter SG (August 1991). Creating the safety culture. *Occup Hazards,* 17–21.

Moore A, Wells R, & Ranney D (1992). Quantifying exposure in occupational manual tasks with cumulative trauma disorder potential. *Ergonomics,* 34,1433–1453.

Nathan PA (April 10, 1992). Hand and arm ills linked to life style. *The New York Times.*

National Safety Council (June 4, 1993). ANSI Z-365: control of cumulative trauma disorders. Draft.

National Safety Council (1993). Does stress have a price? *OSHA Up-To-Date,* 22(6),3.

Pronsati MP (1992). Neck muscles play part in carpal tunnel syndrome. *Adv Phys Ther,* 3,4.

Rice VJ & Rice DM (1993). Helping hands: ergonomic intervention offers employers a comprehensive approach to addressing upper-extremity injuries. *Risk Benefits J,* 16–18.

Rystrom CM & Eversmann WW (1991). Cumulative trauma intervention in industry: a model program for the upper extremity. In *Occupational Hand and Upper-Extremity Injuries and Diseases* (pp. 489–505). Philadelphia: Hanley & Belfus.

Sawyer K (1987). An on-site exercise program to prevent carpal tunnel syndrome. *Profess Safety,* 5,17–20.

Sehnal JP & Christopher RC (1993). Developing and marketing an ergonomics program in a corporate office environment. *Work,* 3(2),22–30.

Simard M & Marchand A (1994). The behavior of first-line supervisors in accident prevention and effectiveness in occupational safety. *Safety Sci,* 17,169–182.

Smith BR (1993). OSHA gathers information for first draft of national ergonomics safety standard. *Occup Health Saf,* 62(1),46–49.

Stankevich BA (1994). Guidelines for videotaping and evaluating cumulative trauma disorders. *Profess Safety,* 39(5),37–40.

Tadano P (1990). A safety-prevention program for VDT operators: one company's approach. *J Hand Ther,* 3(2),64.

The Human Factors Society, Inc. (1988). American national standard for human factors engineering of visual display terminal workstations. Santa Monica, CA: ANSI/HFS 100-1988.

Thomas RE, Butterfield RK, Hool JN, & Herrick RT (1993). Effects of exercise on carpal tunnel syndrome symptoms. *Appl Ergonom,* 24(2),101–108.

Tomal DR (1992). Reduce carpal tunnel syndrome through safety training. *Profess Safety,* 37(12),27–29.

Topf M & Preston R (1991). Behavior modification can heighten safety awareness, curtail accidents. *Occup Health Saf,* 60(2),43.

US Department of Labor (1990). *Ergonomics Program Management Guidelines for Meatpacking Plants.* Washington, DC: Occupational Safety and Health Administration.

Waters TR, Putz-Anderson V, Garg A, & Fine LJ (1993). Revised NIOSH equation for the design and evaluation of manual lifting tasks. *Ergonomics,* 35,749–771.

Wilson PM (1992). An exercise and job modification program in industry. *Work,* 2(3),8–14.

PART V

Specific Programs for High-Risk Populations

Chapter 14

Preventing Cumulative Trauma Disorders in Dental Hygienists

Martha J. Sanders and Claudia Michalak-Turcotte

In the last 10 years, the dental hygiene profession has been plagued by increasing incidence of cumulative trauma disorders (CTDs) affecting new graduates and experienced dental hygienists alike. These disorders include neck and shoulder pain as well as hand and arm pain, all of which interfere with dental hygienists' job performance and the ability to plan a long-term career in dental hygiene.

Health care practitioners are becoming involved in the treatment and prevention of CTDs in dental hygienists (Sanders 1995). Health care practitioners suggest that many of the musculoskeletal problems in dental hygiene activities appear to be related to the instruments and postures used during work. This chapter discusses the dental hygiene practice and strategies to prevent CTDs.

Professional Background and Roles

The dental hygiene profession was first introduced in the United States in 1917 in response to the need for a dental auxiliary person to deliver preventive oral health care services. Since then, the role of dental hygiene has emerged gradually under the general auspices of dentistry.

The primary and most common role of a dental hygienist is to provide preventive oral health care. However, various expanded roles include those of administrator, manager, client advocate, educator, and researcher. The settings for dental hygienists have also expanded from private offices to wellness clinics, school systems, insurance offices, and such specialty practices as periodontal and pediatric clinics.

Entry-level requirements for a dental hygienist are 2 years of schooling and a registry examination. Dental assistants either undergo a 1-year program or learn dental assisting skills on the job. The most advanced degree in dental hygiene is a master's degree.

In terms of legal autonomy, dentists oversee the dental hygienist in private practice, except in a few states, where independent practice by hygienists is legal. Not only does the dentist provide guidelines for the dental hygienist, state and federal regulators (e.g., the Occupational Safety and Health Administration) now mandate that hygienists wear long-sleeved gowns, safety glasses, masks, and gloves. Thus, dental hygienists' control over their work schedule, work environment, and choice of work instruments is often limited.

Job Analysis

A dental hygienist is an allied dental professional who performs oral prophylactic treatment that includes removal of calculus (tartar), stain, and plaque from teeth; intraoral and extraoral inspections; fluoride treatments; and developing radiographs.

In a typical dental treatment session, the dental hygienist first records a medical history, then inspects the mandibles, cheeks, teeth, and gums of the client. The dental hygienist probes the teeth with a dental instrument in a gentle up-and-down stroke

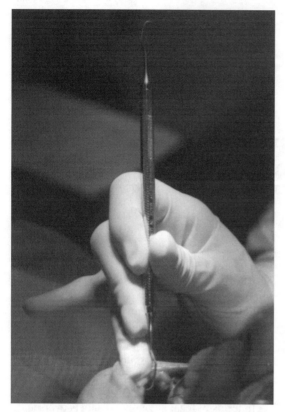

Figure 14.1. A modified pen grasp is used for most dental hygiene instrumentation.

next to each tooth to determine if any gum or bone loss is present. Next, he or she performs scaling to remove deposits of calculus and root planing to smooth the roots of the teeth to deter further calculus deposits from adhering to the tooth. After cleaning the teeth, the dental hygienist may polish the teeth using a vibrating instrument or may simply floss and brush the teeth. Last, the dental hygienist reviews home care or client education and records the treatment session in the medical chart.

The bulk of dental hygienists' time is spent performing root planing and scaling, which are the most hand-intensive procedures. Both functions require proprioceptive feedback from the fingers on the dental instrument to determine the amount of force to use. Scaling requires short strokes, but high forces, to remove calculus. Root planing requires long strokes and larger ranges of wrist motions. Both procedures demand high concentration to clean the teeth thoroughly without hurting the

client. Heavy calculus build-up requires greatly increased prehension forces for the hygienist.

Dental instruments for probing, root planing, and scaling are small-diameter, cylindrical tools with a thin, angled tip at one or both ends. The shaft may be smooth or textured. The grasp used for all instrumentation procedures is a variation of the modified pen grasp (Figure 14.1). The instrument is held between the thumb and index and middle fingers; the fourth and fifth fingers are extended and adducted. The ring finger acts as a fulcrum to leverage the instrument on each tooth.

During root planing and scaling procedures, the fingers are positioned on dental instruments called *scalers* and *curettes*. The fingers guide the instrument on the tooth surface; however, strong wrist and forearm motions power the stroke. Figure 14.2 shows that depending on the location of the tooth, the wrist constantly moves from extremes of wrist flexion to wrist extension, generally within a range of 50 degrees in each direction. The forearm rotates from supination to pronation around the fulcrum of the fourth finger.

Ultrasonic scalers are cylindrical vibrating instruments also used by dental hygienists to remove calculus. The dental hygiene profession recommends that practitioners use ultrasonic scalers rather than hand-scaling to remove heavy calculus. (See Trends in Dental Hygiene for further discussion.)

Most dental hygienists sit during oral examinations and cleaning sessions. They orient themselves at the head or to the side of the client in a position corresponding to hands on a clock (such as the 9 o'clock or 11 o'clock positions) and place the delivery system (instrument table) close by. The head and neck are positioned in flexion, with the shoulders elevated and elbows flexed in order to position the hands at the level of the client's mouth. Dental hygienists maintain this static head, neck, and shoulder flexion for up to 40 minutes at a time.

Dental hygienists treat from eight to 14 clients per day, averaging 50 minutes per appointment (Atwood & Michalak 1992). Dental hygienists also perform other job tasks such as patient scheduling, equipment maintenance, charting, and exposing radiographs. (See Trends in Dental Hygiene for further discussion.) Most of these tasks involve repetitive hand motions.

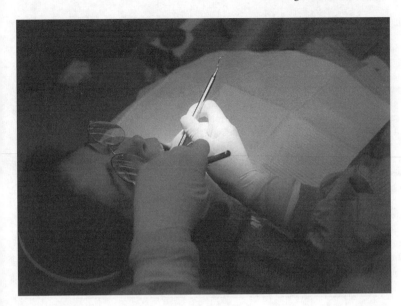

Figure 14.2. Root planing and scaling procedures require that the wrist move in extremes of flexion and extension while the instrument is being grasped.

Risk Factors for Cumulative Trauma Disorders in Dental Hygienists

The job analysis describes the work of dental hygienists as static, yet precise and exacting, requiring intense concentration and the use of a firm, repetitive grasp for the majority of tasks. These factors, among others, place dental hygienists at risk for developing some type of CTD when combined with less-than-ergonomic workstations, instruments, and high standards for care. The following discussion highlights specific factors that may predispose dental hygienists to CTDs. Tables 14.1 through 14.3 provide an outline of biomechanical, ergonomic, and personal risk factors. The factors are organized for ease of discussion notwithstanding that categories overlap.

Biomechanical Factors

Repetition, Force, and Posture

Table 14.1 presents the biomechanical factors that contribute to CTDs in dental hygienists. These factors have been related to CTDs in many industries and are reviewed here in terms of dental hygiene. Repetition, or continual use of the same musculature throughout the day, is cited as a major risk factor, due to the similarity in dental hygienists' job tasks (MacDonald 1987). For example, hygienists use a

modified tripod grasp to examine and clean teeth, write client's progress notes, and grasp radiographs. However, a recent case-control study comparing 20 dental offices with and without claims for carpal tunnel syndrome (CTS) suggests that dental hygienists' hand pain is related more to heavy prehension forces during scaling and awkward position of the wrist during instrumentation than to repetition of the task (Strong & Lennartz 1992). In fact, as the job analysis indicated, dental hygienists often use excessive prehension forces to remove heavy calculus and frequently assume extreme positions of wrist flexion and ulnar deviation during instrumentation.

A static posture creates excessive loads on the neck and shoulder musculature, which may cause muscle strain and fatigue over time (Luopajarvi 1990). Dental hygienists maintain static head and neck positions so as to stabilize the arms and hands for precise work.

Oberg (1993) suggests that this static posture is related to acute and chronic neck and shoulder pain in dental hygienists. Using "posture targeting" and photorecording, Oberg documented the body positions and muscle loads of a dental hygienist. Oberg substantiated that dental hygienists work in a fixed position of neck flexion (approximately 45 degrees) and right-side bending (approximately 30 degrees). Biomechanical computations indicate that substantial loads are placed on the neck and shoulder musculature. In fact, the muscle force needed to

Table 14.1. Biomechanical Risk Factors

Risk Factor	Job Task
Repetition	Constant wrist flexion, extension, and forearm rotation
	Constant grasping with thumb and fingers
Force	Firm grasp on instruments during root planing and scaling
	Firm grasp on ultrasonic scaler, mirror, or writing utensil
Awkward posture	Neck flexed
	Back and shoulders rounded
	Arms flexed or abducted ≥30 degrees
	Elbows flexed ≥90 degrees
	Wrists flexed or deviated in grasping
	Thumbs hyperextended
Static posture	Posture maintained for ≥20 mins
Vibration	Cumulative use of nondampened vibrating instruments (ultrasonic scaler, polishing instrument, or slow-speed handpiece)
Mechanical stresses	Pressure from instrument edges on nerves and blood vessels in fingers
	Tight gloves constrict wrist or fingers
Cold	Hand washing with cold water

maintain the neck in a flexed position (50 N) is twice the muscle force needed to maintain an upright position (25 N).

Other researchers suggest that neck symptoms relate to the degree of neck flexion assumed during work. Neck pain may be associated with static neck flexion of over 20 degrees or static muscle work that exceeds 5–6% of the maximal voluntary contraction (Luopajarvi 1990). Static loading of the supraspinatus muscle may also be related to shoulder pain.

Vibration

Vibration has been associated with symptoms of CTS (McDonald et al. 1988). However, no studies have documented a direct correlation between cumulative use of vibrating instruments and increased risk for CTDs (Ekenvall et al. 1990). At present, most studies indicate that use of a vibration-dampened ultrasonic scaler is preferable to using heavy prehension forces to remove tenacious calculus.

Mechanical Stresses

Mechanical stresses from instrument edges are potential sources of trauma to the neurovascular bundles lateral to each finger. Tight gloves and wrist watches that place direct pressure at the wrist may also contribute to symptoms associated with CTS. During craft activities the use of short-handled tools such as pliers or latch hooks place added pressure on superficial structures (Rhode 1990).

Ergonomic Risk Factors

Table 14.2 outlines other important ergonomic factors to consider in working with dental hygienists. Although most hygienists are trained to minimize stress on hand musculature during instrumentation, some hygienists develop less-than-ergonomic habits over time. The following instrumentation techniques should be addressed and reviewed.

Instrumentation

Instrument procedures should be performed with minimal finger movement and thumb flexion at both joints (Pattison & Pattison 1992). *Excessive finger movements* place high demands on small finger musculature and increase repetitive use of flexor tendons (Meador 1993); *thumb hyperextension* appears related to lateral thumb pain.

Dental hygienists are trained to use indirect vision (use of a small mirror to view the upper and posterior teeth) to maintain an erect posture during treatment sessions. *Direct vision* (without the mirror) contributes to awkward posture, as the operator must flex and rotate the trunk severely to view the teeth.

The use of a *small-diameter instrument* requires a static, firm grip. Although dental instrument diameters vary from less than $\frac{3}{16}$ in. to greater than $\frac{5}{16}$ in., the majority of dental hygienists use instruments between $\frac{3}{16}$ and $\frac{4}{16}$ in. (Atwood & Michalak 1992). These smaller instrument diameters may require increased muscle power for forceful exertions.

Table 14.2. Ergonomic Risk Factors

Risk Factor	Job Task
Instrumentation	Excessive finger movements
	Thumb hyperextension
	Use of direct vision
	Small handle diameter
	Unbalanced instruments
	Dull instruments
	Tangled cords
Workstation	No lumbar, thoracic, or arm support
	Chair too high or too low
	Excessive twisting
	Nonchanging operator position
	Nonchanging delivery system
	Over-reaching or forward bending at waist
Workplace practices	Inadequate time per client
	More than 10 clients per day
	Polishing each client's teeth
	Clients having heavy calculus scheduled together
	Nonchanging tasks
Environment	Inadequate lighting, temperature, space
	Nonsupportive social environment
	Office politics

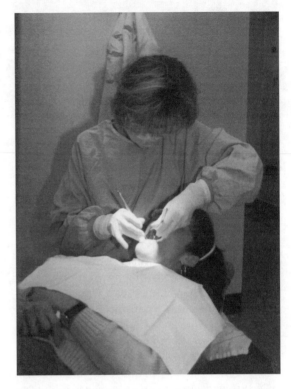

Figure 14.3. Awkward and static neck and shoulder postures contribute to dental hygienists' discomfort during work.

Dental hygienists who use dull instruments must increase prehension forces to remove calculus. Dental hygienists are trained to sharpen instruments as needed; however, studies indicate that most hygienists do not sharpen instruments regularly (Atwood & Michalak 1992; Strong & Lennartz 1992). Unbalanced instruments are instruments whose center of mass is not in the center of the instrument, due to poor manufacturing, dropping, or frequent use. Unbalanced instruments may also require increased prehension forces to maintain their position in the hand.

Workstation

The workstation for a dental hygienist includes the client and operator chairs, the delivery system (instrument tray), and the cleaning and charting area. As a general rule, the dental hygienist should be positioned as close to the client as possible (Figure 14.3). The head and neck should be upright (or minimally flexed), with arms at the side, elbows and hips flexed no more than 90 degrees, and feet flat on the floor. The hygienist's chair should be adjustable and have

lumbar, thoracic, and arm support. Electromyographic studies indicate that use of lumbar support significantly reduces muscle loads on the upper and lower back during dentistry procedures (Hardage et al. 1983). Informal observations indicate that many dental hygienists sit forward on the edge of the chair and therefore do not use the lumbar support available.

Problems arise when the height of the operator's chair (i.e., the dental hygienist's chair) does not match that of the client's chair. If the operator's chair is too high, the dental hygienist must increase neck flexion and lumbar flexion to reach the client. Most likely, the feet will not be flat on the floor. If the chair is too low, the dental hygienist must elevate the arms during instrumentation, thereby increasing static loads on the shoulders.

Finally, dental hygienists should be reminded to face the client rather than sitting sideways during the medical history and patient education periods. Dental hygienists should vary the operator position and delivery system throughout the session so that the same structures are not continually stressed. Hygienists should also avoid over-reaching, which places stress on the low back (Pattison & Pattison 1992; Meador 1993).

Workplace Practices

Activities such as scheduling many heavy calculus clients in 1 day (MacDonald et al. 1988; Rice et al. 1995, unpublished data), increasing the number of workdays (Strong & Lennartz 1992), and increasing the number of clients seen in 1 day (Atwood & Michalak 1992) have been associated with symptoms related to CTDs. Research suggests that dental hygienists who treat more than 10 clients per day may be at higher risk for CTDs. Experts suggest that an adequate amount of time for treatment sessions is 50–60 minutes for adult clients and 35 minutes for children.

Polishing refers to buffing the teeth following cleaning, most often by use of a vibrating instrument. Although clients enjoy the clean feel of polished teeth and often view polishing as a reward at the end of a visit, polishing may be harmful to the client and to the dental hygienist. For the client, polishing removes the enamel from teeth; for the dental hygienist, polishing requires a sustained grip. Dental professionals recommend selective polishing (i.e., polishing only in areas of stain).

Environmental Factors

Factors such as lighting, ventilation, and a comfortable temperature are usually adequate in dental offices. However, these factors, along with the social and organizational factors (e.g., the relationship between the dentist and the dental hygienist) and worker's compensation issues should be addressed.

Personal Risk Factors

Job-Home Stress

The impact of personal factors on dental hygienists' work cannot be underestimated (Table 14.3). The profession consists primarily of women, whose profession demands perfection and who may be balancing several roles outside of work. Health care practitioners treating dental hygienists need to understand their clients' job-home stress and other role obligations. Health care practitioners need to examine a client's entire day with the understanding that hobbies or chores that involve a repetitive or static grasp (e.g., gardening, quilting, latch hook, carpentry, or constantly picking up a child) may also contribute to CTD symptoms.

Further, clients rarely enjoy visiting the dentist and may display anxiety or fear through clenched jaws or hypersensitivity during a session. Client anxiety may have an impact on dental hygienist's anxiety, as the hygienist tends to tense in efforts to avoid inflicting pain on the client.

Hygienist Size

The hygienist's size may be an issue for those who are appreciably larger or smaller than population norms. The adjustable range on chairs must be specifically addressed. Instruments of larger or smaller diameter may be ordered to accommodate hand size.

Work Style

Work style refers to the individual variation in dental hygienists' instrumentation. Those who use excessive prehension forces or excessive wrist deviation during root planing or scaling place higher stresses on the hand and wrist; those who tense the neck and shoulder maintain higher loads on proximal structures.

Job Satisfaction

The satisfaction inherent in the job may play consciously or unconsciously into the perception of pain. Although a recent study showed no correlation

Table 14.3. Personal Risk Factors

Risk Factor	Job Task
Job-home stress	Work-home overload
	Anxious clients
	Hobbies using forceful or repetitive grasp
Hygienist size	Inappropriate instrument size
	Inappropriate chair size
Work style	Exerts excess pressure on instrument
	Excessive deviation of wrist
	Overly tense neck and shoulders
Job satisfaction	Lack of enjoyment, recognition, compensation

between CTD symptoms and job satisfaction (Rice et al. 1995, unpublished data), health care practitioners should understand dental hygienists' motivations to continue work and to prevent injuries.

Cumulative Trauma Disorders Common to Dental Hygienists

Prior to 1985, low-back pain was the most commonly reported source of musculoskeletal pain for dental hygiene practitioners. Since then, CTS and other upper-extremity CTDs have emerged as the major musculoskeletal problems of concern to dental hygienists today (McDonald et al. 1988; Atwood & Michalak 1992; Oberg & Oberg 1993).

Initial investigations of upper-extremity CTDs in dental hygienists examined the incidence and symptoms associated with CTS. Results of a survey of 2,464 dental hygienists in California indicate that 6% have been diagnosed as having CTS and 32% demonstrated one or more of the following symptoms: weak grip, numbness, night pain, and paresthesias. A positive correlation was found between hygienists' symptoms, working more days per week, and treating heavy calculus clients (McDonald et al. 1988; Rice et al. 1995, unpublished data)

Later, a Minnesota study expanded investigations to document the overall musculoskeletal pain in dental hygienists. Researchers found that 63% had experienced back, neck, shoulder, or arm pain in the previous year; those with arm and hand pain lost the most work time (Osborn et al. 1990).

Finally, a study of CTDs in Connecticut revealed that 8% of the sample had been diagnosed with CTS, and an overwhelming 93% of the entire sample had experienced some type of musculoskeletal pain. The most common sites of pain were the shoulder and neck (71%), low back (56%), hand and wrist (65%), and forearm and elbow (27%) (Atwood & Michalak 1992). Internationally, these results compare with researchers from Sweden, who report similar frequencies of neck pain (62%), shoulder pain (81%), and wrist pain (45%) (Oberg & Oberg 1993).

Although CTS may be the most costly and feared condition of dental hygienists, costing up to $21,344 per claim (Strong & Lennartz 1992), neck and shoulder pain may interfere equally if not more so with dental hygienists' quality of work, job satis-

faction, and energy level (Atwood & Michalak 1992). Health care practitioners must be vigilant in examining the entire upper extremity for clinical symptoms and muscle tenderness, as research indicates that neck and shoulder pain may be related directly to a diagnosis of CTS.

Neck

Dental hygienists complain of tightness and spasms of the upper trapezius and scalene muscles, due to static neck flexion, shoulder elevation, and shoulder protraction. Although hygienists strive for a neck-upright position, the actual posture may be flexed, rotated, and side-bent (see Figure 14.3). This flexed posture also may contribute to "double-crush syndrome," or thoracic outlet syndrome, if the dental hygienist habitually reaches behind the body for dental tools (see Chapter 5).

Shoulder

Typically, the shoulders are elevated, protracted, and internally rotated during work. This posture contributes to shortened pectoral muscles and the potential for supraspinatus tendinitis or bicipital tendinitis. These conditions may become a problem for dental hygienists who flex or abduct their shoulders more than 30 degrees (see Figure 14.3).

Elbow and Forearm

Pain at the elbow arises from repetitive forearm rotation, particularly when combined with static grasping, wrist deviation, and excessive elbow flexion (Figure 14.4). Dental hygienists develop lateral epicondylitis because the wrist extensor musculature statically contracts during instrumentation and writing. The condition is aggravated by forceful root planing and scaling with forearm supination (see Figure 14.4) or pronation. Health care practitioners should rule out radial tunnel syndrome for lateral epicondylitis. Less commonly, hygienists develop medial epicondylitis.

Nerve entrapment syndromes, such as cubital tunnel syndrome (ulnar nerve entrapment at the elbow) or pronator syndrome (median nerve entrap-

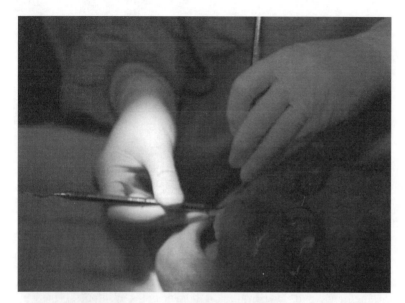

Figure 14.4. Elbow pain may develop from rotating the forearm while grasping the instrument.

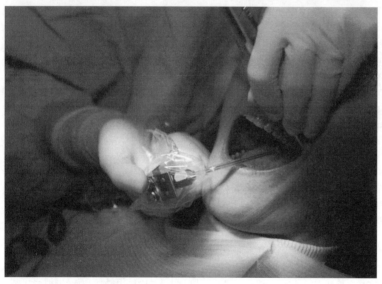

Figure 14.5. In addition to use of instrumentation, other tasks such as spraying or irrigating the mouth may contribute to the development of carpal tunnel syndrome.

ment in the forearm), may occur in hygienists who work with the elbow flexed more than 90 degrees or who rotate the forearm repetitively.

Wrist and Fingers

CTS is the most recognized of all CTDs that affect dental hygienists. CTS may develop from compression of the median nerve during extremes of wrist flexion or extension or from pressure placed on the median nerve when finger or thumb flexor tendons become inflamed (tenosynovitis). Such tasks as ir-

rigating or spraying the mouth with water, developing radiographs, and writing progress notes contribute to this condition (Figure 14.5). Symptoms of CTS include inadvertent shaking of the hands, wrist pain at the end of the day, and finger numbness in the morning or during work (see Chapter 5).

Finger flexor tenosynovitis is more difficult to detect and should be ruled out for CTS. Ganglion cysts, trigger fingers, and cubital tunnel syndrome are other less common conditions that may develop from overuse of the finger flexor tendons and pressure placed on the ulnar side of the hand (see Figure 14.1).

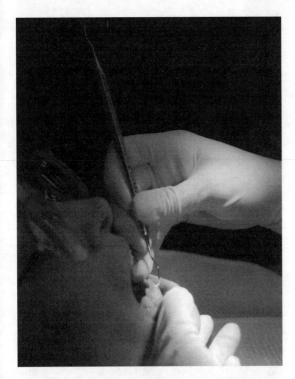

Figure 14.6. Hyperextension of the thumb interphalangeal joint places excess pressure on the collateral ligaments of the thumb metacarpal joint.

Thumb

de Quervain's disease is inflammation of the abductor pollicis longus and the extensor pollicis brevis. Dental hygienists who use excessive thumb extension, abduction, and radial-ulnar deviation of the wrist may be susceptible to this condition.

Thumb pain is a common complaint that has yet to be fully analyzed. Many dental hygienists hyperextend their thumb metacarpophalangeal (MP) or interphalangeal (IP) joints during instrumentation, thereby placing increased stresses on thumb musculature (Figure 14.6). Dental hygienists who hyperextend the MP joint simultaneously hyperflex the IP joint, demanding repetitive use of the flexor pollicis longus. Overuse of the thumb flexor muscles may cause a trigger finger.

Other dental hygienists hyperflex the MP joint of the thumb and extend the IP joint, thereby placing additional stresses on the collateral ligaments, particularly the radial collateral ligament. Overall, the musculature of the thenar eminence (abductor

Table 14.4. Agenda for Continuing Education Workshops on the Ergonomics of Dental Hygiene

I. Introduction
  A. Quality of work-life for dental professionals
  B. Ergonomics: How does it relate?
  C. Cumulative trauma disorders (CTDs): How do they interfere?
II. Musculoskeletal problems in dental professionals
  A. Neck and shoulder pain
  B. Tennis elbow
  C. Carpal tunnel syndrome
  D. Thumb pain
III. Risk factors for CTDs: home and work
  A. Biomechanical risk factors
  B. Ergonomic risk factors
  C. Personal risk factors
IV. Identifying symptoms at work
  A. Self-monitoring
  B. Peer evaluations
  C. Video analysis
V. CTD prevention strategies
  A. Instrumentation
  B. Posture
  C. Work practices
  D. Stretching throughout the day
  E. Personal wellness
VI. General management of CTDs
  A. Decrease pain and inflammation
  B. Local rest
  C. Splint controversy
  D. Stretching throughout the day
  E. General exercise
  F. Healthy lifestyle

pollicis brevis and opponens pollicis) become tight and tender to touch from overuse.

Prevention Strategies for Dental Hygienists

Clearly, the most effective means of handling CTDs is to prevent such disorders. Fortunately, the dental hygiene profession has recognized the imperative nature of integrating good instrumentation and prudent workplace practices into dental hygiene textbooks, curricula, and continuing education (Wilkins 1994; Sanders 1995).

Table 14.4 outlines an agenda for a continuing education workshop developed specifically for dental hygienists. The importance of understanding the dental hygienist's job and familiarity with the instruments cannot be underestimated.

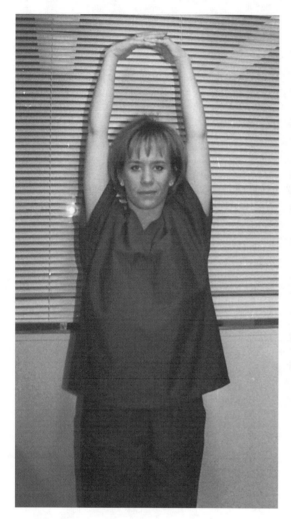

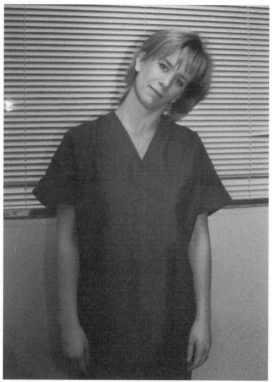

Figure 14.8. Gentle neck circles stretch trapezius, scalene, and sternocleidomastoid muscles.

Figure 14.7. Clasping the hands overhead with the elbows extended stretches the shoulder and elbow musculature.

The workshop format presented has evolved over a number of years to emphasize self-aware-ness, risk factors, workstation ergonomics, and self-help techniques. Dental hygienists are gener-ally aware of the potential for developing CTS but do not always recognize their personal contribut-ing risk factors and early warning signs. Further, many do not realize the importance of arranging the office properly and varying the work positions throughout the day. Each of these areas is dis-cussed and demonstrated, using slides of dental hy-gienists to exemplify the principles discussed. A videotape of a dental hygienist is critiqued by the workshop attendees, who then begin to offer pre-vention strategies themselves.

Stretching Activities

Stretching activities are designed to interrupt the static positions and promote blood flow in body areas used. Stretches are demonstrated and re-viewed in Figures 14.7 through 14.9. Additional stretches recommended are wrist flexion with the elbow extended, wrist rotation, and thumb exten-sion. We recommend performing these stretches after every client (at least one time per hour), hold-ing the stretches for at least 7 seconds, and inte-grating the stretches into the office routine. For example, dental hygienists can stretch the fingers between placing and retrieving instruments (Fig-ure 14.10).

Table 14.5 compiles and reviews the recommen-dations for prevention strategies, including proper instrumentation, posture, workplace practices, and personal health issues. Although these strategies are based on sound theory, no outcome studies have yet documented the effectiveness of the strategies to prevent CTDs.

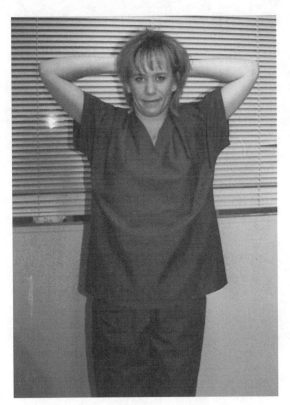

Figure 14.9. Clasping the hands behind the head gently stretches pectoral muscles.

Client Anxiety Control Techniques

An area worthy of further investigation and development is that of client anxiety control techniques. Many dental hygienists discuss the increased muscle tension and anxiety they feel when dealing with anxious clients. Efforts to calm clients may be valuable in the overall picture of decreasing muscle tension and pain in dental hygienists.

The most common technique used to calm clients is diversion and conversation with the clients. Some dental offices use calming music and aesthetic pictures on the walls; some pediatric dental offices use head phones and a sticker program. Verbal preparation as to what the dental hygienist will do next is also helpful to some clients. A new technique to control pain is the use of transcutaneous nerve stimulation during scaling. Finally, in 20 states, dental hygienists can administer local anesthesia to control pain.

Interview for Determining Dental Hygienists' Work Practices

Appendix 14.1 presents an interview that health care practitioners can use when evaluating dental hygienists' with painful conditions. The interview reviews

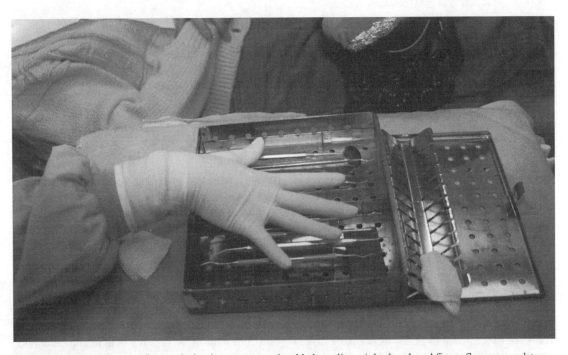

Figure 14.10. Extending the fingers during instrument retrieval helps relieve tight thumb and finger flexor musculature.

Table 14.5. Recommendations to Decrease Cumulative Trauma Disorders in Dental Hygienists

Instrumentation
    Use proper instrumentation techniques
        Avoid thumb hyperextension
        Avoid excessive finger movements
        Keep wrist in neutral position during forearm rotation
        Minimize excessive wrist motions
    Select proper instruments
        Larger diameter, hollow handles, balanced
        Waffle-iron serrations or rubber-coated handles
    Keep instruments sharp
    Dampen vibration components
    Keep cords untangled or use cordless handpiece
    Use ultrasonic scaler and slimlines
    Use indirect vision
    Avoid glove constriction at wrist and thumb
    Vary between intraoral and extraoral fulcrums
Posture
    Minimize twisting and forward bending at waist
    Minimize reach distances
    Minimize elevation of shoulders to $\geq$30 degrees
    Alternate work positions and delivery systems
    Choose an adjustable chair with lumbar, thoracic, and arm support; position chair close to client; feet flat on floor
    Stretch fingers, neck, shoulders, and back periodically
    Extend fingers in placing and retrieving instruments
Work practices
    Allot adequate time for each client
    Alternate scheduling for heavy and light calculus clients
    Recall patients according to individual oral health needs
    Vary tasks (client education, sealants, orthodontic records, radiographs, root planing recalls)
    Provide client anxiety control technique
    Gradually increase work tolerance from part time to full time
    Use selective polishing
    Add buffer times to schedule
Personal health
    Recognize that daily chores and hobbies contribute to cumulative trauma disorders
    Realize that stress affects work performance and pain
    Pay attention to body signals
    Maintain good levels of fitness, relaxation, sleep, and play
    Welcome change and lifetime growth

dental hygienists' work practices, their symptoms, and the effects of neuromuscular pain on work and home life. The interview can be used as a basis for understanding and adapting the work environment if needed.

Trends in Dental Hygiene Practice

The Enlarged Scope of Dental Hygiene Therapy

The scope of the dental hygiene practice has enlarged according to the needs of the client population. Whereas dental hygienists' primary focus was once the prevention of cavities, children now have very few cavities due to the introduction of fluoridated water. Periodontal (gum and bone) disease, however, is still prevalent in the baby boomer population. Thus, the dental hygiene profession has focused efforts on developing techniques to prevent or manage this problem.

Techniques used by dental hygienists to manage periodontal disease include management of the soft-tissue structures around the teeth (scaling and root planing to remove plaque and calculus), good home care techniques, and irrigating (spraying) the tooth below the gum line with rinses that deter a build-up of microorganisms. Dental hygienists are recalling clients earlier for follow-up to prevent the progression of gum disease and build-up of calculus.

Trends in Client Scheduling

Increasingly, dental hygienists have the independence to determine the amount of time needed for clients. Traditionally, clients were recalled every 6 months for a 1-hour examination and cleaning, regardless of whether the client developed heavy calculus more rapidly. Today, more and more dental hygienists are scheduling clients for visits according to their particular oral health needs. This practice will help to prevent periodontal disease and minimize the forces needed for dental hygienists to remove calculus.

The amount of time allotted for dental appointments varies according to the office. Some offices automatically allot 60, 50, or 45 minutes per client. Other offices permit the dental hygienist to determine the amount of time needed. Unfortunately, insurance companies typically pay for only two preventive visits per year, regardless of whether the client needs more visits to prevent problems. Dental hygienists often have the burden of convincing high-risk clients to visit more frequently (although insurers will not pay) through client education or enduring the physical and mental anxiety of completing difficult clients in the allotted time.

Trends in Body Mechanics

In the early years of practice, dentists and dental hygienists worked standing up, with the client seated in an upright position. This position probably contributed to the first reported CTD in dentistry: low-back pain. Over the years, dentistry and dental hygiene have progressed to a sit-down delivery system, with the client in a semireclined supine position. Although less incidents of low-back pain are noted, static loading on the neck and shoulders has contributed to upper-extremity disorders.

Most dentists now work with a dental assistant, which eliminates their need for twisting, bending, and reaching to obtain instruments or to retract oral structures. In contrast, dental hygienists usually work independently. They must retrieve their own instruments, record patients' status, and assume awkward postures with more frequency than do dentists. Further, dental hygienists usually work in a smaller operator chair and with older instruments ("handed-down" from the dentist). Thus, the work environment of dental hygienists is even less ergonomically salient than that of the dentist.

Trends in Dental Instruments

The use of ultrasonic scalers (vibrating instruments with a thin tip to remove calculus) has come full circle since its introduction. Initially, ultrasonic scalers were used routinely to remove heavy calculus. Dental hygienists then switched to hand scaling for more accurate calculus removal and to avoid using another vibrating instrument. Now, clinicians recommend use of the ultrasonic scaler particularly for heavy calculus, and possibly for *all* calculus removal. "Slimlines," a recent development in ultrasonic tips, are designed to remove fine calculus and smooth the root of the tooth.

Overall, the dental hygiene profession has made great strides in recognizing the risk factors for CTDs. Health care practitioners can contribute practical suggestions for the prevention of such disorders.

References

Atwood MJ & Michalak C (1992). The occurrence of cumulative trauma disorders in dental hygienists. *Work*, 2(4),17–31.

Ekenvall L, Nilsson BY, & Falconer C (1990). Sensory perception in the hands of dentists. *Scand J Work Environ Health*, 16,334–339.

Hardage JL, Gildersleeve JR, & Rugh JD (1983). Clinical work posture for the dentist: an electromyographic study. *J Am Dent Assoc*, 107,937–939.

Luopajarvi T (1990). Ergonomic analysis of workplace and postural load. In M Bullock (Ed). *Ergonomic: The Physiotherapist in the Workplace*. New York: Churchill Livingstone.

MacDonald G (1987). Hazards in the dental workplace. *Dent Hygiene*, 61,212–218.

MacDonald G, Robertson MM, & Erickson SA (1988). Carpal tunnel syndrome among California dental hygienists. *Dent Hygiene*, 62,322–328.

Meador HL (1993). The biocentric technique: a guide to avoiding occupational pain. *J Dent Hygiene*, 67,38–51.

Oberg T (1993). Ergonomic evaluations and construction of a reference workplace in dental hygiene: a case study. *J Dent Hygiene*, 67,262–267.

Oberg T & Oberg U (1993). Musculoskeletal complaints in dental hygiene: a survey from a Swedish county. *J Dent Hygiene*, 67,257–261.

Osborn JB, Newell KJ, Rudney JD, & Stoltenberg JL (1990). Musculoskeletal pain among Minnesota dental hygienists. *J Dent Hygiene*, 63,132–138.

Pattison G & Pattison AM (1992). *Periodontal Instrumentation* (2nd ed). Norwalk, CT: Appleton & Lange.

Rhode J (June-July 1990). Ambidextrous gloves: can they contribute to carpal tunnel syndrome? *Dent Today*, 19–20.

Sanders M (March 1995). Wellness in the workplace: the ergonomics of dental hygiene. Presented at Professional Learning Services Conference, Norwalk, CT.

Strong DR & Lennartz FH (1992). Carpal tunnel syndrome. *CA Dent Assoc J*, 20(4),27–39.

Wilkins EM (1994). *Clinical Practice of the Dental Hygienist*. Malvern, PA: Williams & Wilkins.

Appendix 14.1

Interview for Determining Dental
Hygienists' Work Practices

Personal Data

Name: _____   Date: _____

Address: _____

Phone: _____ Age: _____ Gender: _____

Diagnosis: _____

History of current diagnosis: _____

_____

_____

Chief complaint: _____

_____

Medical History (please check and comment)

❐ Diabetes _____

❐ Hormone abnormality _____

❐ Kidney disorder _____

❐ Endocrine disorder _____

❐ Rheumatoid arthritis _____

❐ Previous surgeries _____

❐ Wrist fracture _____

❐ Acute trauma _____

❐ Family history of carpal tunnel syndrome _____

❐ Pregnancy _____

❐ Motor vehicle accident _____

❐ Other musculoskeletal diagnosis _____

Previous treatment for the present condition: _____

_____

_____

Employment History

Number of years practicing dental hygiene: _____

Types of dentistry practiced: _____

_____

Types of dentistry at present job(s):

Primary _____ Secondary _____

Number of years at present job(s):

Primary _____ Secondary _____

Number of days worked per week:

Primary _____ Secondary _____

Number of hours worked per day:

Primary _____ Secondary _____

Tasks performed at present job(s): _____

_____

_____

Workplace Practices

Average number of clients per day: _____

Amount of time allotted per client:

Adults _____ Children _____

Percentage of clients with the following degrees of calculus:

Light _____

Moderate _____

Heavy _____

Do you alternate scheduling clients with light and heavy calculus? _____

Percentage of clients on whom you use the ultrasonic scaler: _____

Percentage of clients whose teeth you polish: _____

Frequency of sharpening instruments: _____

Handle shape used most frequently (check):

❏ Round
❏ Hexagonal
❏ Octagonal

Handle size used:

❏ Smaller than $\frac{3}{16}$ in.
❏ Larger than $\frac{3}{16}$ in.

Primary mode of instrument delivery:

❏ Side
❏ Rear
❏ Front

Do you rotate instrument delivery systems?

❏ Yes
❏ No

Handle serration used most frequently (check):

❏ Smooth
❏ Long, parallel
❏ Crosswise
❏ Intermittent bands
❏ Waffle-iron
❏ Rubber-coated
❏ Other: _____

Primary operator position:

❏ 9 o'clock
❏ 12 o'clock
❏ 3 o'clock

Do you rotate operator positions?

❏ Yes
❏ No

Please draw a sketch of your office set-up.

Musculoskeletal Symptoms

Please check if you have had any of the following conditions:

❏ Pain or swelling in the hands or wrist
❏ Numbness or tingling in the hands or wrist
❏ Tendency for your fingers to "lock"
❏ Weakness in your grip
❏ Discomfort in the elbow or forearm
❏ Discomfort in the shoulder
❏ Discomfort in the neck area

Please indicate the location of your discomfort. Feel free to include locations other than your primary diagnosis.

What is the frequency of your discomfort?

❏ Morning
❏ During work
❏ After work
❏ Evenings
❏ Interferes with sleep

Which extremities?_____

❏ Dominant
❏ Nondominant
❏ Both

Have you ever noticed any of the following during work?

❏ Increased discomfort toward the
    end of the day
❏ Increased discomfort after clients with
    heavy calculus
❏ Difficulty in maintaining my grasp
    of instruments
❏ Difficulty in detecting calculus
❏ Difficulty in judging the amount of pressure
    being used
❏ Dropping objects inadvertently
❏ Increased overall fatigue at the
    end of the day
❏ Shaking of my hands

Do any other activities induce similar discomfort?

❏ Typing   ❏ Use of utensils
❏ Lifting or carrying   ❏ Sports
❏ Brushing teeth   ❏ Scrubbing
❏ Writing   ❏ Opening jars

What methods have you used to alleviate your discomfort?

❏ Shaking wrists   ❏ Taking more breaks
❏ Ice   ❏ Aspirin
❏ Heat   ❏ Splints
❏ Stretching   ❏ Seeing fewer clients
❏ Changing positions   ❏ Vacation

Which of the above methods are effective?

_____

_____

Briefly describe a typical day for you. _____

_____

_____

_____

_____

What are your hobbies? _____

_____

_____

How frequently do you perform your hobbies? _____

If you have experienced musculoskeletal discomfort, do you feel that it has interfered with other aspects of your life? (Please check those that apply.)

❏ Household chores   ❏ Driving
❏ Dressing   ❏ Writing
❏ Grooming and bathing   ❏ Social recreation
❏ Cooking   ❏ Hobbies
❏ Child care   ❏ Energy level
❏ Social recreation   ❏ Positive attitude
❏ Job satisfaction   ❏ Relationships

Please describe aspects of your job that you enjoy and those that you do not enjoy.

_____

_____

_____

_____

Summary comments: _____

_____

_____

_____

Therapist's name: _____ Date: _____

Chapter 15

Cumulative Trauma Disorders in the Performing Musician

Caryl D. Johnson

When the repetitious motions of playing musical instruments exceed conditioning, the motions can cause accumulated microinsults to tissues and create cumulative trauma disorders (CTDs). "Play through the pain" has been as much a part of the rigorous training and attitude of performing musicians as it has been for athletes. Teachers, like coaches, encourage strict self-discipline and practice as the routes to success. Only recently have performing musicians become more willing to admit to chronic pain or injuries.

In this chapter, the term *performing musicians* refers to amateur musicians and conservatory students as well as professional musicians. All of these individuals spend sizable amounts of time playing their instruments. Professional musicians play varying amounts of time each day, usually from 3 to 10 hours. Amateur musicians frequently spend 3 hours daily with their instruments and may spend even more time on weekends. Conservatory students play their instruments at least 5 hours per day, 7 days per week.

Most CTDs in these patients are related to length or quality of playing time. Length of time at the instrument can condition the body, but excessive or inconsistent playing time can transform conditioning into injury. Quality of playing time is determined by many factors—the workplace or practice place, instrument quality, technical level of the performer, musical demands on the performer, and other stress-producing circumstances. A lengthy or stressful period at the instrument can set the stage for cumulative trauma.

Each instrument generates unique qualities of sound, but the processes of generating sound, changing pitch, sustaining sound, articulating sound, and stopping sound occur with all instruments. Any one of these mechanisms may be the implicated factor in an injury, but more often a combination of these factors is culpable. The work of playing a musical instrument includes generating sound on the instrument and, for many instruments, holding the instrument against gravity. Specific muscles controlled by complex neurologic interactions carry out this work. The efficiency of this neuromuscular activity evolves from training and conditioning. However, when the work is carried out using incorrect technique or when it exceeds the body's conditioning, injury can result.

Performing musicians must spend part of every day in training. They need to warm up, rehearse with other players or practice, learn new music, prepare for performance, and perform. To meet the rigors of training and performing, they inflict repeated trauma on their body parts and accumulate small injuries. These small injuries, when balanced with recovery time, lead to conditioning. (*Conditioning* for a performing musician includes repeating note patterns and movement sequences that are needed to train neuromuscular responses and to increase endurance.) However, if repeated microinsults are not followed by sufficient recovery time, injuries result.

Factors that Contribute to Cumulative Trauma Disorders in Performing Musicians

Fatigue

Nearly all CTDs of the performing musician are manifestations of fatigue or inadequate recovery time after fatigue, whether physical or mental. A performer who is mentally or physically tired is liable to incur an injury. The key word to remember when considering CTDs in musicians is *beyond*: Performing musicians are prone to going beyond the bounds of what is reasonable and healthful: *beyond* instrument conditioning, *beyond* whole-body conditioning, and *beyond* training (i.e., using poor or insufficient technical training to perform the chosen task).

Training and Conditioning

Training and conditioning are carried out to prepare the body for the actions required to play the instrument. Training parameters are those of the traditional technical approaches to each instrument. These parameters determine body and hand position, the motions used to produce sound, and the image of desirable sound. Conditioning for speed, endurance, positioning, strength, pressure, and breathing takes place during practicing and playing. When the performer exceeds his or her conditioning, the performer becomes fatigued. If the performer plays *beyond* fatigue, he or she eventually alters his or her normal performance techniques and begins to use recruited, less efficient muscle combinations. This is a frequent cause of injury.

Time and Intensity

The length or the emotional intensity of a performance can exceed conditioning, cause fatigue, and lead to injury. Music takes place in time, and training for endurance on an instrument is a priority. However, in certain work settings, the length of some performances or practice sessions is far beyond normal endurance limits. (For instance, certain operas by Wagner last 6 hours or more.)

Music is also an expressive art. Many compositions or playing situations require sustained emotional intensity from the players. Emotional fatigue can alter neuromuscular control. Either length of time or degree of emotional intensity can generate injury.

Stress and Performing

Performing is stressful. Stage fright, or at least "stage nerves," are very real, as are the neurologic responses to this psychological stress. Along with autonomic manifestations such as perspiration and dry mouth, involuntary muscle contractions (especially in the face, neck, and shoulders) make controlled playing more difficult. Cocontraction of additional muscle groups decreases control of fine-motor response. Stress can be a path to injury if it decreases endurance and control.

Static Posturing

Maintaining an instrument in one place for long periods of time causes muscle fatigue, muscle recruitment, and tension in the neck, shoulders, and arms. This posturing also eventually decreases venous return. Fatigue, muscle recruitment, and diminished venous return can lead to injury.

Repetition

Repetition is an important way to learn and perfect performance, but it can easily be carried to damaging extremes. Repeating a unit of music embeds this pattern of notes in the mind and in the "muscle memory." Repetition is also a way of strengthening the execution of a given pattern of notes and of perfecting muscle timing. However, mindless or excessive repetitions can exceed conditioning and cause injury.

Instrument Transport

Most instruments are carried by performers to work or school and home again. If the instrument is small, this is not a burden. If the instrument is large and requires a heavy case, transporting it may be an important factor in fatigue. An injury can result from repeatedly lifting a large instrument into and out of a car or from lifting it over the subway turnstile.

Work Settings

Work environments can contribute to CTDs if they are not ergonomically sound. In most orchestras, the musicians are seated while playing. As part of evaluating orchestral players, one should check the following factors:

- Chairs used—their height, support, and the space between them
- Viewing angle to music
- Viewing angle to conductor
- Sufficiency of lighting
- Space for moving parts of instrument or body

Injuries by Instrument Group

As more performing musicians with CTDs present themselves for treatment, therapists have increased opportunities to treat and help prevent such injuries. However, in order to treat these patients effectively, the therapist must have a knowledge of instruments, of instrument techniques, and of the physical demands presented by different instruments.

Woodwind Instruments

The flute, piccolo, clarinet, oboe, English horn, bassoon, and saxophone all consist of a tube or column of air that vibrates, amplifying the sound initiated by a mouthpiece or *fipple*. Early forms of these instruments were wood tubes, and most still are made of wood—hence the term *woodwinds*. Pitch changes depend on the length and width of the column. Many of these instruments now have a mechanical key system that facilitates changing pitch. Volume is changed by faster (harder) or slower blowing. Sound stops when air no longer vibrates within the column. All commonly used woodwinds are held to the mouth for playing. All woodwind instruments can be carried by the player in hard or semirigid cases. Certainly the larger instruments require more strength to carry.

Problems related to playing woodwinds are frequently the result of static posture and holding the instrument for extended periods of time. Fatigue in the shoulder, elbows, and wrist may lead to CTDs such as bursitis, tendinitis and, in older players, degenerative joint problems and calcific tendinitis.

Several of the woodwinds (i.e., clarinet, oboe, saxophone) rest on the right thumb while they are being played, which causes stress to ligaments and painful metacarpophalangeal and carpometacarpal joints. Such joint stress, if allowed

to continue for years, can lead to attrition injuries of ligaments at either joint or to degeneration of the carpometacarpal joint.

Ligament attrition injuries also can result from the repeated finger and thumb abduction required to play larger woodwind instruments (e.g., contrabassoon). On these instruments, the keys are very far apart and the instruments are longer and thicker than other woodwinds.

Brass Instruments

The trumpet, trombone, French horn, and tuba are brass instruments and consist of cylindric and conic tubes of brass that vibrate to amplify the sound initiated by the player's lips. Pitch can be changed two ways: by changing the air pressure or by changing the length of the tube. Tube length is altered by adding or removing units of the tube or by using valves to add or subtract units of tube length.

Few players of brass instruments suffer from CTDs of the upper extremities. All brass instruments are brought to the mouth for playing, but none requires intricate finger skills or unusual reaches. In most musical pieces, these instruments are not played for long periods, and so players have opportunities to lower their instruments, change their position, and rest.

Percussion Instruments

Percussion instruments include drums, the timpani, the xylophone, and cymbals. Percussion instruments have one or more parts that resonate when struck. Sticks, mallets, brushes, and even hands are used for striking an instrument to make sound. Tuning and pitch changes on percussion instruments are made deliberately by the player (as when the musician tunes the timpani) or by striking specially tuned parts of the instrument (chimes, keys, metal bars, etc.).

Cumulative trauma for these performers usually results from repetitious playing, forceful playing, and performing for extended periods. CTDs seen in percussion players include de Quervain's disease from repeated use of drumsticks. The use of sticks on the timpani and certain other drums requires rapid alternation of radial and ulnar deviation. If the player has faulty technique, he or she may stress wrist extensors and the abductor pollicis longus when playing for long periods. Tendinitis of the forearm extensors can result from repeated forceful strikes of the cymbal. This action also causes an impact to shoulders.

Playing with a rock band requires forceful loud strokes of sticks for long periods. The drumstick is pivoted on the second and third fingers and slaps the palm. These repeated forceful strokes of sticks cause soft-tissue trauma to the palm and trigger fingers.

Many jazz and rock percussionists do not play in the same location every night. They often transport instruments, amplifiers, keyboards, and electrical equipment to each job. This may be a secondary rather than primary cause of cumulative trauma, but it should be considered as a possible contributing factor to injury.

Keyboard Instruments

The structural element shared by the piano, electronic keyboard, and organ (to name a few such instruments) is a keyboard that controls pitch change on resonating strings, pipes, or speaker cones. The player usually sits in front of the keyboard(s) and reaches forward to touch the keys.

Placement of the player in relation to the keyboard, pedals, and music is frequently a factor in cumulative trauma problems among these musicians. When evaluating a keyboard performer at his or her instrument, the therapist should check elbow and wrist angles. Some positions place forearm muscles at a disadvantage. If the player sits too close to the keyboard, the elbows will be excessively flexed and the wrists may remain ulnarly deviated. If the musician sits too low, the wrists may be actively extended rather than in neutral. In both of these examples, additional muscle activity and tension cause inefficiency and fatigue. If back and trunk posture is poorly supported, distal fine-motor actions can be less effective and more costly in terms of energy expenditure, which often results in cumulative and compound injuries.

Compression neuropathies can result from repeated excessive elbow or wrist flexion or excessive wrist extension These neuropathies include cubital, radial, and carpal tunnel syndromes.

Repeated practicing of extended reaches can fatigue or injure soft tissues in the hand. Recovery from such an injury (e.g., palmar ligament injury, tendinitis) is protracted and requires careful monitoring.

Lateral epicondylitis results from repetitive use of extensor tendons of both the fingers and the wrist. de Quervain's disease is another common finding in keyboard performers. It relates to forceful thumb use in abducted and extended positions.

Stringed Instruments

The violin, viola, cello, double bass, or guitar is basically a resonating box with strings stretched tightly across it. The strings are set to vibrating by a bow, a pick, or a finger. Pitch is changed by stopping the string, which changes its length. The instrument body is the box, which resonates and amplifies the sound of the string. Violins and violas are held near the left shoulder, guitars and lutes are held in front of the trunk, and cellos and double basses rest on the floor.

Chronic shoulder pain is common among players of stringed instruments. The traditional position for playing violins and violas probably is the most frequent cause of CTDs in string players. These instruments are held in front of the left shoulder and under the chin by the left arm, which is in forward flexion and internal rotation. This arm position is physically demanding and causes many cumulative inflammatory disorders.

Right-handed guitarists play with the left hand supinated and the right pronated. The left hand moves in varying amounts of wrist flexion to reach and stop the strings. Some performers also use a flexed right wrist. Sustained flexion in either wrist can make facile or continuous finger flexion both difficult and fatiguing. Tendinitis of the flexor tendons is not uncommon.

Compression neuropathies also are seen in stringed instrument players. Cubital tunnel syndrome is caused by repetitive elbow flexion. Carpal tunnel syndrome can result from repetitious finger flexion with the wrist flexed.

Tendinitis of the wrist extensors results from playing beyond conditioned endurance levels and is seen in either hand.

Evaluating the Injured Performing Musician

Evaluation of the injured performing musician begins with obtaining a useful history (Appendix 15.1), including personal, medical, and instrumental facts. Characterization of the pain or problem (e.g., whether it is acute or chronic) is essential. The patient should be asked to describe the pain, including its location, duration, and other descriptive notes. A pain log may be useful but only if it includes logging of the pain in relation to instrument use.

The next step in the evaluative process is the physical examination, which should include the following checks:

- Observe patient's build and posture in relation to instrument
- Note unusual findings in skeletal development
- Examine skin for callous or signs of inflammation
- Note use of glasses, straps, pads, or any extra-instrument items
- Note localized swelling
- Measure grip strength, lateral pinch strength, three jaw chuck, and tip pinch strength
- Measure any limitations of active range of motion (AROM) or greater-than-normal AROM of joints
- Observe and note joint stability, laxity, or other-than-normal alignments

The patient should also be examined at the instrument. The therapist should try to provide a playing situation that is close to normal for the patient. The patient must be observed from all angles—front, side, back, and oblique. The musician should be asked to play a customary warm-up, something slow, something fast, and any piece or section of a piece that might have caused the presenting problem. During the patient's playing, the therapist should make the following observations:

- Skill level
- Instrument technique as it compares to standard technique
- Posture changes during playing
- Dynamic joint alignment
- Tension mannerisms

The therapist should reconsider the presenting problem or diagnosis while listening and observing: Can causative factors be recognized from observation?

Principles of Treatment

Rest

Rest is essential to recovery from inflammatory conditions. Splints can be used to isolate and rest injured tissues but must be monitored regularly. It is important to rest only the involved tissues. Patients are urged to maintain active use of all uninvolved parts of their bodies. Rest and a non-steroidal or even a steroidal anti-inflammatory drug regimen usually compose the first step of a treatment protocol.

Whole-Body Exercises

Whole-body postural exercises can be introduced at the earliest stage of treatment. They maximize preservation of previous specialized conditioning and maintain muscle health. Exercises that emphasize breathing, trunk alignment, and release of static tension should be selected.

Isometric Exercises

Isometric exercises are used to begin graded resistance to the involved area. Because they place less stress on tendons, tone and strength can be returned to the muscle portion of the musculotendinous unit.

Progressive Resistive Exercises

Progressive resistive exercises are the last step of treatment. They are used for conditioning and coincide with steps to return to a full playing regimen.

Case Report

AE is a 31-year-old, right-handed piano student who suffered an acute injury to his left hand and forearm 1 week before being seen for his first visit. He believed the injury to be the result of extra practicing on one piece he was preparing to perform.

He was referred by a hand surgeon for evaluation, splinting, and treatment. The physician had placed him in a plaster volar mold wrapped in place with an Ace bandage, immobilizing his forearm, wrist, and hand. The thumb had not been immobilized. The physician's referral reported negative x-ray findings.

History taking provided the following pertinent information:

The patient is a pleasant but very worried young man of moderate height and weight. He is a full-time "preprofessional" student with minimal academic classes but many performing responsibilities at his conservatory. He has studied piano for 25 years, with a series of excellent teachers in both the United States and abroad and is an experienced performer who is outgoing, assertive, and confident at the instrument.

He described his problem and its occurrence in this way: He was practicing a difficult contemporary piece for the piano in which there is a long section requiring the left hand to cross over the right and jab loudly accented notes above and between those notes being played by the right hand. He decided he would work out one part, repeating it until he could do it easily. As he usually does, he was practicing at full volume, late at night, after a full day of classes and practicing. He was tired but determined to learn this particular section. He stopped because his arms felt fatigued and a little painful on the ulnar border of his left wrist. Both hands felt a little more tired than usual.

The next morning, when he awoke, the patient had extreme pain in his left wrist, in his hand, along the ulnar border of the forearm, and around the lateral epicondyle. He tried to rest his hand and did not practice that day, but the painful symptoms worsened. The next day he tried to practice and thought, at first, that the pain was better, but in the evening it became worse than ever. The following day he went to the nurse and was referred to a "hand doctor."

The patient reported no previous episodes of such pain, although he previously had felt aches in his forearms after long hours of practice. He plays a classical piano repertoire. He has made no recent changes in his musical life. AE's goal is to become a concert artist. He is currently preparing for a performance that will fulfill part of the requirements of his school. Customarily, he practices 5–7 hours daily. AE does some additional work to earn money, but none of it is demanding physically. He has made no recent changes in lifestyle. AE reports that he never exercises. His family is musically inclined; a brother is a cellist. Just 2 months ago, his father died.

The physical examination showed no vascular or skin changes. His left wrist was painful to touch on the dorsum and when moved beyond midrange. Pain increased in resisted finger extension and wrist extension. He was more uncomfortable when he moved actively into ulnar deviation. There was minimal diffuse swelling around the wrist, the carpometacarpal joint of the thumb, and in the distal forearm, with tenderness to pressure over the dorsal wrist extensor compartments. Strength measurements were deferred. AROM measurements were normal except as limited by pain in full wrist flexion with no resistance and full pronation against minimal resistance.

Lateral epicondylitis and extensor tendon synovitis were diagnosed in AE. Treatment was begun with immobilization in a molded wrist cock-up splint, placing the wrist in 60 degrees of extension, neutral radial-ulnar deviation, and extending two-thirds of the length of the forearm. The splint was worn at all times except during meals and for three 15-minute periods each day when AE was to move through an active range of motion. He was begun on naproxen (Naprosyn) and told to discontinue practicing or playing the piano. His teacher was contacted, and the diagnosis and treatment plan were explained to her.

Two days later, he was seen again. His splint was checked, and he began regular treatments with heat and massage to the forearm, wrist, and hand, and shoulder AROM exercises (no weight or resistance). He was also reinstructed not to avoid the left arm but to use it as normally as possible even when wearing the splint. This first phase of treatment was continued for 3 weeks. By the end of the first week, AE's symptoms were beginning to resolve. He was seen three times per week for symptomatic treatment.

At the end of 3 weeks, AE was to wean himself from the splint under a protocol that began with removal of the splint for 1 hour at each mealtime and gradually increased this splintless time until, by the end of the fourth week, he donned the splint only when he felt pain. During the second 3 weeks, he began guarded isometric exercises to the involved muscle groups and increased the number of repetitions of his shoulder AROM exercises. His nonsteroidal anti-inflammatory drug was continued through the second 3-week period.

The fourth week after beginning treatment, AE was allowed a guarded return to the keyboard. Limitations on practice included length of time at the keyboard (30 minutes) and which pieces were to be practiced. Piano practicing was preceded by shoulder AROM exercises used as a warm-up. He maintained this regimen daily including Sunday. Visits to the therapist were reduced to once weekly until 6 weeks into treatment.

At the end of 6 weeks, AE began phase three of treatment: graded resistive shoulder AROM exercises, with a resistance of 1 lb, and AROM of involved muscles against gentle manual resistance by the therapist.

From this point, the patient progressed to increased resistance for his upper-extremity exercises, to increased lengths of time and a more difficult repertoire at the keyboard, and to increased strengthening of the injured muscles. At approximately 3 months after injury, the patient was cleared for a full 5-hour practice routine, was performing his exercises regularly with 3-lb weights, and was preparing a recital. Except for occasional twinges of discomfort, he was without problem and had learned a lesson: that he was not able to practice in awkward or unconditioned hand positions for unlimited hours without injuring himself.

Summary of Important Considerations

Evaluation and a correct diagnosis are all important in treating CTDs in this population. Treatment is planned and carried out on the basis of these findings. Because work conditions cannot usually be changed, the patient must be taught to adapt, to condition, to pace his or her energy consumption, to anticipate stresses, and to condition alternative muscle patterns.

The most difficult issue is determining when it is safe for the patient to resume playing. Generally, the shorter the time between injury and treatment, the sooner can the patient safely return to playing. The timing of a safe and successful return to the instrument depends on (1) all the factors causing the injury, (2) the extent of the injury, (3) the length of time before treatment, (4) the length of time the patient continued to play while injured, and (5) rates of healing.

Return to playing estimates can be made as follows: For a simple CTD—an acute injury involving one type of tissue—one can expect to see a normal healing rate for the tissue involved. After following the steps of treatment outlined earlier, the patient can usually be promised an expeditious return to the instrument. For a complex CTD—a chronic injury in which more than one type of tissue is involved, or an injury related to faulty technique—the timing of return to playing is not easy to foresee, as the rate of healing cannot be predicted. The steps of treatment must be carried out patiently; each involved tissue must repair itself. Technical changes may have to be made. Repertoire is chosen to match tissue recovery and conditioning level. Functional use must be preserved, and the patient requires continuing support and encouragement. The timing of a full return to a normal playing schedule will be individual and unpredictable.

Suggested Reading

Charnass ME & Barbaro MN (1987). Occupational cubital tunnel syndrome in instrumental musicians. *Neurology*, 35(4),74.

Edwards RHT (1988). Hypotheses of peripheral and central mechanisms underlying occupational muscle pain and injury. *J Appl Pathol*, 57,275–281.

Fry HJ (1986). Overuse syndrome of the upper limb in musicians. *Med J Aust*, 44(4),182–183.

Fry HJ (1987). Prevalence of overuse syndrome in Australian music schools. *Br J Indust Med*, 44(1),35–40.

Hochberg FH (1990). The upper extremity difficulties of musicians. In JM Hunter, LH Schneider, EJ Mackin, & AD Callahan (Eds). *Rehabilitation of the Hand* (3rd ed, pp. 1197–1209). Philadelphia: Mosby.

Johnson C (1992). Treating the hands that make music. *J Hand Ther*, 5(2),58–60.

Lippmann HI (1991). A fresh look at the overuse syndrome in musical performers: is "overuse" overused? *Med Prob Perform Art*, 6(2),57–60.

Lockwood AH (1989). Medical problems of musicians. *N Engl J Med*, 320,221–227.

Lowe C (1992). Treatment of tendinitis, tenosynovitis, and other cumulative trauma disorders of musicians' forearms, wrists and hands . . . restoring function with hand therapy. *J Hand Ther*, 5(2),84–91.

Mackinnon SE & Novak CB (1994). Clinical commentary: pathogenesis of cumulative trauma disorder. *J Hand Surg [Am]*, 19,873–883.

Prokop LL (1990). Upper extremity rehabilitation: conditioning and orthotics for the athlete and performing artist. *Hand Clin*, 6,517–524.

Sataloff TR, Brandfonbrener AG, & Lederman RJ (Eds) (1991). *Textbook of Performing Arts Medicine*. New York: Raven Press.

Stern PJ (1990). Tendinitis, overuse syndromes, and tendon injuries. *Hand Clin*, 6,467–476.

Appendix 15.1
History Form for Use When Evaluating a Musician with a Cumulative Trauma Disorder

Personal Data

Patient name: _____Date: _____

Date of birth: _____Age: _____Gender: _____

Instrument(s): _____

Referred by: _____

Referred for: _____

Medical Data

Patient description of problem (including duration and intensity of symptoms): _____

_____

_____

If patient has been referred, what was given as the diagnosis?_____

_____

_____

Was the patient ever evaluated or treated by other medical professionals? _____

When? In what sequence? Was any previous treatment successful? _____

_____

_____

_____

Is patient being treated at the present time? _____

Body type:_____

Posture: _____

Does patient have a history of neck or back problems? _____

Does he/she exercise regularly? _____

Physical Examination Findings

_____

_____

_____

_____

Professional/Musical History

Type of performer (i.e., student, amateur, teacher, professional performer; full- or part-time):

_____

_____

Performing employment status (i.e., freelance, concertizing, theater pit, church, combination):

_____

Years playing this instrument: _____

Employed by: _____

Professional responsibilities and schedule or school where enrolled (include academic and music schools):

_____

_____

Schedule of academic and performance activities: _____

_____

Teachers/training/technical background: _____

Style of music played: _____

Professional/musical goals of patient: _____

_____

Any change of teacher, technique, work load, instrument setup, style that coincided with onset of symptoms:

_____

Recent increases in practicing (may relate to competitions, performances, auditions, etc): _____

_____

Practicing habits (including comments on regularity, location, time of day, instrument, use of practice time):

_____

_____

Does patient believe the problem relates to a specific piece of music or a specific technical challenge?

_____

Psychosocial/Lifestyle History

Does the patient have a family that includes other performers?_____

_____

Does the patient have a nonmusic job? Could it relate to his/her problem?_____

_____

Has the patient suffered any recent trauma, emotional or physical?_____

_____

Evaluation with Instrument

Technical correctness and proficiency: _____

_____

Posture and body mechanics: _____

_____

Can patient demonstrate techniques that he/she feels cause his/her problem? _____

_____

Chapter 16

Video Display Terminal Workers

Judith Pelletier Sehnal

The Automated Office Environment

The use of visual display terminals (VDTs) in the workplace has traditionally been associated with clerical job functions. However, as technology moves forward, computers are quickly becoming standard equipment in offices, schools, retail businesses, laboratories, design outfits, and other environments. Grandjean (1987) has distinguished the following five kinds of jobs that are characterized by predominant modes of interaction with the VDT:

1. Data-entry work
2. Data acquisition
3. Conversational or interactive communication
4. Word processing
5. Computer-aided design (CAD) or computer-aided manufacturing (CAM)

Although it is possible to identify specific jobs that would fall exclusively within each of the preceding categories, many VDT-related positions require the performance of combinations of a variety of job functions, crossing the job categories as listed here.

VDTs now are used by more people in a larger variety of capacities than ever before. It has been estimated that by 1997, 50% of American workers will be using VDTs at work (Scalet 1987). Today many businesses far exceed this estimate within their companies.

The proliferation of computers in the workplace is due at least in part to their versatility and capacity for detailed operations. Computers and software can handle many operations previously performed by manual procedures. These manual procedures are now considered time-consuming and inefficient. Computers add value to business operations by increasing productivity, quality, and customer service.

With an increase in the frequency and intensity of VDT use and in the number of workers using VDTs, the incidence of work-related illnesses and injuries in this environment has increased as well. With more VDT users seeking treatment, occupational therapists are seeing more clients with VDT-related cumulative trauma disorders (CTDs). Although therapists provide the necessary treatment, they recognize the need for preventive services. This chapter provides background on CTDs in the automated office environment and reviews proactive and reactive approaches to addressing this issue.

The Changing Office Environment: Why Cumulative Trauma Disorders Occur

A commonly asked question is why computer operators develop CTDs when, historically, those using typewriters did not experience these problems. The answer to this question is multifaceted.

Keyboard Design

The design of the keyboard is one factor in the incidence of CTDs among computer operators (Barry 1993; Bureau of National Affairs, Inc. 1994). Standard typewriter keyboards and most contemporary keyboards conform to the QWERTY keyboard layout, referring to the letter-number-symbol sequence of the keys. The top row of alphakeys in this layout begins on the left with the letters *QWERTY*. This layout was designed to distribute keystrokes over the entire keyboard and thereby prevent jamming of keys as typists' keyboard skills and speed increased. Thus, manual and even electric typewriters provided a built-in system to pace workers. In addition, the typewriter requires inputting interruptions for paper replacement and correction of errors. Finally, many typists were trained on technique and appropriate use of the typewriter.

The standard computer keyboard still conforms to the QWERTY layout. However, the advanced technology of computers can handle unlimited inputting speed. From a biomechanical perspective, this presents a dilemma in that faster typing and inputting speeds are supported technologically by the system but not physically by key layout. This technology has also eliminated the opportunity for work interruptions and changes of posture related to paper changes and error corrections. In addition, the keys of the computer keyboard are closer to the work surface, making the work surface more accessible to the wrist and forearms for support. The result is a greater propensity for awkward and sustained postures during computer keyboard use.

Work Practices

The VDT itself probably is no more demanding of workers than older equipment replaced or supplemented by computerization, such as manual typewriters, accounting machines, keypunch machines, and switchboards. However, the capacity of computer equipment allows people to work faster and, perhaps, more intensely.

Because task variety is reduced, yielding to increased repetitiveness of some job tasks and decreased postural changes, VDT-related physical discomfort is likely to arise from long periods (more than several hours per day) of highly routine duties. Problems of visual or postural discomfort reported by VDT users are probably not related to any intrinsic property of VDTs but rather to how the VDT is used. Individual characteristics of stature, work habits, the nature of the job, and the design of the equipment and workplace each play a role in affecting worker comfort.

Job Design

In addition to the differences between typewriter and computer keyboard use, the advent and development of computer technology has changed significantly the way many jobs are done. Work practices, work methods, sequence of tasks, and intensity of visual attention are some factors that have changed. Today's computer-intensive jobs tend to require less physical body movement and more cognitive attention and concentration.

When Pascarelli began to treat computer operators, he likened their symptoms to those experienced by the musicians he had been treating for years (Pascarelli & Quilter 1994). He found that the same ills that plagued musicians also plagued computer operators, including improper technique, poor fit between human and instrument, and lack of physical conditioning and postural awareness. His treatment approach includes both retraining computer operators to avoid further damage at work and rehabilitation to improve posture and overall fitness.

Psychosocial factors weigh heavily in the development and management of CTDs and in ergonomics (Gennusa 1994). Technological advances may be accompanied by different kinds of fears that can be expressed in a variety of ways, including physical symptoms. VDT workers may feel a reduced or limited sense of competence, control, or power. These concerns affect motivation and job satisfaction and can be very stressful.

Educating workers about health and wellness issues in the workplace and what they can do to achieve a comfortable environment is directed toward empowering workers to take responsibility for themselves and have some control over the work environment. Workers should be sensitive to their own limitations, whereas supervisors should be alert to differences among employees. Problems must be dealt with individually on a case-by-case basis. Complaints of discomfort must not be ignored.

Video Display Terminal Job Description

Many types of businesses are well-suited to VDT operations, and some have become extremely VDT-dependent. Among the more common such industries are insurance, banking, mail-order sales, clerical work, and telephone operations. Job titles used in these and other occupations commonly associated with VDT use are listed in Table 16.1.

As technology continues to advance, this list of job titles associated with VDT use continues to grow. New hardware and software products are expanding traditional computer applications. For example, according to local newspaper accounts, some police departments are exploring the use of portable computers by officers to provide improved access to criminal databases on the road. It is reasonable to expect that in this current climate of technological development, the use of computers in traditional and other settings will continue to expand.

Job functions specific to VDT operations can be identified through a functional job analysis. Individuals who use computers for any purpose are required to perform a combination of the following job tasks:

- Inputting information
- Operating input devices (keyboard, mouse, trackball, pen, tablet)
- Calling up information from the computer and reading it from the display
- Reviewing information on the screen
- Referencing source documents
- Entering or recalling text or graphic information, controlling text for errors, keying in corrections, and designing layout
- Paying attention visually
- Scanning visually (display, source documents)

The frequency, duration, and intensity of inputting and other job functions varies from job to job and from setting to setting. It has been estimated that a typist, typing 60 words per minute for 7 hours, may actually perform 126,000 repetitions with the hands (Ross 1994). Data-entry work is characterized by continuous inputting, whereas customer service and sales work more commonly require intermittent inputting. Work speed in data entry is high; it is not uncommon for a worker to perform 8,000–12,000 keystrokes per hour (Grandjean 1987).

Employers and regulatory bodies that have attempted to develop guidelines for ergonomic programs have used definitions of *light, moderate,* and *heavy VDT use* to identify, prioritize, and target high-exposure jobs. In many cases, these definitions are based on hours of use per day. In fact, the U.S. Occupational Safety and Health Administration (OSHA) has proposed the use of time intervals as a measure of risk (US Department of Labor, OSHA

Table 16.1. Job Titles Associated with Video Display Terminal Use

Telephone operator
Customer service representative
Telemarketing representative
Facilities designer or planner
Architect
Graphic artist
Stenographer
Airline reservationist
Librarian
Journalist
Engineer
Clerical support staff
Secretary
Billing clerk

1994). Some companies have determined that ergonomic exposure in jobs requiring 4 or more hours of input per day is sufficient to warrant attention. The jobs listed in Table 16.1 easily meet this criterion in most settings. Nevertheless, ergonomic exposure or risk in jobs that do not meet this criterion must still be considered. Factors such as intensity of inputting and intermittent versus steady input must also be considered.

In addition to actual VDT use, there are other tasks common to VDT-intensive jobs that may contribute to ergonomic risk. Some of these tasks are telephone use, writing, filing, and calculator use. Sorting, stapling, staple removal, and hole punching are other job functions that may pose ergonomic risk in the office environment.

Video Display Terminals and Cumulative Trauma Disorders

Cost

Potential cost exposures for VDT-related claims are significant. Most VDT-oriented operations have experienced at least one VDT-related injury. The average cost of claims generated by VDT-related injuries or illnesses ranges from $6,000 to $35,000. Although many claim cost estimates include medical expenses paid and anticipated, most do not include costs associated with time away from work or employee replacement or training.

There is little direct information available on the incidence and cost of upper-extremity and VDT-related CTDs. Statistical data available from the U.S. Department of Labor, Bureau of Labor Statistics (BLS) report the incidence of CTD and lost and restricted time related to CTDs as a whole. Categories of CTDs are not specified, although data by business type is available. According to BLS data, the number of reported CTDs rose from 23,000 in 1981 to 223,600 in 1991 (a ninefold increase over 10 years). These figures represent 18% of all occupational illnesses in 1981 and 61% of all occupational illnesses in 1991, respectively (Webster & Snook 1994). This trend has continued. The BLS *Survey of Occupational Injuries and Illnesses, 1992* (US Department of Labor, BLS 1994) indicated that most workplace illnesses were disorders associated with repeated trauma (approximately 282,000), such as carpal tunnel syndrome (CTS). The 1994 national survey (US Department of Labor, 1996) reported a 10% increase in repeated trauma cases from 1993 (302,400) to 1994 (332,000). The 1994 total represents nearly two-thirds of workplace illnesses. Median days away from work were highest for carpal tunnel syndrome (30 days). Furthermore, trade, finance, and service industries together accounted for almost all of the 1991–1992 increase in injury and illness rates (Murray 1994). These are the industry groups in which we see phenomenal growth in automation and VDT ergonomic exposure.

Table 16.2. Cumulative Trauma Disorders Commonly Associated with Work in the Automated Office Environment

Nerve
  Carpal tunnel syndrome
  Cubital tunnel syndrome
Neurovascular
  Thoracic outlet syndrome
  Raynaud's syndrome
Musculoskeletal
  Bursitis
  Neck sprain or strain
  Back sprain or strain
Tendon
  Tendinitis
  Epicondylitis
    Golfer's elbow
    Tennis elbow
  Tenosynovitis
  de Quervain's disease
  Trigger finger
  Rotator-cuff tendinitis
Other
  Ganglion cyst

Note: Categorized by system involved.
Source: Developed by J Sehnal for The Hartford, 1993.

Common Workplace Injuries and Illnesses

A variety of CTDs have been associated with working in an automated office, and particularly with VDTs. Common CTDs that may be associated with work in the automated office environment are outlined in Table 16.2 (also see Chapter 4).

The incidence of these disorders by occupation has not been definitively established. However, Leavitt and Taslitz (1993) refer to three studies that address incidence and risk. In one study of 2,876 telephone operators, 86% reported neck or back pain, 78% indicated arm or shoulder pain, and 14% developed cysts on hands or wrists; in 9%, CTS was medically diagnosed. A study of 533 communications workers reported upper-extremity musculoskeletal disorders in 22%, with the hand-wrist area most frequently involved

(12% of participants). A 5-year study of 15 occupational groups, including butchers and meatcutters, found data-entry operators to be at the second greatest level of risk for developing CTS, followed by dental hygienists.

CTDs associated with the automated office environment most commonly affect anatomic structures of the fingers, the hand, the forearm, and the upper arm (Kroemer 1992). Disorders of the neck and back, which have gone more or less unreported in the past, are surfacing now with greater frequency. The causal relationship between muscular activity and CTDs remains uncertain. If a causal relationship between work activities and CTDs is presumed, the exact job factors are not well defined (Kroemer 1992).

Adverse health effects of VDT operators include visual problems and musculoskeletal discomfort and disorders. Visual problems reported among these workers include eye strain, burning or itching eyes, blurred or double vision, deteriorations of visual acuity, and headaches (Bergqvist & Knave 1993). The back, neck, shoulders, and wrists are frequently the most common musculoskeletal complaints, many of which are associated with poor sitting postures. Other factors include equipment, workstation, and job design (Karwowski et al. 1994).

Common injuries in the automated office environment include *all* the disorders listed in Table 16.2. CTS has, unfortunately, become a catch-all category but clearly is not the only disorder that occurs in this environment. In fact, there are many cases in which the general aches, pains, and discomforts that are reported cannot be specifically diagnosed. In the author's practical experience, nonspecific diagnoses such as tendinitis are most common in this group of workers, followed by CTS and de Quervain's disease.

From a risk-management perspective, it is advisable to focus on proactive early identification of those symptoms and related exposures. Without an active, effective program, the preventable and treatable aches and pains may go unrecognized and develop into more serious problems that may be more difficult or perhaps impossible to remedy.

Symptoms

The symptoms of CTDs are listed in Table 16.3. Symptoms occur at varying levels of intensity, from mild to severe. Any symptom at any level should be heeded as a possible warning sign, particularly if it occurs with any degree of severity, regularity, or consistency. In the office worker, the earliest indication of a potential developing CTD can be discomfort. The discomfort may begin or persist during periods of heavy workload. Discomfort and pain may be generalized or specific and may develop over varying periods of time. Additional symptoms usually occur in a specific identifiable body location.

The occurrence of symptoms usually indicates that something is wrong. Symptoms may occur on or off the job. Pain, for example, may occur at night when the worker is more relaxed. Sleep disruption can be a sign of the severity of the symptom.

Treatment

Symptoms that are allowed to progress without intervention will ultimately develop into injuries.

Table 16.3. Symptoms of Cumulative Trauma Disorders

Discomfort
Pain
Tingling
Numbness
Swelling
Weakness
Loss of dexterity

There are three approaches to intervention. The first is *prevention*. Issues of comfort in the workstation must be addressed before symptoms develop. This can be done through engineering design and training programs supported by routine follow-up.

A second approach is *symptomatic treatment*. Workstation modification or alternative work assignments may be necessary as physical corrections. Medical intervention may include modalities (e.g., application of ice), medication (anti-inflammatory drugs), splints, work restrictions, or rest. Wrist splints may be effective for night use. However, when splints are used in the workplace, symptoms may be masked or diverted to other areas of the body. Close communication between the therapist and involved medical providers is necessary.

The third approach is *surgery*, a treatment method that, in many instances, can be avoided through effective training programs or effective intervention at the first report of symptoms. *Early* identification of symptoms and *early* intervention are necessary. Surgery is a last-resort treatment.

From an occupational health perspective, the most effective intervention for all work-related disorders is prevention. A proactive health and safety program with a strong emphasis on ergonomics is an effective tool. Early identification of worker discomfort and hazardous conditions is a key ergonomic program element and requires a clear understanding of the symptoms and risk factors associated with work-related disorders.

When reported early enough, most cases of work-related injury or illness involve short-term discomfort and not permanent injury. "Almost all of these complaints can be alleviated or avoided by proper attention to the workstation, the work environment, and the design of work" (Scalet 1987).

Table 16.4. Risk Factors in the
Automated Office Environment

Static posture
Awkward posture
Repetition
Force
Physical contact
Temperature extremes

Risk Factors

The adverse health effects of many workplace hazards do not become immediately apparent but may take years to develop. We cannot yet predict specific injuries and time frames with 100% accuracy, but we are able to identify common risk factors associated with CTDs in the automated office environment. These risk factors are outlined in Table 16.4 (see Chapter 7 for further discussion).

Static Posture

Static posture over long periods of time should be avoided. Static positioning has become an issue of equal importance to repetitive motion in office work. Numerous office workers spend many hours each day performing work at the VDT, with little opportunity to move around or change position. During inputting, motion is greater in the distal joints of the upper extremity, although the proximal musculature statically supports the distal movements. When the hands and fingers are not actively keying, the entire upper extremity often is in a static "ready" position. Stiffness and fatigue occur in response to static postures, even when good principles of body mechanics are applied. Task variation and workstation exercises can be effective in reducing or eliminating static postures. It is important that employees vary tasks as much as their jobs will allow, in order to achieve changes of position. Employees should take scheduled breaks. It has been advised that employees who regularly work at VDTs for 4 or more hours daily be encouraged to perform some alternate tasks each hour.

Awkward Posture

The rules of good body mechanics suggest that neutral body postures are most efficient and effective.

This is true in all environments, not merely in automated offices. Work habits, poorly designed furniture and equipment configuration, and other factors contribute to posture. Neutral body posture at the VDT workstation and the optimal position of equipment and furniture are outlined in Ergonomic Guidelines for Video Display Terminal Operators. Particularly important body areas to evaluate are shoulders and wrists. Shoulders should be relaxed and symmetric, not elevated. Arms should be near the sides of the body. Wrists should be neutral, not extremely extended, flexed, or deviated toward either side.

When VDT components or other workstation equipment is not appropriately aligned, the result may be asymmetric or other awkward postures. For example, the primary visual reference (monitor or document) should be positioned in alignment behind the keyboard to facilitate symmetric body posture. The keyboard must be centered in front of the user. An appropriately adjusted, organized, and orderly work area will facilitate good body mechanics and minimize possibilities of awkward positioning.

Repetition

The most common occurrences of repetitive movements involve the fingers, wrists, and neck. High-frequency keystroke is responsible for repetitive finger movements in many input-intensive jobs. Repetitive wrist movements can be observed as operators reach for some keys, particularly function keys. Repetitive neck movements occur as the visual reference point changes from monitor to document to keyboard.

Amounts of actual input vary from job to job but, in many cases, inputting is intermittent. Repetitive movements in these jobs, as well as in VDT-intensive jobs, can be related to other than VDT job functions. For example, stapling, staple removal, hole punching, filing, and sorting tasks all require significant repetitive movements of various joints.

Force

Force is another factor that creates muscle fatigue and stress. Applying too much force to the keyboard creates unnecessary pressure and shock to the complex hand, wrist, and arm structures, including tendons and nerves. Force can also be a factor in non-VDT job tasks, including stapling, staple removal, hole punching, and filing. In addition, many workers use unnecessarily tight grips on pens and pencils. Light touch and skillful use of many fingers may reduce muscle fatigue and strain significantly.

Physical Contact

Prolonged physical contact with the work surface or equipment can impair blood circulation and nerve function. Common examples of physical contact include wrists "planted" on the work surface or edge of the keyboard during inputting, forearms resting on the edge of the work surface, elbows resting on the armrests of the chair, and front edge of the chair seat pressing on backs of thighs or on the backs of legs at the knee.

Temperature Extremes

Temperature and humidity are important environmental elements that clearly influence worker comfort. Frequent changes and extremes of temperature and humidity must be avoided. Temperature variation in the office environment is generally not marked. However, temperatures that are out of the range of normal comfort can affect posture. In addition, cold temperatures can restrict circulation. The net result is increased susceptibility to discomfort or, ultimately, the development of common work-related disorders listed earlier.

Components of an Ergonomics Management Program

In its Ergonomics Program Management Guidelines for Meatpacking Plants, OSHA (US Department of Labor, OSHA 1991) has identified four major components of an effective ergonomics program: (1) work-site analysis, (2) hazard prevention and control, (3) medical management, and (4) training and education. These guidelines are comprehensive and applicable to a number of industry groups. The components can, however, be broken down more specifically, as follows:

1. Work-site or workstation assessment: Review injury and illness records and workstation assessment to identify risk factors and problem jobs.

2. Risk prevention and control measures: Institute engineering and design changes to eliminate existing exposures and to prevent potential exposures (may involve changes in work methods, workstation design, tool and equipment specifications, work practice, administrative practice, facility and equipment maintenance).

3. Medical management: Implement a plan for early identification of symptoms and injuries and illnesses, assuring timely and appropriate medical care, and integrating workplace intervention and return to work.

4. Training: Provide education to all employees, including new hires, supervisors, and managers, on the following topics: proper and safe work practices (including use of equipment and tools), awareness of ergonomic hazards and corrective measures, and health and safety (ergonomic) roles and responsibilities of all employees.

5. Equipment, furniture, and job design: Conduct ongoing review and adjustment of equipment, furniture, and job specifications; ergonomic review of proposed equipment and furniture purchases, new job functions, and changes in job functions.

6. Management participation and support: Actively involve all levels of management in safety and health management and visible support of the ergonomic program (policy, procedure, budget).

7. Employee involvement: Monitor ongoing feedback from employees regarding health, safety, and other job issues, and ensure employee representation on the company's health and safety committee.

8. Follow-up: Conduct ongoing program evaluation and follow-up work-site analysis to ensure program effectiveness.

There are various methods of providing training. A train-the-trainer approach is outlined in Table 16.5. Using this approach, individuals are selected to be trained as local resources who will be responsible for providing ergonomic awareness training to VDT users and for performing routine workstation assessments. Trainee selection is critical to the effectiveness of such a program. It is important that the individuals selected (1) have a genuine interest in the subject, (2) have an ability to relate well to others, and (3) have management support to carry out training and workstation assessment responsibilities.

Table 16.5. Proposed Agenda for
Train-the-Trainer Program

8:30–8:45	**Introduction**
	Facilitator(s), participants
	Participants' expectations of session
	Objectives, roles, and responsibilities
8:45–9:30	**Ergonomics training program**
	Program components
9:30–9:45	**Ergonomics**
	Definition
	Research facts
	Trends in the workplace
	Effects: productivity, quality, safety, profit
9:45–10:15	**Basic sciences and ergonomics**
	Anatomy and functional relationships
	Anthropometry and furniture and equipment design
	Body mechanics
	Ergonomic risk factors
10:15–10:30	**Break**
10:30–12:00	**Basics of workstation ergonomics**
	Workstation components and configuration
	Workstation assessment
	Checklists and other forms
	Workstation assessment demonstration (analysis of videotape/on-site assessment)
12:00–1:00	**Lunch**
1:00–2:30	**Basics of workstation ergonomics (continued)**
	Problem solving: simple practical changes
	Accessory use
	Follow-up and referral
2:30–2:45	**Break**
2:45–3:30	**Facilitation and training techniques**
	Presentation
	Typical questions and responses
3:30–4:00	**Discussion and questions**

Source: Developed by J Sehnal for The Hartford, 1992.

Workstation Assessment

Process

The first step in developing an effective workstation-assessment program is to understand job tasks and workstation components. A typical workstation is composed of a variety of pieces of furniture and equipment. Some components of a typical worksta-

Table 16.6. Components of a Typical Workstation

Chair
Desk, work surface
Monitor
Central processing unit
Keyboard
Telephone
Calculator
Shelves
File cabinets
Waste can
Power cords
Document holder
Lighting
Manuals
Paper
Pencils, pens
Baskets (in/out)
Footrest
Eyewear
Wristrest

tion are listed in Table 16.6. Each of these components has its own characteristics, dimensions, and function. Some are used in isolation, others in various combinations. Information regarding where each piece is located and how it is used provides the basis of ergonomic workstation assessment.

A workstation assessment is an evaluation of how a job is performed, taking into account the physical characteristics of the workstation as they relate to the performance of job functions. A complete workstation assessment requires observation of the worker and workstation as the job is being performed. This observation must cover at least one full work cycle. The following factors are considered during the workstation assessment:

- Components of the physical workstation (including furniture, equipment, tools, and materials)
- Location, dimensions, and adjustability of the workstation components
- Job functions
- Work flow (including schedules, breaks, overtime, productivity standards)
- Body posture

The purpose of a workstation assessment is to identify job performance factors or workstation features that may contribute to or create injury exposures and to recommend corrective actions to eliminate or minimize these exposures and risk of injury. It is important to observe the person performing job functions at the workstation. The focus of a workstation assessment is primarily on the person's body posture and secondarily on the workstation configuration and how it is used.

The workstation-assessment and adjustment process is a common-sense approach to comfort at the workstation. Problem solving involves a certain element of trial and error, and one problem frequently has several possible solutions. Because the feasibility and practicality of alternative solutions varies, it is necessary to evaluate the advantages and disadvantages of each possibility before choosing and implementing one option.

Key elements in the workstation-assessment process are communication and timely response to requests for assistance and adjustments. A recognized and organized method of recording and communicating recommended workstation changes must be established. It is imperative that the employee understand the reasons for adjustments and be involved in the problem-solving process. Optimally, the supervisor should also be actively involved in this process. At the very least, results of the workstation assessment must be communicated to the supervisor.

Protocol

A typical protocol for the workstation-assessment process in a corporate VDT ergonomics program is described in this section. Workstation assessments can be done proactively to identify exposures and implement corrective actions prior to the potential development of symptoms. Reactively, a timely workstation assessment must be performed in response to any report of symptoms or injury. The initial assessment should be performed within 2–3 days of the injury report. Finally, use of workstation assessment efficiently fulfills ongoing surveillance requirements of an effective program. Periodic workstation or workplace reviews, with implementation of necessary corrective actions, are effective in proactively maintaining an exposure-free environment and a healthy work force.

In this author's experience, follow-up workstation assessment is effective within 2 weeks of the initial assessment. Subsequent follow-ups can be scheduled at intervals determined individually by need. Follow-up can be discontinued after two symptom-free reviews or when maximum symptom improvement has been reached *and* no further workstation or job performance changes are required.

Follow-up is critical to the success of workstation assessment. The education and assessment involved in an ergonomic program must be ongoing. How this is achieved will probably differ somewhat at each location. In most cases, when an employee reports discomfort, the supervisor (if not already notified) and the local ergonomics resource person should be notified.

After the initial individual workstation assessment is completed, it is necessary to verify that the recommended changes were made. The changes must be reviewed within 1–2 weeks to determine their effectiveness. If the recommended changes were not made, it is necessary to determine why. The situation should be reassessed and action taken to ensure that the necessary changes are made. Follow-up assessments need not be as detailed or time-consuming as the initial assessment, but they must be thorough. Follow-up assessments can be documented on a workstation-assessment form or in another format.

Feedback on the effectiveness of changes is a necessary component of the follow-up process. Both the employee and the supervisor are expected to provide this feedback. The medical department or personnel department may be included to complete the communication loop in the organization.

When symptoms are reported early, workstation or work-style changes are, in most cases, effective in eliminating those symptoms. However, some cases are not so easily resolved. These may require multiple workstation assessments and modifications.

In summary, critical components of an effective workstation-assessment protocol are as follows:

- Communication
- Timely response
- Ongoing education
- Feedback
- Follow-up

Documentation

Documentation of all workstation-assessment activity is required, because the initial workstation as-

Table 16.7. Ergonomic Guidelines for Video Display Terminal (VDT) Operators

---

Optimal body position for seated VDT work
1. Trunk upright with ears, shoulders, and hips in vertical alignment
2. Shoulders in symmetric, nonelevated position
3. Arch in back supported by back of chair or cushion insert
4. Feet flat on floor or on a footrest
5. Thighs supported evenly on chair and approximately parallel with floor
6. Upper arms close to the sides of the body
7. Forearms approximately parallel to floor
8. Wrists in neutral position

Optimal equipment position
1. Top line of monitor screen slightly below eye level or lower
2. Monitor screen at approximately 20–26 inches from user's eyes
3. Keyboard and monitor positioned in alignment in front of user (when monitor is primary visual reference)
4. Keyboard (height) positioned such that home row (ASDF) is approximately at elbow level
5. Mouse (height) positioned at elbow level and as centrally as possible
6. Document holder located near monitor at same height and distance as is screen from user
7. Work surface at height to allow appropriate arm, wrist, and hand position while also allowing adequate leg space
8. Chair: seat and backrest height and angle adjusted to allow comfortable posture
9. Shelf height and location within comfortable reach
10. All frequently used equipment, manuals, and so on within comfortable reach

---

Note: The preceding criteria are provided as generic guidelines for comfortable and safe VDT operation. Variations in specifications may be acceptable and should be determined individually.
Source: Developed by J Sehnal for The Hartford, 1993.

sessment establishes the basis for subsequent follow-up assessments. In addition, documentation provides an auditable paper trail as demonstration of ergonomics program activity and implementation.

A sample of a detailed workstation-assessment form is provided in Appendix 16.1. This form provides a mechanism to document current job function, body positions, workstation features, comments relative to ergonomic concerns, possible causes, and possible solutions, and recommended changes. It can be used to document workstation assessments performed in response to reports of medical symptoms. When this form is also used to document subsequent follow-up workstation assessments, it is possible to compare forms and evaluate the effectiveness of interventions.

Recommendations are recorded on the workstation-assessment form. Changes that require assistance for implementation can be recorded on a work request form. Distribution of the workstation-assessment form and the work request form can assist in the communication process.

Workstation checklists can be used as self-assessment tools. A sample is provided in Appendix 16.2. This kind of checklist can be completed by every employee at the time of initial ergonom-

ics awareness training and at least annually thereafter. The checklist should be reviewed by the supervisor with the employee to ensure that the review is accurate and complete and that necessary corrective actions have been taken.

Checklists and forms can be used to record observations of each workstation. Detailed observations are a major source of information. The process requires recorded observation of individuals performing their work. Employee feedback regarding how they feel at their workstations is valuable information. Involving employees in problem solving and including them in developing recommendations for changes is very effective.

Ergonomic Guidelines for Video Display Terminal Operators

Application of principles of good body mechanics eliminates or minimizes risk of injury in any workplace. Suggestions regarding posture and position of equipment in the office environment are based on principles of good body mechanics for seated work. The ergonomic guidelines for VDT operators outlined in Table 16.7 are useful to VDT operators as

Table 16.8. Workstation Assessment: Possible Causes of Awkward Postures

Observation	Possible Causes
Elbows away from side of body	Work surface too high
	Keyboard too far away
Feet on base of chair	Chair too high
Sitting on leg crossed under other leg on chair	Chair too high
	Seat-pan angle inappropriate (i.e., too far down)
Sitting forward on chair away from back	Seat-pan angle inappropriate (i.e., too far down)
	Chair too high
	Keyboard too far away
	Screen too far away
Wrist resting on sharp edge or surface of desk	Keyboard too far away
	Work surface too high
Wrist in extension	Wrist resting on work surface
	Keyboard angle too steep
Head and neck extended	Screen too high
Excessive turning or twisting of head and neck or trunk	Asymmetric position of video display terminal or components
	Poor chair support
	Unsatisfactory position of hard copy
	Unsatisfactory position of equipment or files

an educational tool and to those performing workstation assessments as an evaluation guide.

Common Observations During Workstation Assessment

The workstation-assessment process calls for identification of deviations from neutral postures as well as identification of conditions that might be contributing to reported symptoms. Some typical postural observations and their possible causes are presented in Table 16.8. Typical discomforts or symptoms and contributing causes are presented in Table 16.9. Note that these lists are not exhaustive and are not intended to be used to determine "cookbook" solutions. The observations and possible causes are examples of those commonly determined through the workstation assessment.

Furniture and Equipment

Work Surfaces and Chairs

As you embark on workplace or workstation assessments and job analyses, you will note that work surfaces supporting VDTs vary greatly. In

many situations, VDTs have been installed on existing work surfaces that may have been designed for clerical, non-VDT job functions. Typically, standard clerical desks are nonadjustable at 28.5–30.0 in. in height. Work surface heights within this range may be suitable for a large percentage of the population performing non-VDT tasks, but these heights are excessive for many workers performing VDT functions.

In other situations, VDT furniture marketed for its purported ergonomic design may or may not be suitable for its users or for some job functions. In any case, a complete assessment requires a thorough examination of the work surface and other components of the workstation in order to identify dimensions, adjustability, and other features.

The features observed in the types of chairs being used will vary as much as the variations observed in work surfaces. The chair is perhaps the most critical element in the workstation as it provides the basis for proximal support and good posture.

Video Display Terminals

The design and specifications of the VDT equipment itself must be considered in the workstation assessment. Size or dimensions and location of VDT components relative to the work surface

Table 16.9. Workstation Assessment: Possible Causes of Symptoms

Observation	Possible Causes
Neck or shoulder discomfort or pain	Screen too high
	Hard copy too far from screen
	Screen off to side with keyboard central
	Work surface too high
	Elbows bump armrests
	Keyboard or work too far away
Back discomfort	Chair too high or too low
	Backrest not used
Lower-leg circulation cut off	Feet not supported
	Seat pan too deep
	Chair too high
General pain at back of wrist, top of forearm	Excessive wrist extension
	Keyboard too far away
	Keyboard too high
	Keyboard angle too steep
Wrist discomfort on little-finger side	Overstretching to reach function, cursor, enter keys
	Striking keys with excessive force
	Elbows away from body
Numbness or tingling of little finger or on little-finger side of hand	Pressure on elbow
	Pressure on underside of forearm
	Resting forearm, elbow, or little finger on work surface
Pain through thumb or thumb side of wrist	Repetitive spacebar strike
	Striking keys with excessive force
	Folding paper and using thumb to crease
	Writing with excessive grip force
	Writing with awkward thumb angle
Eye strain	Screen too high
	Screen too far or too close
	Poor resolution or clarity
	Poor visual acuity
	Reflection due to screen angle
	Reflection due to screen position
	Glare

and the VDT user influence posture and comfort. The height, width, depth, and, in some cases, the weight of each of the components should be determined.

The current trend toward computer multi-tasking has led to an increase in the size of monitors. Screen size usually is indicated as the diagonal measure in inches, similar to the system used for measuring televisions. The greater height and width of the monitor influences angle of vision (height of screen) and position of other equipment on the work surface (width of screen). Of perhaps more significance is the depth of the monitor. The average-size monitor (15-in. screen) measures approximately 16–18 in. in depth. In some cases, an additional 1–2 in. of work surface space is required for connecting cables off the back of the monitor. This size monitor can be positioned on a 30 in.–deep work surface while maintaining a comfortable eye-to-screen distance. However, 17-in. (and larger) monitors measure 20–22 in. in depth. If positioned on a 30 in.–deep work surface, the eye-to-screen distance is reduced significantly and, in some cases, the remaining work surface space is not adequate for the keyboard. Workers respond by using self-determined fixes, which commonly result in asymmetric positioning of the monitor or keyboard (or both). When this happens, body posture is seriously compromised.

Ergonomic Accessories

A variety of standard office accessories, when used appropriately, can be effective in improving comfort in the workplace. Document holders, computer tables, telephone headsets, electric staplers, glare screens, staple removers, task lights, and a variety of pens are found in many offices. Other special accessories have been designed to address ergonomic concerns. Some of these are wristrests, footrests, and pencil grips. Workstation factors and job functions must be considered in the determination of need for or potential effectiveness of ergonomic accessories. Requests for ergonomic accessories may be indicative of another related or possibly unrelated ergonomic need for change and, therefore, proactive workstation assessment is in order. If not used appropriately, an accessory can be ineffective or even injurious.

Products that meet ergonomics and safety standards can be made available through company purchasing systems. Additionally, many office and ergonomic accessories are now available from vendors in the community. Some of these products are listed in Table 16.10. Many office and computer supply houses, as well as medical and rehabilitation suppliers, carry these products.

A wristrest is a common comfort aid designed to provide wrist support to computer operators. It is particularly useful during intermittent inputting. There are many designs or styles on the market. Wristrests are most beneficial when the keyboard and work surface are at an appropriate height. An appropriate height is achieved when the user or operator is able to type with his or her forearms relatively parallel to the floor, wrists in a neutral position, and upper arms close to the body. Wristrests are designed to help users avoid direct body contact (arms, wrists) with the work surface.

Whereas a wristrest is intended to provide wrist support at least intermittently, it is not intended to encourage users to position or "plant" their wrists on the wristrest during all phases of inputting and typing. There should be some clearance between the wrists and the wristrest during actual typing and inputting.

Table 16.10. Common Office Products that Can Be Effective Ergonomic Accessories

Abdominal belt
Backrest
Cleaning pad (for glare filter)
Video display terminal foam cleaner
Document holder
Document holder accessories
Electric hole punch
Electric stapler
Monitor risers
Pens
Footrest
Glare screen
Headsets
Forearm cushion
Mouse pad
Pencil grip
Staple remover
Task light
Terminal stand or table
Wristrest

Ergonomic Guidelines for Workstation Design

The optimal workstation design applicable to *all* situations does not exist. Given the need for some standardization of furniture and equipment specifications in some organizations, particularly large ones, however, it is possible to make some general recommendations regarding work surfaces intended to support VDTs as well as chairs and other equipment intended to support the individuals performing VDT-intensive jobs. Some of these general recommendations also appear in Table 16.7.

The VDT work surface height should be adjustable in a range of 23–28 in. The work surface should position the keyboard such that the home row (*ASDF*) is approximately level with the elbow. A nonadjustable VDT work surface of 26–27 in. is acceptable if appropriate body position can be achieved through chair height adjustments or accessory use. Operator-adjustable work surfaces are recommended for shared or multiuser workstations and may also be an advantage in frequently changing environments.

The depth of the VDT work surface must be adequate to allow aligned symmetric position of the keyboard and monitor. A minimum of 30 in. is required for VDTs with standard-size monitors that are up to 18 in. deep and 36 in. for VDTs with larger monitors that exceed 18 in. in depth. In some situations, a work surface less than 30 in. deep can be adapted to accommodate the VDT.

The width of the VDT work surface must be adequate to support the keyboard and other necessary equipment, including mouse, mouse pad, paperwork, document holder, telephone, and calculator. A minimum of 36 in. is required to support both the keyboard and the mouse.

Noninterfering and accessible storage space is required for the processing unit. In general, work surface space should be adequate to support all necessary equipment and supplies, placing frequently used items within comfortable reach.

As stated previously, the chair is perhaps the most critical component of the workstation because a stable, comfortable seated posture provides the basis of support for body movements, distal joint positions, and task performance. Critical chair features include the following:

- Easily height adjustable (range of 15–21 in.)
- Smooth rolling casters
- Locking back
- Height-adjustable backrest
- Tension adjustment for chairs that recline
- Model available with and without arms
- Model available in smaller or larger size
- Independently adjustable seat and back angles
- Swivel
- Five-spoke base

Other chair features, including seat-pan tilt, height-adjustable armrests, and width-adjustable armrests, increase the individual adjustability of the chair.

Adequate and accessible work-surface space for non-VDT job functions is also required for many jobs. This work surface should also be height-adjustable (range, 24–30 in.). Adequate and accessible filing and storage space, as required by specific job functions, must be available.

The criteria for workstation design can be met in a variety of ways and by various types of furniture. The caveat to any generic guideline is that the specific workstation design may need to be tailored to meet the needs of the specific job. The optimal goal is to build maximum adjustability and flexibility into a generic workstation design such that various job functions and individual staff variances can be accommodated.

Current Video Display Terminal Issues

Office ergonomics has evolved into a distinct specialty that is distinguished from industrial ergonomics. As demonstrated in this chapter, there are some unique features to the application of basic ergonomic principles in the office environment. Automation of an office, particularly one that may have been designed primarily for nonautomated functions, creates a situation in need of ergonomic attention. The focus of office ergonomics has largely been directed toward the VDT and how it is used in the workplace.

Computer technology is changing at a rapid pace. Computers have proved to be effective and, in many cases, necessary tools in a variety of settings. As computer applications expand and hardware changes, we are faced with ever-changing challenges from an ergonomic perspective. The basic principles of workstation ergonomics, including application of good body mechanics and the assurance of comfort at the workstation, are universal to all applications. Four of these new and challenging applications are addressed here.

Input Devices

The primary recognized input tool has been the keyboard because it is, perhaps, the most commonly used tool. More recently, the mouse has also been recognized as a key input tool and as a potential contributor to work-related discomfort and ergonomic risk factors. Many of the newer computer programs are mouse driven, and this accounts for increased use of the mouse as a primary input device. Other input devices gaining rapid popularity are trackballs, joysticks, and pens. Some laptop designs incorporate trackballs or mini-joysticks into their keyboards or inputting systems. Newer technology of pentops offers additional versatility in application. These pentops may engage a pen, keyboard, or mouse for inputting. Finally, improvements in technology have rendered voice-activated (or voice-recognition) systems productive methods.

From an ergonomics perspective, each of these tools offers its own set of advantages and disadvantages. No tool is universal for all applications and, ergonomically, the perfect input device does not yet exist. Key factors in determining the appropriateness of a particular tool in a particular application are how it is used, along with frequency, duration, and intensity of use. It is important to know whether this tool is the primary or only input device used. Are neutral postures maintained during use, and is the individual comfortable during and after use? Each tool must be evaluated carefully, with consideration of how, where, and by whom it is to be used.

Keyboards

A variety of so-called ergonomic keyboards are currently on the market. According to the sales literature, these keyboards eliminate awkward postures demanded by standard keyboards, and they prevent the development of various CTDs. The presumption that keyboards cause CTDs is unproved. Perhaps these ergonomic keyboards would be more appropriately referred to as *alternative keyboards*.

The new alternative keyboards conform to a variety of designs that meet different combinations of ergonomic criteria. Some mimic the standard keyboard layout with variation in key placement. For example, one model splits the standard keyboard layout, angling two groups of keys. Another model actually splits the keyboard into two adjustable pieces. Other features offered by various models include:

- A curved base with angled keys
- A detached numeric keypad
- A trackball located in the wristrest
- Concave keypad sections
- A foot pedal for keystroke assignment
- A split keyboard with articulating sections
- Detachable palmrests

Other keyboard designs vary considerably from the standard keyboard. One model, called a chord keyboard, resembles a small musical instrument. It is cylindric and hand held. The fingers lie over buttons that activate the keyboard for inputting. Another model consists of two boxlike units, one for each hand. A glove-shaped depression in each unit supports the hands. The fingertips lie in three-dimensional "wells" where they are surrounded by magnetic switches. These switches are activated by the fingertips in various combinations for inputting. Obviously, there is a learning curve associated with the use of these types of keyboards by new users.

The cost of these products varies as much as the design. A recent review identified prices in the range of $89–2,095.

The true benefit of these keyboards has yet to be scientifically determined. There is little doubt that an individual operator may find one keyboard more comfortable than another. However, few data exist to support the use of alternative keyboards as a means to correct physiologic problems. Support for manufacturers' claims that their keyboards provide relief to the many who "suffer through grueling keyboard aerobics" day after day or that their keyboards will prevent keyboard-related injuries requires more research.

Nevertheless, there have been several lawsuits implicating keyboard design in the development of various CTDs. Injured users maintain that keyboard manufacturers have known for many years that conventional keyboards are responsible for exposures that lead to such disorders and that the manufacturers deliberately withheld warnings of the dangers. They also claim that alternative keyboard designs existed that could have prevented users' injuries. In fact, data supporting these claims do not exist. As a result, the courts have ruled in favor of the manufacturers in the cases to date. Despite continued controversy on the subject, some manufacturers have decided to put warning labels on keyboards in an effort to reduce the probability of product liability lawsuits.

A combination of factors, including posture, workstation design, work practices, and the ways in which the workstation is used, contribute to operator discomfort or symptoms of CTDs related to keyboard use. The keyboard is best considered as any other accessory. Each situation requires individual assessment to determine the appropriateness or effectiveness of a particular product. The VDT workstation must be considered as a system. Many factors, including furniture, equipment (e.g., keyboards), workstation design, the general work environment, work organization and practices, and performance pressures, must be considered in order to truly prevent or eliminate risks associated with CTDs. More definitive research is necessary to determine the true effect of the new keyboard designs. Until that research is available, alternative keyboards must not be considered a generic solution to a very complex problem.

Portable Computers

With the growth of a mobile workforce and ongoing technological advances, the portable computer market is expanding rapidly. Certainly, the mobility of portable computers, laptops, and pentops is a significant advantage for many. However, some users have reported physical discomforts that seem to be related to the use of portable equipment. Risk factors identified through observation of portable-computer users include static postures, awkward postures, and limited keyboard and mouse work space. As with conventional desktop VDT operation, a variety of factors, including equipment design, workstation configuration, work space, work organization and practices, and performance pressures, combine to create these risk factors.

Again, a variety of factors, one of which is how the equipment will be used, must be considered. Ongoing ergonomic evaluation of portable computers and their use is necessary. This evaluation should address equipment design and function, how the equipment is used in and outside of the workplace, and carrying case design and function. The following criteria must be considered:

Factors common to all computers

- Size (including profile)
- Screen size
- Screen resolution (including backlighting and color)
- Screen adjustment controls: location, function
- Keyboard construction and sensibility (touch)
- Keyboard layout
- Joystick or alternative
- Compatibility for left- or right-handed users
- Usability: overall comfort, posture during use

Factors specific to portable computers

- Weight
- Screen sensibility, pentops ("feel," pen control)
- Pen: size (diameter, length), accessibility, sensibility (touch), port (stability), battery requirement
- Stand (for desktop use): availability, stability, height adjustability, angle adjustability

- Battery: size, weight, accessibility
- Mouse, trackball compatibility
- Carrying case: size, equipment accessibility
- Cable connections: ease of use, accessibility, noninterference with position of components
- Ease of desktop connection
- Usability: static holding

Although the success of portable equipment depends in part on design factors, user technique and training are also significant factors. Portable computers are designed for portable use. Conventional desktop monitors and keyboards may be more appropriate for use in the office. Some circumstances may require availability of conventional equipment for use in the office.

Telecommuting

As many companies realize the benefits of portable computers, some are also realizing benefits from a relatively new and innovative work option called *telecommuting*. Telecommuting offers employees flexible work arrangements in which they work out of their homes or other remote locations. One author describes telecommuting as "moving the work to the workers, instead of the workers to work" (Smart Valley 1994).

Telecommuting work arrangements lend themselves to many types of jobs. Telecommuting can work well in word processing, data entry, information management, writing, and research. Some companies have instituted telecommuting for customer-focused jobs such as technical support staff, customer service, catalog sales, and travel agents. Less traditional approaches include human resource, finance, engineering, marketing, and manufacturing applications (Hamilton 1987).

Although many telecommuting situations have evolved on an informal basis, some companies are developing and implementing formal telecommuting programs. In some cases, federal legislation such as the Clean Air Act Amendments of 1990, the Americans with Disabilities Act, and the Family Leave Act has sparked the initiative to develop these programs (Romano 1994). As these programs are being developed, employers have recognized the need to address some issues that could become potential obstacles if not adequately handled. Among these issues are technical requirements, legal issues, security issues, tax issues, and ergonomic issues. For this reason, it is necessary to establish guidelines governing conditions of participation, equipment use, and liability issues (Best 1986; Beiswinger 1994).

The application of principles of ergonomics in a telecommuting situation varies little from other applications. Development of specific ergonomic guidelines for personal computer use must be developed. These guidelines should provide recommendations for optimal body position and workstation configuration. The principles discussed elsewhere in this chapter apply. The following factors must be considered:

- Furniture, equipment, tools, materials, and other components of the physical workstation
- Location, dimensions, and adjustability of the workstation components
- Job functions and tasks
- Work flow, schedules, breaks, overtime, productivity standards
- Body posture

Implementation of an ergonomics program in a telecommuting situation can be, in some ways, more challenging than in a traditional office environment. Unless the company selects and provides furniture for remote installation, there is likely to be more variety and less adjustability in what is being used. In addition, monitoring and enforcement of the ergonomics program can be more difficult in a remote rather than an on-site location. Nevertheless, an active ergonomics program is necessary in the telecommuting environment to maintain a healthy work force and to manage worker's compensation issues.

References

Barry J (1993). A review of ergonomic keyboards. *Work*, 3(4),21–25.

Beiswinger GL (1994). The home office: a practical guide. *D&B Reports*, 43(1),38–40.

Bergqvist U & Knave B (1993). Eye discomfort and work with visual display terminals. *Scand J Work Environ Health*, 20(1),27–33.

Best F (1986). No place like home. *Management World*, 15(6),9–12.

Bureau of National Affairs, Inc (1994). Keyboard design examined. *Job Saf Health*, 433,1–2.

Gennusa CR (August 1994). Psychology plays important role in ergonomics of the workplace. *Adv Occup Ther*, 5.

Grandjean E (1987). *Ergonomics in Computerized Offices*. New York: Taylor & Francis.

Hamilton C (1987). Telecommuting. *Personnel J*, 66(4),91–101.

Karwowski W, Eberts R, Salvendy G, & Noland S (1994). The effects of computer interface design on human postural dynamics. *Ergonomics*, 37,703–724.

Kroemer KHE (1992). Avoiding cumulative trauma disorders in shops and offices. *J Am Ind Hygiene Assoc*, 53,596–604.

Leavitt SB & Taslitz NJ (1993). *Computer-Related Injuries: Legal and Design Issues*. Chicago: The BackCare Corporation.

Murray TE (1994). Survey of occupational injuries and illnesses for 1992. *Workers' Compensation Report*, 11,1. New York: American Insurance Services Group, Inc.

Pascarelli E & Quilter D (1994). *Repetitive Strain Injury: A Computer User's Guide*. New York: Wiley.

Romano C (1994). Business copes with the clean air conundrum. *Manage Rev*, 83(2),34–37.

Ross P (1994). Ergonomic hazards in the workplace. *AAOHN J*, 42,171–176.

Scalet EA (1987). *VDT Health and Safety Issues and Solutions*. Lawrence, KS: Ergocyst Associates, Inc.

Smart Valley, Inc (1994). *Smart Valley Telecommuting Guide* (Ver 1),1. Palo Alto, CA.

US Department of Labor, Bureau of Labor Statistics (1994). *Survey of Occupational Injuries and Illnesses, 1992* (Summary 94-3). Washington, DC: Bureau of Labor Statistics.

US Department of Labor, Bureau of Labor Statistics (1996). *Characteristics of Injuries and Illnesses Resulting in Absences from Work, 1994* (USDL-96-163). Washington, DC: Bureau of Labor Satistics.

US Department of Labor, Occupational Safety and Health Administration (1991). *Ergonomics Program Management Guidelines for Meatpacking Plants* (OSHA 3123). Washington, DC: US Government Printing Office.

US Department of Labor, Occupational Safety and Health Administration (1994). Draft Ergonomic Protection Standard Summary of Key Provisions. [Unpublished document.]

Webster BS & Snook SH (1994). The cost of compensable upper extremity cumulative trauma disorders. *J Occup Med*, 36,713–717.

Suggested Reading

Carlson CR (1990). An experiment in productivity: the use of home terminals. *J Inform Systems Manage*, 7(4),36–41.

Human Factors Society, Inc (1988). *American National Standard for Human Factors Engineering of Visual Display Terminal Workstations* (ANSI/HFS 100-1988). Santa Monica, CA: Human Factors Society, Inc.

Jauchem J (1993). Alleged health effects of electric or magnetic fields: additional misconceptions in the literature. *J Microwave Power Electromag Energy*, 28(3),140–155.

National Safety Council (1993). *Ergonomics: A Practical Guide* (2nd ed). Chicago: National Safety Council.

Sauter SL (1990). *Improving VDT Work: Causes and Control of Health Concerns in VDT Use*. Lawrence, KS: The Report Store.

Sehnal JP & Christopher RC (1993). Developing and marketing an ergonomics program in a corporate office environment. *Work*, 3,22–30.

Tillman P & Tillman B (1991). *Human Factors Essentials: An Ergonomics Guide for Designers, Engineers, Scientists, and Managers*. New York: McGraw-Hill.

Venturino M (Ed) (1990). *Selected Readings in Human Factors*. Santa Monica, CA: Human Factors Society, Inc.

Woodson WE, Tillman B, & Tillman P (1992). *Human Factors Design Handbook* (2nd ed). New York: McGraw-Hill.

Appendix 16.1

Workstation-Assessment Form

WORKSTATION ASSESSMENT

NAME: _____ Position: _____ Tel. _____ Bldg/Flr _____

Date of Referral: _____ by _____ Dept. _____ Supv. _____ Tel. _____

Date of WSA: _____ by _____

Chief Complaint: _____

Right Handed: _____ Left Handed: _____ Ambidextrous: _____

CURRENT POSITION Start Date _____   FT   PT   Schedule: _____ Overtime: Yes   No

DUTIES: input: _____% writing: _____% other _____ frequency: _____

touch typist: yes___ no ___   prior typing training: yes ___ no ___   schedule: _____

special skills: _____

other: _____

scheduled breaks: yes ___ no ___ taken consistently _____ when _____

workstation shared: yes ___ no ___ with whom _____ supv. _____ when _____

OBSERVATION CHECKLIST*	f/u	f/u		COMMENTS: (concerns, causes, possible solutions)
	Date	Date	Date	
1. Posture				
Neck				
Shoulders				
Back				
Arms				
Wrist				
Legs				
Feet				
2. Chair				
Height				
Seat				
Back				
3. Desk				
Height				
Work space				
Leg room				
4. Equipment				
VDT location				
VDT height				
VDT angle				
Keyboard location				
Keyboard angle				
Document holder				
Telephone location				
Tel. receiver/headset				
Calculator location				
Calc. height/angle				
Mouse				

5. Other

_____   _____
_____   _____
_____   _____

*Use + for OK, - for problem

WORKSTATION   How long have you been at current workstation? _____
Please draw a diagram of your workstation.

		DATE		f/u 1 DATE		f/u 2 DATE	
		current	rec.	current	rec.	current	rec.
WORKSURFACE							
_____	Height						
(type)							
CHAIR	Height						
_____	Seat pan						
(type)	Back						
KEYBOARD	Location						
	Position						
DISPLAY	Height						
	Position						
EQUIPMENT	Footstool						
	Wrist rest						
	Doc holder						
	Glare screen						
	Headset						

RECOMMENDATIONS

Date	f/u Date	f/u Date	
			Work station adjustments as indicated
			Work practice change:
			Ergonomic accessories:
			Other:
			Follow-up:

cc: **Employee** _____ **Supervisor** _____ **Personnel/EHC** _____

f/u = follow up.
Source: Developed by J Sehnal for The Hartford, 1991.

Appendix 16.2
Workstation Checklist

Chair

Is individual sitting up straight?	❏ Yes	❏ No
When sitting, are thighs parallel to floor?	❏ Yes	❏ No
When sitting, are feet resting firmly on floor?	❏ Yes	❏ No
Is seat pan adjusted so that front of seat pan is up?	❏ Yes	❏ No

Actions taken: _____

Video Display Terminal (VDT) Screen

Is top line of screen slightly below eye level?	❏ Yes	❏ No
Is VDT screen glare-free?	❏ Yes	❏ No
Is VDT screen clean?	❏ Yes	❏ No

Actions taken: _____

Keyboard, Calculator, Mouse

Is keyboard as close to edge of desk as practical?	❏ Yes	❏ No
Is keyboard angle adjusted to middle or lowest position?	❏ Yes	❏ No
Is keying done without pen, pencil, or other tool in hand?	❏ Yes	❏ No
Is mouse at keyboard height and close to keyboard?	❏ Yes	❏ No

Actions taken: _____

Body Position

Are shoulders in a relaxed position?	❐ Yes	❐ No

While inputting information, are:

Forearms parallel to floor or slightly angled?	❐ Yes	❐ No
Wrists in neutral (close to straight) position?	❐ Yes	❐ No
Upper arms close to side of body?	❐ Yes	❐ No
Is body position changed throughout the day?	❐ Yes	❐ No

Actions taken: _____

General

Are equipment, supplies, files, and manuals easily accessible?	❐ Yes	❐ No
Is the floor area free of clutter?	❐ Yes	❐ No
When talking on phone, is phone supported by hand instead of neck?	❐ Yes	❐ No

Actions taken: _____

Name of employee and extension: _____

Name of supervisor and extension:_____

Date: _____

Source: Developed by J Sehnal for The Hartford, 1992.

PART VI
Outcome Assessment

Chapter 17

Outcome Assessment of Prevention Programs

Richard K. Schwartz

A Pragmatic Approach to Program Evaluation

Outcome assessment is an evaluative process. It is most simply described as a process used to determine the extent to which organizational or program goals have been met. Possible outcomes range from finding that goals have *not* been met to finding that goals have been exceeded. Done well, outcome assessment can provide valuable insights into the strengths and weaknesses of program activities, suggest changes that will enhance the program's effectiveness in the future, and determine the economic impact of the program. Done poorly, outcome assessment may measure accurately how certain indicators, such as incidence rates or program costs, have changed over time but may fail to provide any insight into the impact of a prevention program on the organization and its employees.

There are no formulas, checklists, or methodologies that mandate clearly those prevention options most suitable for particular groups, industries, job categories, or regions. It is imperative that those who undertake cumulative trauma disorder (CTD) prevention programs document a given program's effectiveness, lack of effectiveness or, ideally, relative effectiveness compared to other options. Both quantitative and qualitative evaluations are necessary. Because those who enact and those who conduct CTD-prevention programs are unlikely to have formal training in outcome evaluation research and methods, outcome

assessment is rarely conducted, and the evaluation of prevention programs is often simplistic and biased. It is best to include as a member of the program team a trained outcome evaluator; at the very least, one team member should have a thorough understanding of the issues and approaches available. Those persons interested in developing such skills independently would benefit from consulting Borich and Jemelka (1982) on the evaluation of programs and systems, Cascio (1991) on determining costs related to human behaviors in organizations, and Hayes (1988) on how one can extrapolate the immediate data from a sample and make inferences about larger systems and organizations. This chapter's focus is the importance and complexity of outcome evaluation studies. Procedural instruction in methods, which range from social survey data analyses to financial analyses to advanced linear-model inferential statistics, are beyond the scope of this chapter.

The outcome evaluation process requires that an organization clearly define the goals of the prevention programs being evaluated. It is essential to delineate indicators of successful programs before program implementation. This generally occurs in two stages. The first stage entails the compilation and maintenance of an accurate CTD injuries and losses database. This means not only incorporating data that will describe human behaviors (i.e., types of injuries, lost time, trends over time) but also developing information that allows the organization to evaluate the short-term and long-term costs associated with injuries. Why is this so important? In my experience, CTD injury incidence rates often increase rapidly during the first several years of a successful ergonomics and prevention program. This increase in the number of cases does not necessarily mean that the programs fail initially. Rather, by documenting that the severity of accidents and injuries declines and that total dollars lost diminishes even with increasing numbers (incidence), it is possible to show that workers' awareness has been enhanced by the program and workers have been encouraged to report signs and symptoms of cumulative trauma earlier than they had been formerly. Earlier detection and intervention are essential steps in the prevention of CTDs and thus indicate that behaviors have changed in a desirable manner.

The second stage involves assessment of the needs of the organization and establishment of measurable prevention program goals. This second stage requires that baseline or historical measures be compiled to give a picture of human activity and costs at the beginning of the program. This may include cost-accounting and bottom-line approaches, as described for stage one. These measurements permit trend and projection analyses to be conducted, so that the benefits of a program for any given year are measured not only in comparison to the previous year but also in comparison to what a trend analysis predicts the costs of injuries would have been to the company or organization if no intervention was conducted. Cost-benefit analyses are another important element in a comprehensive program evaluation. The final stage of the outcome evaluation process involves qualitative assessments to determine the effects of prevention programs on job satisfaction, employee stress, morale, and attitudes of employees toward supervisors, managers, and the employer.

Outcome assessment is not a hard science. It is more than the collection of statistical and informational techniques used to measure performance. This requires both qualitative and quantitative evaluation. Properly conducted outcome assessment always indicates the congruence between what is *valued* by an organization and how the organization actually *behaves:* It answers the question, "Are we really doing the things we should be doing to meet our goals and fulfill the mission of the organization?"

Compiling a Cumulative Trauma Disorder Injury Information System

The starting point of any approach to risk reduction is an injury information system containing all relevant data that the company has about each injury and each injured employee. Such data are compiled from Occupational Safety and Health Administration (OSHA) 200 logs, from illness and injury reports, and from occupational health records. The creation and maintenance of such an electronic database makes it possible to pinpoint specific categories of employees, specific types of injuries, and even specific locations where interventions are most needed. Table 17.1 is data from such a database and shows how information that is readily available can be formatted for storage, retrieval, and statistical analyses. Although only a single page of this database is shown here, the actual database records more than 600 injuries reported over a 4-year period and is updated annually.

The database has two important epidemiologic features. First, it permits a given workforce to be compared with state and national data in terms of incidence, severity, and risk factors for specific injuries. Second, it permits both descriptive and inferential statistical analysis of the company's injuries over time. Both types of information are extremely useful in targeting the most important problems for intervention and in assessing the impact of all interventions over time by comparing preintervention data with postintervention data.

Figure 17.1 shows how gender effects on the length of time lost per injury can be profiled over an extended period by comparing the average days of lost time per injury in each year. An analysis of variance shows that there are no significant differences from one year to the next at the $p = 0.05$ level but that the averages for male and female workers differed significantly in 1993. Such a comparison can be used to determine whether a safety program has a selective effect or whether there is a tendency toward increasingly severe injuries within a given category. Although the information from an injury and illness database can be useful, it also can be misleading if considered in isolation. For example, if one finds consistent gender differences in injury rates, lost time due to injuries, or a certain type of injury, it could be misleading to *attribute* such differences to gender; an equally, if not more, plausi-

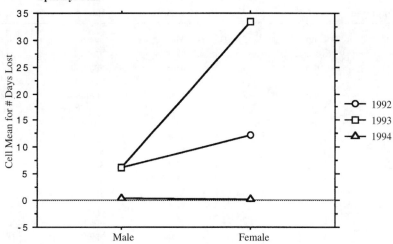

Cell Line Chart
Grouping Variable(s): Gender
Split By: Year

ANOVA Table for Number of Days Lost

	df	Sum of Squares	Mean Square	f-Value	p-Value
Gender	1	4778.81	4778.81	2.33	.1292
Residual	119	243647.52	2047.46		

Model II estimate of between-component variance: 58.02

ANOVA Table for Number of Days Lost
Split By: Year
Cell: 1992

	df	Sum of Squares	Mean Square	f-Value	p-Value
Gender	1	217.81	217.81	.11	.7455
Residual	51	104288.07	2044.86		

Model II estimate of between-component variance: —

ANOVA Table for Number of Days Lost
Split By: Year
Cell: 1993

	df	Sum of Squares	Mean Square	f-Value	p-Value
Gender	1	10245.33	10245.33	4.52	.0380
Residual	56	127071.56	2269.14		

Model II estimate of between-component variance: 292.06

ANOVA Table for Number of Days Lost
Split By: Year
Cell: 1994

	df	Sum of Squares	Mean Square	f-Value	p-Value
Gender	1	.08	.08	.40	.5447
Residual	8	1.52	.19		

Model II estimate of between-component variance: —

Figure 17.1. Effect of gender on length of time lost per injury. (ANOVA = analysis of variance.)

Table 17.1. Sample Data from Injury/Loss Database Used for Planning and Assessment of Cumulative

Case No.	FT/PT	Years Employed	Status	Age	Gender	Race	Accident Date
101	FT	10	Emp	31	Male	Spanish	4/30
102	FT	—	Term	37	Male	Spanish	5/24
103	FT	18	Emp	43	Male	Spanish	5/18
104	FT	4	Term	33	Male	Caucasian	11/25
105	FT	1	Emp	23	Male	Spanish	5/28
106	FT	3	Emp	27	Male	Caucasian	3/6
107	FT	4	Emp	29	Male	Spanish	2/25
108	FT	—	LOA	21	Male	Spanish	5/2
109	FT	—	Emp	44	Male	Spanish	5/12
110	FT	12	Emp	32	Male	Spanish	5/11
111	PT	—	Emp	19	Male	Spanish	10/6
112	FT	9	Emp	36	Male	Spanish	6/3
113	FT	9	Emp	31	Male	Spanish	8/28
114	FT	2	Emp	29	Male	Spanish	4/17
115	PT	4	Emp	26	Male	Spanish	10/2
116	FT	11	Emp	59	Male	Spanish	1/25
117	FT	—	Term	21	Male	Spanish	3/22
118	FT	3	Emp	26	Male	Spanish	8/15
119	FT	4	Emp	29	Male	Spanish	5/8
120	FT	1	Emp	38	Female	Spanish	7/20
121	FT	2	Emp	23	Male	Caucasian	6/29
122	FT	7	Emp	34	Male	Spanish	4/19
123	PT	—	Term	29	Male	Spanish	3/9
124	PT	—	Emp	39	Male	Spanish	6/1
125	FT	11	Emp	33	Male	Spanish	5/25
126	FT	8	Emp	30	Male	Spanish	8/25
127	PT	—	Term	22	Male	Black	11/22
128	PT	1	Emp	22	Male	Spanish	1/7
129	PT	1	Emp	28	Male	Caucasian	10/7
130	FT	7	Emp	29	Male	Spanish	3/24
131	FT	—	Term	25	Male	Caucasian	4/30
132	FT	13	Emp	32	Male	Spanish	8/17
133	FT	—	Emp	33	Male	Spanish	11/29
134	PT	3	Term	19	Male	Spanish	10/16
135	FT	3	Emp	42	Male	Spanish	12/18
136	FT	2	Emp	24	Male	Spanish	4/23
137	FT	—	Emp	24	Male	Black	6/15
138	FT	4	Emp	26	Male	Spanish	10/5
139	FT	7	Emp	27	Male	Spanish	1/4
140	PT	—	Emp	19	Male	Spanish	8/11
141	FT	8	Emp	34	Male	Spanish	12/10
142	FT	—	Term	30	Male	Spanish	1/18
143	PT	1	Emp	20	Male	Spanish	9/13
144	FT	12	LOA	51	Female	Spanish	1/28
145	PT	—	Term	19	Male	Spanish	12/7
146	FT	8	Emp	48	Male	Black	1/13
147	PT	2	Emp	24	Male	Spanish	2/16
148	FT	8	Emp	25	Male	Caucasian	8/18
149	PT	—	Term	55	Female	Spanish	3/23
150	FT	11	Emp	46	Female	Caucasian	8/10

FT = full-time; PT = part-time; Emp = currently employed; Term = terminated; LOA = leave of absence; UE = upper extremity; LE = lower extremity.

Trauma Disorder Prevention Programs

Days Lost	Accident Year	Department	Job Title	Location	Accident Code
33	1991	Ice Cream	Supervisor, foreman	San Antonio	UE Contusion
33	1990	Meat	Sanitation, maintenance	San Antonio	Laceration
33	1989	Meat	Meatcutter	San Antonio	UE Strain
33	1988	Meat	K-Pak operator	San Antonio	Laceration
32	1990	Meat	Sanitizer	San Antonio	UE Strain
32	1991	Meat	Boneguarding	San Antonio	UE Strain
31	1990	Milk	—	San Antonio	Back Injury
31	1989	Meat	Sanitizer	San Antonio	Back Injury
29	1989	Meat	—	San Antonio	UE Contusion
29	1989	Meat	Breaker, boner	San Antonio	UE Strain
29	1990	Bakery	General laborer	San Antonio	Back Injury
29	1990	Milk	Cheesemaker	San Antonio	LE Strain
28	1989	Meat	Boner, trimmer	San Antonio	Back Injury
28	1991	Meat	Order selector	San Antonio	Back Injury
28	1990	Meat	Product handler	San Antonio	LE Contusion
28	1989	Meat	Mechanic	San Antonio	UE Contusion
27	1989	Meat	Order selector	San Antonio	UE Strain
27	1991	Meat	Scale operator	San Antonio	Back Injury
27	1989	Meat	Breaker, boner	San Antonio	Laceration
27	1990	Ice Cream	General laborer	San Antonio	Back Injury
26	1989	Milk	Sanitation, maintenance	San Antonio	LE Strain
26	1988	Meat	Scale operator	San Antonio	UE Strain
25	1988	Bakery	Machine operator	San Antonio	UE Contusion
25	1989	Ice Cream	General laborer	San Antonio	UE Strain
24	1990	Meat	Supervisor, foreman	San Antonio	Back Injury
24	1989	Ice Cream	Supervisor, foreman	San Antonio	LE Strain
24	1990	Meat	Order selector	San Antonio	UE Strain
24	1991	Meat	Sanitizer	San Antonio	UE Contusion
24	1988	Ice Cream	General laborer	San Antonio	Laceration
23	1988	Bakery	Machine operator	San Antonio	Back Injury
23	1988	Ice Cream	Mechanic	San Antonio	Back Injury
23	1990	Meat	Meatcutter	San Antonio	Back Injury
22	1990	Meat	Boner, trimmer	San Antonio	Groin
22	1990	Meat	Sanitizer	San Antonio	LE Contusion
22	1989	Meat	Boner, trimmer	San Antonio	Laceration
22	1990	Meat	Order selector	San Antonio	Back Injury
22	1991	Meat	Sanitation, maintenance	San Antonio	UE Strain
21	1991	Bakery	Order selector	San Antonio	LE Contusion
21	1988	Meat	Meatcutter	San Antonio	UE Strain
21	1988	Meat	Order selector	San Antonio	Laceration
21	1989	Milk	CIP	San Antonio	UE Contusion
21	1988	Meat	Order selector	San Antonio	Back Injury
20	1989	Milk	Production	San Antonio	Laceration
20	1988	Bakery	Packaging	San Antonio	LE Contusion
20	1990	Meat	Sanitizer	San Antonio	Trunk Contusion
20	1989	Milk	General laborer	San Antonio	Laceration
20	1989	Bakery	Production	San Antonio	Back Injury
19	1990	Meat	Order selector	San Antonio	UE Strain
19	1989	Bakery	Grocery worker	San Antonio	UE Strain
19	1990	Ice Cream	Production	San Antonio	LE Contusion

ble explanation might be height, strength, or weight differences (as gender differences in these three areas are common). Although statistical associations should not be confused with causal relationships, a database of the losses associated with occupational illnesses and injuries can enhance the value of the injury and illness database greatly by revealing prevention programs' financial and behavioral effects on the organization.

Determining Company Losses

Although an injury database is a sine qua non of effective outcome assessment, it would be misleading to equate injuries and accidents with losses. This is especially true when evaluating CTDs because initial injuries are almost always both less severe and less expensive than subsequent injuries to the same employee. A single surgical case for a ruptured intervertebral disc could easily cost more than $100,000 in compensation, medical costs, administrative costs, and disability settlement. In contrast, 20 back sprains that are treated conservatively onsite by an occupational health service and that entail no physician visits, only over-the-counter anti-inflammatory and analgesic medications, and minimal lost productive time may average less than $50 per case, for a total cost of no more than $1,000. The adverse impact of injuries on an organization cannot always be measured solely in direct injury costs. For example, consider the case of a lead technician on a project who is out of work for several weeks at a cost of $1,000–2,000 in medical and lost-time expenses. If this worker's absence delays the shipping of a critical product and causes the company to default on a major contract, the actual losses in present and future business from that account could be enormous.

Assessment of losses requires that additional data concerning productivity, medical, and administrative costs of occupational injuries and illnesses be integrated into the assessment database for later analysis and interpretation. This risk-management data system integrates direct and indirect costs of prevention with other outcome measures to permit comprehensive statistical analysis of program activities and outcomes. Table 17.2 shows some of the data required in addition to the injury data provided in Table 17.1.

Risk-Management and Loss-Control Information Systems

The concept of risk management defies a single definition. In some contexts, the risks to be managed are those related to natural disasters such as tornados, floods, and drought, whereas in other contexts, risks are related to uncertainties about the demand for goods and services, to delays in production schedules, or to unanticipated taxation or governmental regulation. A risk-management program designed to reduce the adverse impact of worker's compensation claims, injuries, and lost time must be driven by risks related to employee health and safety. Organizations are faced with decisions concerning two categories of risk: pure risk and speculative risk (Mehr 1983). *Pure risks* are risks that lead to losses without opportunity for any net gain. Included among these are losses due to injuries, illnesses, lost time, and litigation brought against an employer on behalf of an employee. *Speculative risks* offer the opportunity for both losses and gains and include the hiring of new employees, decisions to offer a new product or service, and investment of organizational resources. Although pure and speculative risks may appear to be independent, persons responsible for loss-prevention programs, including those responsible for CTD prevention, appreciate relationships between the two that affect management decisions. For instance, a wellness program requiring a fitness center and trained staff is a speculative risk. If it decreases a single year's incidence rate for worker's compensation injuries without lowering worker's compensation insurance premiums, it may be said to reduce pure risk yet still be a net financial loss. However, if both occupation-related and non-occupation-related injuries and illness are reduced to a significant extent by such a program, premiums for both worker's compensation and health insurance may be decreased, and assets beyond the amounts required by the fitness center may be conserved, resulting in a net "profit" to the cash flow of the organization.

The concept of risk management has often been identified closely with the transference of risks from one party to another through the purchase of insurance. For many organizations, the risk manager is little more than an insurance manager. At its best, risk management is a process whereby certain risks that cannot be controlled are transferred and those

Table 17.2. Sample of Additional Data Needed for Prevention Program Planning and Assessment

Case No.	Years at Company	Age Group*	Tenure Group	Volume Rank Order	Output Volume	Total Incurred Loss	Average $/Day Lost
95	1.00	Younger	New hire	3	Unknown	$104.00	$52.00
96	3.00	Younger	1–5 yrs	4	Unknown	—	—
97	1.00	Younger	New hire	2	High	$83.00	—
98	1.00	Younger	New hire	3	Unknown	$163.00	—
99	1.00	Younger	New hire	1	High	$50.00	—
100	21.00	Older	>15 yrs	2	High	$15,147.00	$136.45
101	1.00	Middle aged	New hire	3	Unknown	$196.00	—
102	0.50	Middle aged	New hire	6	Low	$177.00	—
103	5.00	Middle aged	1–5 yrs	6	Low	—	—
104	5.00	Middle aged	1–5 yrs	3	Unknown	$9,999.00	$136.97
105	18.00	Middle aged	>15 yrs	6	Low	$2,017.00	$77.57
106	1.00	Middle aged	New hire	3	Unknown	$246.00	—
107	18.00	Middle aged	>15 yrs	5	Low	$129.00	—
108	1.00	Middle aged	New hire	3	Unknown	$89.00	$44.50
109	12.00	Middle aged	11–15 yrs	6	Low	$5,000.00	$2,500.00
110	3.00	Older	1–5 yrs	6	Low	$173.00	—
111	18.00	Older	>15 yrs	5	Low	$10.00	—
112	1.00	Middle aged	New hire	2	High	—	—
113	5.00	Younger	1–5 yrs	3	Unknown	—	—
114	9.00	Middle aged	6–10 yrs	2	High	—	—
115	0.25	Middle aged	New hire	1	High	—	—
116	17.00	Middle aged	>15 yrs	2	High	—	—
117	18.00	Older	>15 yrs	—	—	—	—
118	1.00	Middle aged	New hire	3	Unknown	—	—
119	0.33	Middle aged	New hire	3	Unknown	—	—
120	1.00	Younger	New hire	3	Unknown	—	—
121	15.00	Older	11–15 yrs	4	Unknown	—	—

*Younger = <30 years; Middle aged = 30–45 years; Older = >45 years.

that can be controlled are retained, and programs are enacted to reduce or eliminate the behaviors and events that lead to losses.

The notion that risks should be assumed and not transferred is novel and heretical and makes good business sense! Risks need not be transferred to be managed effectively. Indeed, on the contrary, the transference of risks via insurance has led to the concept of acceptable risks and acceptable losses, even when the dollars to effect such transfer of risk represent a huge opportunity cost. This is especially true in cases in which losses are unnecessary, being attributable to human behaviors that can be modified, and in cases in which the causes and patterns of losses are known in advance. Risks may be managed proactively through the decision to assume responsibility for the prevention of undesirable events

that lead to losses. Regardless of the type of risk or whether a prevention program depends on transferred risks (insurance) or retained risks (management programs), two classes of losses—direct and indirect—must be measured and accounted for to assess prevention program outcomes.

Direct Injury Costs: Indemnity

Organizations that carry worker's compensation insurance or use insurance products to cover losses due to CTDs are charged a premium in advance of each covered period to indemnify or reimburse such losses, either in whole or up to some prestated limit or cap. This premium usually covers (1) usual and customary medical expenses incurred in the treatment of occupation-related illness and injury; (2) compensation expenses, including the payment of a significant portion of wages that the worker otherwise would lose if unable to work; (3) administrative costs of documentation; (4) reserves that must be deposited in an account and remain available for future payments as the claim develops over time; and (5) actuarial adjustments, including experience modifiers (i.e., multiples of a standard premium for a group at risk that are used to pass along unexpected losses to future policy premiums). These amounts, large as they may be, that are paid from premiums are only a fraction of the actual premium cost. Profit for the insurance company, commissions for the agents, and state insurance taxes are also included in the premium. Some states now permit employers to provide themselves with worker's compensation and disability insurance (self-insured) by forming "captive" or "self-funded" insurance plans, subject to state and federal regulation plans. The actual determination of costs associated with CTDs is complicated further by the fact that some companies use an Employee Benefit Trust [ERISA 501(c)(9) Plan] or other fiduciary mechanism that allows them to place assets into a tax-free trust fund that earns interest, which can be reinvested in the fund.

This challenging and potentially confusing description of insurance issues is provided merely to illustrate that the true costs of identical programs under different conditions are not equal. Those firms paying worker's compensation insurance premiums must count 100% of the cost of their prevention programs, including staff, consultants, and materials, as well as all premiums paid as the true cost of their prevention effort. Companies that are self-insured under an ERISA plan may actually deduct from the true costs of their prevention programs the interest earned on that portion of the trust fund used to pay for the prevention program, which, in effect, leads to a lower cost for identical programs (Tax Management, Inc. 1992).

Because not all those who are interested in and capable of offering CTD-prevention programs are necessarily knowledgeable about cost accounting, tax laws, and insurance coverages, a caveat is in order: Determining the actual costs of a program requires special expertise. Simple approaches will most likely be inappropriate. A financial analyst, accountant, chief financial officer, or attorney is an important ex-

pert to consult when developing the measures to be used in prevention program outcome assessment.

Sources for the data required to calculate direct costs of programs and losses are the risk manager, chief financial officer, accountant, and insurance provider. Loss runs from the insurance company will detail medical indemnity, amounts paid to date, amounts reserved for future claim development, and what remains encumbered at any given point in time after an occupational illness or injury.

Indirect Injury Costs

The true costs to companies of injuries and accidents go far beyond the obvious medical, rehabilitative, and even compensation costs. For each day an employee is unable to work, there is lost productivity, disruption in the work schedules of others who must temporarily replace the injured worker, and documentation costs for the company that eventually may include costs of determining liability and other legal services. If the employee cannot return to work, there are the costs of hiring and training a replacement and then a productivity differential in the output or work capacity of the new employee that seldom equals that of the injured person being replaced. Incremental increases in cost per unit of goods or services produced and the cost of compensatory overtime or replacement of workers are significant costs that can and must be determined to evaluate a CTD prevention effort. Settlements with injured workers and short-term and long-term disability status must also be considered. In addition, there may be tax-supported state, local, and even federal disability benefit costs financed by taxpayers in each jurisdiction. There will be lost tax revenues such as unpaid social security contributions, Federal Insurance Contribution Act funds, state and federal income taxes, and sales tax revenues that would have been generated by a healthy worker and returned to society to meet our common needs.

Other Costs

Not all costs can be converted directly to simple indicators such as dollars. One of the most insidious costs of CTDs is that these injuries affect the morale and attitudes of subpopulations of workers, often within small work groups. The stresses of working short-handed, having to adjust to the absence of a valued employee, and placing demands for attention on immediate supervisors may be significant. Such stresses can lead to increased errors, quality deterioration, interpersonal tensions, and decreased productivity. These effects are often anticipated by managers who are aware of the corporate cultural milieu, but they prove difficult to measure.

The Goal-Setting Process: Foundation of Outcome Evaluation

Outcome evaluation is most effective when built into a prevention program at its inception. Adding an unplanned outcome assessment to a program will limit its usefulness. Outcome assessment should begin during the earliest stages of program planning and continue throughout the lifetime of the program. It is my experience that organizations more often conceptualize evaluations as activities to be performed only at periodic intervals, and most often these organizations prefer that such evaluation periods be as brief and infrequent as possible. However, outcome assessment is linked inextricably to the goals of the program being assessed. Therefore, the first step in outcome assessment is to define the goals of a particular prevention program. This is also the first step in program development.

Clearly, if they are to be measured, program goals must be *measurable*. The essential question that is repeatedly asked is, "To what extent has our prevention program fallen short, hit the mark, or exceeded our expectations?" An approach to defining and prioritizing program goals that is worthy of consideration is formally known as *needs-discrepancy analysis*. It is based on the work of Borich (1990) at the University of Texas at Austin. This approach has proved especially useful in large organizations in which a committee or group has been charged with the task of developing a comprehensive prevention program. A particular advantage of this approach is that it develops the consensus of a large group (12–30 people at a time) without permitting excessive discussion, argumentation, or turf battles among the participating stakeholders. *Stakeholders* are those who have a direct interest in the prevention program—its administration, funding, or outcomes. Ideally, a stakeholders' group will include represen-

tatives of all major organizational constituencies from upper management to direct labor and support staff. A minimum of 10 participants is required to minimize systematic bias within the planning group.

Needs-discrepancy analysis is predicated on the belief that goals are established to organize activities that will change the behavior of an organization. If there existed no discrepancy between the present and the desired state of affairs within the organization, there would be no need for a prevention program.

The group leader or facilitator for these sessions begins by asking all stakeholders to take a seat in a circle facing one another. The leader then instructs participants that the first meeting is to be a brainstorming session. This process will generate an exhaustive list of both currently existing and desirable but undeveloped activities designed to realize the organization's injury and illness prevention and occupational health mission. The leader should summarize the ground rules as follows: Each participant will speak in turn. No participant is allowed to comment on or react to what any other participant says. The leader will call on each person in turn, proceeding around the circle, asking each to identify and describe the single most important problem related to CTDs (or any similar problem) faced by the organization. Each person's comments are recorded. Then, after everyone has had a turn to speak, the leader proceeds around the circle once again asking the same question. This continues until there are no new responses. The leader then repeats the process, this time asking participants to identify and describe any activities that they believe are essential to an injury and illness prevention program. At the end of this second round of brainstorming, the meeting is adjourned *without discussion* among participants.

This process encourages all stakeholders to listen to one another and prevents any participant from intimidating, questioning, or negating the perceptions of any other participant. The facilitator or leader uses the transcripts to develop a *needs-analysis survey,* a comprehensive list of perceived needs in the form of a dual-rating scale (Figure 17.2).

The second stakeholders' meeting requires participants to rate on two scales each item developed on the needs analysis survey. The first of these scales, which appears in the left-hand column of Figure 17.2, assesses the extent to which the activity currently is being performed. The second scale, which appears in the right-hand column of Figure

Ergonomics Training Program Survey

Richard K. Schwartz, MS, OTR
Consulting Services
1800 NE Loop 410, Suite 416
San Antonio, TX 78217

	To What Extent *Does* XXXXXXX Currently Do the Following?					To What Extent *Should* XXXXXXX Be Doing the Following?				
	To a great extent	To some extent	Very little	Not at all	Don't know	To a great extent	To some extent	Very little	Not at all	Don't know
1. Provides job-safety analyses for each position to identify potential risks and hazards.										
2. Provides training on how to prevent repetitive-motion problems.										
3. Provides adequate breaks or rest periods to minimize fatigue.										
4. Provides appropriate chairs for those who work primarily in a seated position.										
5. Provides opportunities for changing positions while working.										
6. Offers accommodations to employees returning to work after injuries or illness.										
7. Responds to concerns raised by the Ergonomics Committee.										
8. Analyzes accidents or injuries and illnesses to determine whether there are underlying patterns.										
9. Enforces existing safety and health policies.										
10. Provides an administrative environment responsive to the needs and concerns of employees.										
11. Provides appropriate tools and equipment to perform work assignments.										
12. Provides adequate space to work.										
13. Trains employees for the tasks they are assigned.										
14. Provides for rotation of duties or tasks assigned to a given employee.										

Figure 17.2. Needs analysis survey.

17.2, assesses the extent to which the activity is valued. After all stakeholders have completed the formal survey (which should take approximately 40 minutes to 1 hour), the leader explains the entire process to participants.

Between the second and third meetings, the surveys are analyzed statistically and presented graphically to represent the group's assessment of needs (Figure 17.3, top). A schematic representation of the four data quadrants (Figure 17.3, bottom) indicates which goals are (1) high need and high priority (highly valued), (2) high need and low priority (less valued), (3) low need and low priority, and (4) low need and no priority (not valued). These results are then used to prepare a prioritized list of all project goals (Table 17.3), which will serve as a road map for program-planning activities.

A final session is usually devoted to creating a list of task-oriented objectives and a timetable to serve as an action plan for this project.

Regardless of the methodology used to determine goals, the ability to evaluate outcomes depends on the ability to appropriately define how goal achievement will be measured. These measures include both objective and subjective indicators of program accomplishments, as will be discussed.

Conducting Outcome Evaluations

Issues in Outcome Evaluation

It has been noted that those who do not know where they are going are most likely to end up someplace else. Although it may seem facetious to assert that this is the most common flaw in outcome evaluation and program assessments, this aphorism highlights the inescapable fact that outcomes must be predefined, in terms of measurable objectives, in one or more of the following ways:

- *In relation to previous outcomes:* requires analysis of differences over time within samples and populations. For example, the costs of losses for an entire organization, a department, or a work group could be compared from one year to the next.
- *In relation to normative data from a comparison population:* requires the identification of a criterion for success (benchmarking). For ex-

ample, if the CTD incidence rates and standard distribution are known for those organizations within a specific Standard Industrial Code group, then the organization's incidence rate for any period can be compared to the industry as a whole.

- *In relation to cost-benefit and return-on-investment:* for example, determining the ratio of net dollars saved in comparison with total dollars invested in a program or activity.
- *In relation to the judgment of putative experts:* that is, those responsible for conducting the program.

Whereas the first three of these methods of assessment require objective and measurable results from data that must be as free as possible from evaluator bias, the final type of assessment clearly relies on judgment data that is both subjective and intentionally representative of the biases of a single expert (such as the chief financial officer or director of human resources) or a panel of such experts. Many who attempt to perform outcome assessment in general, and subjective assessments in particular, are confused by the fact that subjective assessment is bound by the same rules of evaluation, statistical analysis, and inference as is objective outcome assessment. The major difference between these types of evaluation is not the procedural rigor or the need for reliable and valid measurement but simply the nature of the data itself.

Qualitative Measures of Outcome

Organizational behavior and the behavior of individuals in organizations are not always rational. The opinions, needs, beliefs, perceptions, and desires of people are often called into play in organizational decision-making processes. Despite their qualitative or subjective nature these factors can be described and used to interpret programmatic outcomes. It may be extremely useful to know, for example, that the vast majority of supervisors on production lines that have few injuries believe that workers' input is "very important" while supervisors on production lines with numerous injuries believe that workers' input is "unimportant." Being able to quantify, rank, describe, and correlate such subjective information can provide reliable and valid predictors of organi-

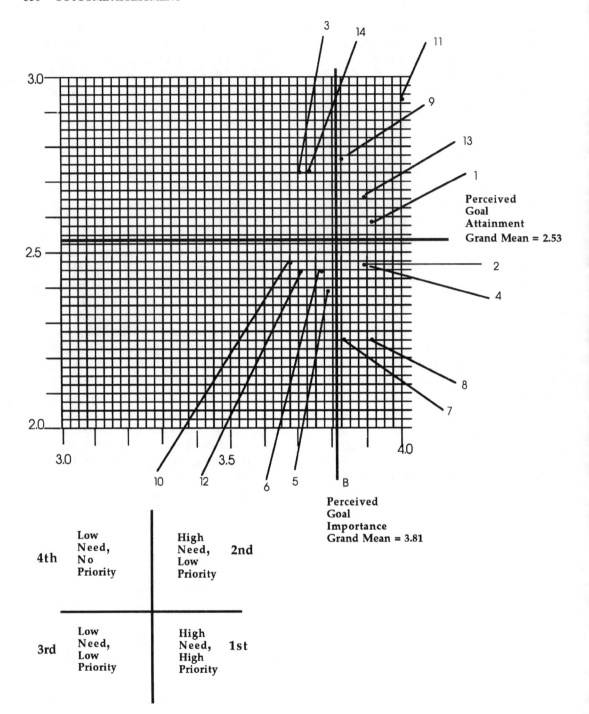

Figure 17.3. Needs assessment.

Table 17.3. Ergonomic Needs Test Results: Rank Ordering of Program Priorities by Importance

Highest priorities
    Analyze accidents or injuries to determine whether there are underlying patterns (Item 8)*
    Respond to concerns raised by Ergonomics Committee (Item 7)
    Provide training on how to prevent repetitive-motion injuries (Item 2)
    Provide appropriate chairs for those who work primarily in a seated position (Item 4)
Moderate priorities
    Provide job safety analyses for each position to identify potential risks and hazards (Item 1)
    Provide opportunities for changing positions while working (Item 5)
    Offer accommodations to employees returning to work after injuries or illness (Item 6)
    Provide adequate space in which to work (Item 12)
    Provide administrative environment responsive to needs and concerns of employees (Item 10)
Low priorities (current strengths)
    Provide appropriate tools and equipment with which to perform work assignments (Item 11)
    Enforce existing safety and health policies (Item 9)
No need exists
    Provide adequate breaks or rest periods to minimize fatigue (Item 3)
    Provide for rotation of duties or tasks assigned to a given employee (Item 14)

*See appropriate survey item number in Figure 17.2.

zational or employee behavior even when such behaviors are not rational. Examples of the types of data that may be collected before, during, or after prevention program activities include the following:

Narrative Records

One of the simplest methods of outcome evaluation is a journalistic or narrative record of prevention program activities. For example, a log of the ways that specific work-related complaints of symptoms or discomforts are addressed over time, including both the preintervention and postintervention periods, can be used to identify changes in the number and quality of complaints (Appendix 17.1). It can also be used for expert review of the treatment interventions to determine whether such complaints decrease or increase following intervention. If dates

at which recommendations were implemented are specified, the timeliness of responses can be evaluated to determine whether interventions are being accomplished relatively quickly and periods of exposure to hazards are growing shorter.

Case Studies

Case studies have the advantage of providing in-depth accounts of how specific problems are addressed by the prevention program. The major strength of case studies is that they can provide a longitudinal description that is both interesting and informative. The major weakness, however, is that they can be biased and select only certain kinds of information to report while systematically ignoring other information.

Interviews

Interviews are the single best method for establishing a program context and perspective that is independent of the inherent limitations of a particular study design. The potential sophistication of this approach generally is not well appreciated. For example, interviews may be structured (fixed-format questions addressed to each respondent) or unstructured (think-aloud protocols in which each person recounts all that is going on during work). Interviews may be given to individuals, entire groups, or representatives of groups. Interviews may be overt or covert, in that the interviewer can make known the purpose and nature of the interview or can keep the interviewee from knowing that the interview actually is taking place. Interview data can be recorded in journal format, on audiotape, on videotape, at fixed intervals, or randomly using what is termed a *systematic time sampling strategy* (Borich 1990).

Focus Groups

A simple, direct assessment of outcomes can be obtained by forming a small group of experts in the prevention of CTDs and charging them with the responsibility of performing on-site, direct observation analysis of a group or organization. The group should be independent experts or evaluators rather than individuals known to one another. The first step in using a focus group for assessment requires that the program goals and objectives be shared with the focus group. The group then develops a list of natural-language questions concerning the program that will guide the group's observations. Examples of the kinds of questions focus groups might address that are not likely to be answered by objective data include the following:

1. Who seems to benefit most from the program? Least?
2. Do employees really seem to have a better understanding of CTD risk factors after training than they had before training?
3. After training, do employees show any noticeable changes in work postures or body mechanics?
4. Will those supervisors who initially are resistant support the program to make it work for their employees or undermine the program to show their opposition?

The second step in the focus group evaluation process requires that the group spend 1–2 days talking with workers while gathering information and observing activities that the group members deem relevant. At the end of their visit, the group members will meet and provide verbal feedback, which should be followed by a written report of recommendations for changes and improvements in the program. Such a group may meet at fixed intervals, such as semiannually or annually, or before and after the program implementation in a pre- and post-test comparison design. It is useful to assign at least one key management person in the organization to be available to the group, to clarify impressions, answer questions, and provide access to whatever information the group requires. A special strength of this approach is that the experts often ask questions that were not initially anticipated, whereas a distinct weakness is that the limited observation periods may give a biased rather than a representative sample of employee behaviors.

Checklists and Attitude Rating Scales

Although the data gathered from checklists and attitude scales is subjective, the format often permits statistical analysis across a representative sample of employees or, in some cases, from an entire group or organization. The clear advantage of such an approach is that it provides a common set of issues and reactions from individuals, permitting comparison of attitudes, values, and beliefs across demo-

graphic groupings or actual work groups or with other settings. Such checklists and scales can be completed either by trained observers or by individual program participants. A weakness of the approach is that comparisons can be made only between groups on any single item. Comparisons of one item to another are problematic as there is no way of knowing which items are more important or more highly valued.

Quantitative Measures of Outcome

Many excellent texts can be consulted for those who wish to learn the models, methodologies, and step-by-step techniques for performing program analysis using objective data. Anderson et al. (1989) provide an excellent perspective for business data, whereas Borg and Gall (1983) present clear direction for the analysis of educational and behavioral data. Because these and other texts treat this subject in great deal and with more expertise than can be offered here, the focus of this section is on defining objective variables that are especially useful in the assessment of CTD-prevention programs.

Equally important is consideration of the vast array of computational tools available to analyze data and develop statistical inferences. Should one use simple two-variable models or multivariate analysis? Should one rely on strong associations or correlations or require more rigorous causal analysis? What type of experimental design is appropriate: randomized clinical trials, crossover design, blocking? Hayes' book (1988) would be an excellent starting point for those with some background in statistics. However, for most readers, such issues are too technical and esoteric. What is more important than being able to conduct these analyses is having an awareness of the tools and options available. Consultation with a research methodologist, statistician, or evaluation consultant may save much time and energy and avoid pitfalls that could fatally flaw an outcome evaluation.

Many obvious outcome measures warrant little or no comment. Among these are injury and illness incidence rates (i.e., per 200,000 hours worked), program costs (discussed later), lost workdays, medical and indemnity costs, employee turnover rates, absenteeism, numbers of nursing or other medical visits, complaints, near-misses, injuries,

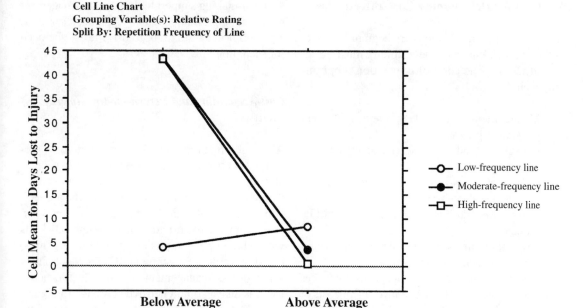

Figure 17.4. Days lost as a function of frequency of repetitive motion when controlled for employee performance rating.

nonsurgical cases, and surgical cases. Other measures, such as the cost of specific or aggregated employee-related losses per unit of production or services, are illustrated in the case studies at the end of this chapter.

Some independent outcome measures, such as time from onset of injury until return to work, may not reveal much about a program, but when combined with demographic and behavioral data such as age, gender, ethnicity, employment tenure, number of previous jobs, educational level, smoking history, and prescription drug use, the possibilities for more meaningful analysis expand greatly. One of the most useful methodologies for combining outcome measures with demographic and behavioral data is trait-treatment interaction (Berliner & Cahen 1973). For example, we would assume the success of a program if the average time between injury and return to full duty after unilateral carpal tunnel surgery to the preferred hand declined from 4 months before the implementation of an early-return-to-work accommodated-duty program to 1 month after the implementation of such a program. Yet secondary analysis that evaluates the influences of gender, age, tenure, or smoking history on such an outcome might reveal that smokers still averaged 4 months per case but that nonsmokers averaged only 3 lost

workdays per case for surgery. In such an instance, the secondary analysis is more helpful in evaluating and revising the program than was the primary analysis.

An even more interesting outcome analysis is that which shows that frequency of repetitive motions may *not* be a risk factor for upper-extremity CTDs, including tendinitis, carpal tunnel syndrome, and de Quervain's disease. Figure 17.4 shows that how an individual scored on his or her employee performance evaluation better predicted how much time would be lost on average for upper-extremity CTD complaints than did the number of repetitive motions performed on average per shift. Most interesting were the following findings:

1. Only those workers whose performance was rated below average showed increased lost time that was associated with frequency of repetition
2. For those workers who ranked above average on employee performance evaluations, the highest average days lost to injuries was among workers having the lowest frequency of repetitions
3. Those employees who ranked above average and whose work entailed the highest frequency of repetitions composed the only group that did not have any lost-time injuries

Methods for Determining Cost-Effectiveness

Businesses and organizations are beginning to recognize that risk-management dollars must be invested wisely. The costs of prevention programs may include:

- Management costs to design and implement prevention programs
- Consultancy and fee-for-service agreements for professional services
- Clerical and data-processing services to document and evaluate programs
- Release time during which employees will be trained
- Physical resources, space, and materials to conduct safety activities and training
- Incentive plans and direct payouts to employees
- Opportunity and alternative investment costs or income that could be earned by funds invested in prevention programs if such funds were invested in other activities of the company

The benefits of prevention include:

- Decreased lost time related not only to injuries but also to a wide range of health problems
- Decreased medical and workers' compensation costs
- Reductions in reserves or insurance costs
- Decreased employee turnover
- Increased average productivity

Not every alternative approach to injury prevention and risk management is equally cost-effective, and some may actually be cost-ineffective. Although cost-effectiveness data associated with injury prevention programs has not been reported in the literature, issues are emerging that should be studied: Are those programs most cost-effective that target workers with the highest risk of injury? How often must training, safety inspections, and other prevention activities be conducted to maximize the return on dollars invested in prevention? Beyond the benefits of prevention programs to individual employers, what are the economic benefits of such programs to society at large?

Economic data and evidence of cost-effectiveness of prevention programs are needed for two reasons. First, such information provides an excellent decision-making support tool to assist management in allocating prevention dollars. Second, it serves as a powerful marketing tool to drive home the need for such programs.

Cost-Accounting and Return-on-Investment Analysis

Although often thought of as a methodology, prevention is, first and foremost, a way of conceptualizing work processes, environments, tools, equipment, and labor that emphasizes the appreciation and consideration of human beings as valuable biomechanical and biocomputational tools with which to accomplish corporate or organizational objectives. Prevention of CTDs is not only a safety or risk-management or human factors activity; it is also a comprehensive approach to organizational problems that can and must permeate every activity within the system (Schwartz 1995).

A key question that an organization with a CTD-prevention program must ask is, "What is the opportunity cost in present and future dollars of *not* providing such programs?" A CTD-prevention program should pose alternative solutions to problems and permit the attribution of costs and benefits to the various alternatives. This means that even when assumptions must be made and information is not complete, there is a methodology for accurate estimation of return on investment (ROI) from each alternative. As a decision-making tool, outcome assessment provides a framework within which engineering and procedural activities can be translated into a cost-accounting model and evaluated technically and from a bottom-line and investment-risk perspective. Information such as anticipated payback periods for capital investments (how long it will be until the benefits realized from a particular activity equal the additional cost of the activity); effects of changes in human behaviors on cycle time, errors, and labor costs; and analyses of value added to a product or service by a particular improvement in the methods used to produce that commodity or service are essential to the evaluation of specific outcomes anticipated from CTD-prevention programs.

Those seeking to implement a responsible prevention program must be prepared to compete for

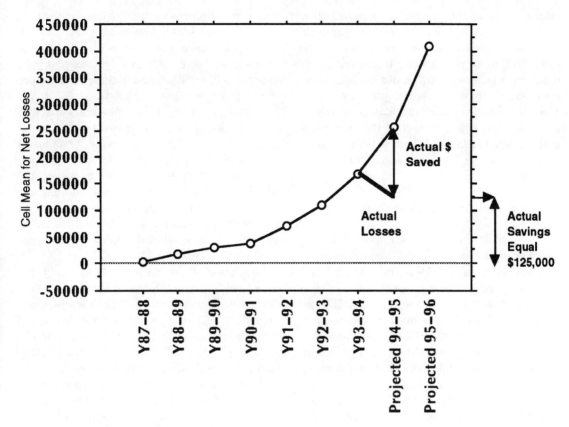

Figure 17.5. Injury cost trend analysis.

the dollars required for the implementation. These dollars must be justified with respect to the desirability of the projected outcomes, and they must be justified as a better investment of resources than competing alternative activities that desire to use these same scarce resources. Finally, a worst-case analysis should be conducted to minimize the risk of the prevention program itself becoming a deficit operation. In those instances in which the certainty of outcomes is difficult to predict, small pilot studies are a more responsible and less risky alternative than full-scale program implementation. This methodology caps losses and permits the development and refinement of both the prevention program activities and those evaluation activities that will be used to assess program outcomes. The case studies at the end of this chapter illustrate both cost-accounting and ROI analysis.

Injury Cost Trend Analysis

A risk-management and ergonomics program designed to reduce the adverse impact of worker's compensation claims, injuries, and lost time must be assessed in relation to long-term, historical trends, not simply in terms of the absolute value of dollars spent or saved from one year to the next. Figure 17.5 shows that for one company, actual losses due to worker's compensation claims resulting from CTDs were approximately $175,000 in 1993–1994. To evaluate the impact of the prevention program established in 1993, a trend analysis based on a simple regression model was used to generate a curve that would predict the expected levels of losses in 1994–1995 and 1995–1996. The actual losses in 1994–1995 declined by nearly $50,000 to the neighborhood of $125,000. However, these savings from one year to the next do not accurately reflect the true value of the prevention program to the organization. The actual *value* of saving $50,000 in 1 year is the difference between actual and predicted losses for 1994–1995, as the program clearly reversed a trend of nonlinear increases in losses that had been growing progressively worse over the previous 7 years. Thus, the outcome measure that most accurately indicates the economic impact of this prevention program is the $125,000 difference between trend-predicted losses for 1994–1995 and actual losses for 1994–1995.

Productivity and Labor Costs Analysis

Even in profitable organizations in which there is insignificant risk of injury and minimal repetitive motion, prevention of CTDs is important. In fact, it could be argued that the more successful a company or group is in reducing losses due to CTDs, the more prevention and ergonomic approaches are the *only* ways to increase the ROI of capital and labor. Ergonomic interventions designed to reduce the physical and psychological demands on workers result in energy conservation, work simplification, stress reduction, and time and motion reduction, thereby allowing workers to be more efficient and effective. Ergonomics is an important tool in quality enhancement, cycle time reduction, and optimization of the marginal value of labor dollars invested in production or services (Schwartz 1994).

The literature on multiphasic health screening has failed to find that comprehensive screening and testing of all employees is a cost-effective means of controlling risk. However, there is reason to believe that screening for certain types of specific health limitations may be an additional tool in a total risk-management strategy. Medical costs for the treatment of injuries and diseases have been escalating for the past decade. Corporations pay approximately 70% of the health care dollars spent each year in the United States. In 1989, less than 6% of the gross national product was spent on the military. In this same year, more than 11.5% of the gross national product, or $599 billion was spent on health care. It is no surprise that medical cost containment has become the number-one priority of many corporations.

One example of a screening tool that may lower total risks is pre-employment screening for illegal drug use. Such screening is undertaken not to elim-inate from consideration for hire those individuals with significant health problems but rather to discourage the application of persons who abuse drugs. Drug screening also sends a strong message that the company will not condone the abuse of scheduled drugs and the attendant health risks.

Another screening tool is physical capacities testing to determine a minimal skill level, such as the ability to lift a 50-lb load from 12 to 48 in. off the ground. Such screening may identify those persons who are unable to meet strenuous job demands. If these tests are job specific and are conducted as postoffer, preplacement tests, they are both appropriate and legal under the Americans with Disabilities Act (Equal Employment Opportunity Commission 1993).

Simulation of alternative duties that are being considered for an employee may reveal which duty can be best tolerated with the highest levels of productivity. Direct analysis of labor costs per unit of production or unit of service provides a powerful indicator of improved efficiency in worker performance as a result of a prevention program.

Reduced employee turnover, with its associated reduction in hiring and replacement costs, is another example of a labor cost that can be used as an outcome indicator in evaluating a prevention program. In one 2,800-employee firm in which the author has worked for more than 4 years to establish a comprehensive loss-control and risk-management program based on prevention principles, the savings for the first 2 years of the program exceeded $1,400,000. In the third year of the program, actual losses were less than $300,000, and there appeared to be no way to equal the savings of the previous years. However, an astonishing trend began to emerge. Whereas turnover of employees had averaged more than 19% annually for many years, it suddenly dropped in the third year to less than 10% per year, and the savings attributable to reduced hiring, replacement, and training costs was approximately $1,300 per position; multiplied by 260 fewer-than-expected employee turnovers, the estimated savings totaled $338,000. The employees' perceived that the same work that had been done in the past now was easier to accomplish because of ergonomic interventions and training and was safer because of the prevention program activities, and this perception was a major factor in retaining employees who were otherwise at high risk for leaving the company.

Employee Interviews and Surveys

It must be recognized that many corporate decisions are not made solely on the basis of financial considerations. In U.S. industry today, there are very powerful moral and humanitarian considerations that support prevention concepts for other than economic reasons. It should not be assumed that an adversarial relationship always exists between managers and workers. Likewise, it should not be assumed that only economic costs and benefits of prevention must be studied.

Figure 17.6 depicts a survey form that was distributed to more than 900 employees of a government agency to determine the effects of an office ergonomics and CTD-prevention program. A parallel version of this survey was administered simultaneously to 140 supervisory and management personnel in the same settings, and the perceptions of these groups were compared. Figure 17.7 is an example of one of the more interesting findings from this survey process. Significant differences by role and by location were noted when respondents were asked to describe the aches, pains, and discomforts experienced at work. It was found that supervisors had significantly fewer complaints on average than either their employees or their own supervisors (i.e., chiefs). This was valuable information in assessing the role of supervisors in the prevention program, as supervisors (because they rarely complained) were viewed favorably by their chiefs and unfavorably by employees, who believed that supervisors were insensitive to employee complaints (perhaps because these supervisors did not experience the same stressors as their employees).

The role of qualitative outcome assessment in general and the effects of prevention programs on morale specifically were described earlier. Evaluation of such outcome measures provides insight into psychosocial and group dynamics that are influenced, both for better and worse, by CTD-prevention programs.

An Explanatory Note

A search of the literature on injury and illness prevention programs, outcome analysis, and CTDs and ergonomics is unlikely to uncover instruction related to outcome evaluation of prevention programs.

The reader may wonder whether anyone else has attempted such evaluation or whether it is merely an esoteric and academic exercise of little or no use to actual organizations.

Most organizations are extremely reluctant to allow outsiders access to information that is a business asset. The great value of such evaluations to employers, the costs of bringing in outside consultants, and the competitive advantage of using information to improve the organization all mitigate against sharing these studies. An honest picture of organizational behaviors, organizational losses, waste, and harm done to humans is vital to comprehensive outcome evaluation. Outcome evaluations are typically conducted using data that are restricted, confidential, and potentially damaging to the organizations profiled by such data. These data also are potentially "discoverable"—that is, they could be subpoenaed as evidence in litigation and used against those who had the courage and foresight to conduct an honest self-appraisal. No organization wants to air its dirty laundry in public. One *can* find in the literature the successes of prevention programs, but these often are published long after the programs have been in place and only after they have been scrutinized, and often sanitized, by attorneys and executive officers.

The figures cited earlier in this chapter and those in the case studies that follow are actual data from the author's clients that have been merged and disguised. Evaluation is both art and science. Knowledge of spreadsheets, databases, statistics, and accounting is insufficient to conduct useful outcome assessments. There will always be those who use such information tools in a procrustean manner, avoiding the issue of appropriateness of approach and the need to assess continually and to refine the techniques. Those looking for quick-and-dirty, turnkey systems for outcome evaluation are bound to be disappointed, as these do not exist currently and it is unlikely that they ever will.

Case Studies

The numeric data reported in the following "fictitious" case studies are actual data from a number of different clients which have been integrated and dis-

MICS Training Program Assessment

This information is requested to permit us to evaluate the impact of this training program. Please answer all questions. Thank you.

1. Name: _____ 2. Job title:_____

3. How many hours do you work during a typical week? _____

4. Do you have other paid employment in addition to your work here?
   Yes _____ No_____
   If yes, what type of work do you do at your other job?

   _____

5. How physically demanding is your work? Mark the place along this line that shows how physically demanding your job is.

   0   1   2   3   4   5   6   7   8   9

   _____

   Not at all   Extremely
   demanding   demanding

6. How mentally demanding is your work? Mark the place along this line that shows how mentally demanding your job is.

   0   1   2   3   4   5   6   7   8   9

   _____

   Not at all   Extremely
   demanding   demanding

7. How tired are you at the end of a typical workday? Mark the place along this line that shows how you feel at the end of the workday.

   0   1   2   3   4   5   6   7   8   9

   _____

   Not at all   Extremely
   tired   exhausted

8. How helpful to you was the ergonomics program (presentation or personal consultation with a trainer)?

   0   1   2   3   4   5   6   7   8   9

   _____

   Not at all   Extremely
   helpful   helpful

9. Please describe any aches, pains, or discomforts that you experience either during your work or after your work. _____

   _____
   _____

Figure 17.6. Ergonomics training program assessment.

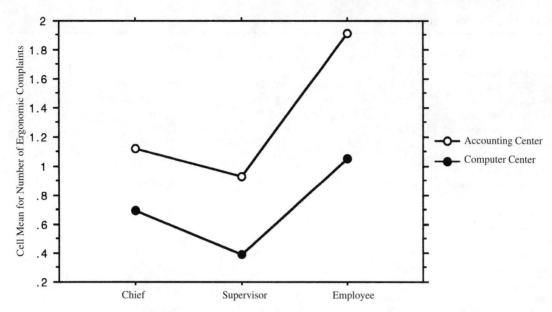

Figure 17.7. Cumulative trauma disorder complaints by role and location.

Case 1: Somebody Else's Business

Somebody Else's Business is a high-tech company that manufactures tiny PITA units, which do almost nothing, but they look great and everybody wants them. Although there are hundreds of workers, there are only four jobs:

- Whomees, paid $8/hour, nonexempt
- Knowitalls, averaging $50,000/year, salaried exempt
- Bosses, who divide up half of the profits evenly
- Supervisors, who average $32,000/year, salaried exempt, plus divide one-fourth of the profits evenly

The remaining one-fourth of the profits are divided among the shareholders. There are currently 1,500 whomees, 300 knowitalls, 100 supervisors, and 5 bosses. All the whomees stand all day to do their work. Because all the workstations are a fixed height, the short workers must hold their arms in awkward positions to work, and the tall workers

guised to maintain confidentiality. All examples used are thus real-world examples, albeit not presented in their original context.

must stoop over to work, thus having to position their hands and wrists in awkward positions. *They want chairs, good chairs, expensive chairs.* All the knowitalls, supervisors, and bosses already have such chairs.

Context Data

See Table 17.4 for context data on Somebody Else's Business.

Cost-Accounting Analysis of Cumulative Trauma Disorder Losses

Direct Labor Costs

- $8.00/hour + 0.21% indirect labor costs including benefits = $9.68/hour
- 40-hour work week = 2,080 paid hours annually
- Productive hours per year = 2,080 − 80 (10 vacation days) − 80 (10 holidays) − 4 (sick time taken from Table 17.4 for 1993, in which 754 days [6,032 hours] were used by 1500 workers; i.e., 6,032/1,500) − 105 (breaks) − 105 (meals) − 52.5 (daily meetings) − 24 (annual training hours) = 1,629.5 average productive hours/whomee.

Table 17.4. Context Data for Somebody Else's Business

Variable	1991	1992	1993
Total no. of employees	2,600	2,695	2,955
Total hours worked	4,161,367	4,599,692	4,770,436
Total payroll	$53,025,094	$59,361,552	$68,786,234
Avg. hrs/yr/employee	1,600.52	1,706.75	1,632.60
Avg. earnings/employee	$20,394	$20,171	$23,540
Turnover percentage	23.17% (N = 602)	19.71% (N = 531)	19.50% (N = 569)
Est. turnover costs/position*	$3,000	$3,200	$3,400
Est. total turnover costs*	$1,806,000	$1,699,200	$1,934,600
Overtime costs paid	$2,914,338	$3,676,553	$4,027,735
Total lost-time injuries	125	116	112[†]
Total injury lost workdays	2,395	2,487	1,922
Total sick days	840	540	754
Grand total lost workdays, all causes	3,235	3,027	2,676
Injury costs	$414,855	$1,039,055	$455,504
Total medical insurance claims	$6,040,430	$7,283,554	$6,930,096
Avg. medical claims/employee	$3,128	$3,570	$3,177
Gross revenue	$223,350,000	$261,088,000	$267,897,000
Net profit or (loss)	$14,674,000	$15,666,000	$11,569,000

*This is a very conservative estimate. It is likely that turnover costs exceed $7,000/position.
[†]This includes 45 back injuries (40.2%) and 9 carpal tunnel and repeated strain injuries (8.0%).

- Actual labor costs = 2,080 ÷ 1,630 × $9.68 = $12.35/scheduled productive hour and $18.53/overtime production hour.

Fifteen hundred production employees worked 2,445,000 hours and produced 26,789,700 PITAs, or 10.956 PITAs per production hour, which sold at $10.00 each wholesale and yielded $109.56 revenue per production hour. The average whomee earned $20,798 regular wages and $2,570 in overtime wages, for a total average income per whomee of $23,368.

- Total wages for whomees = 1,500 × $23,368 = $35,052,000 = $1.31/PITA
- Total losses attributable to whomees = $4,765,500 in non-occupation-related medical claims + $1,934,600 in turnover costs + $299,967 in injury costs = $7,000,067 = $0.26/PITA
- Losses/production hour = 0.26 ÷ 1.31 = 19.8%

Corporate Perspective on Losses (Earnings/Gross Sales Ratio)

- Revenue needed to support each dollar of loss = $267,897,000 ÷ $11,569,000 = $23.16

Return-on-Investment Analysis of Proposal to Purchase Chairs: A Pilot Study of Ergonomic Chairs

On production line A4, on which 25 whomees (or 1.667% of the workforce; i.e., 25/1,500) work, total losses for the previous year are $116,667, the average loss per whomee being $4,666/year.

- 1.667% of workforce produced 446,495 PITAs
- Gross revenue from PITA production = 446,495 × $10 = $4,464,950
- Cost of each new chair = $500 + $40 tax + $22 administrative overhead = $562 per chair

Scenario One. Let us suppose that new chairs will increase productivity 4% and decrease losses 50%.

- 4% increase in productivity = 446,495 × 0.04 = 17,860 additional PITAs = $178,600 added revenue
- 50% decrease in losses = $116,667 × 0.50 = $58,333
- Combined net gain = $178,600 + 58,333 = $236,933 = $9,477/whomee/year
- Time to payback (ratio of chair costs to net gain per employee) = $562 ÷ $9,477 = 0.059 years = 21.53 production days.
- Total gain on investment (assuming chairs last 5 years) = ($236,933 × 5) – cost of chairs (25 × $562) = $1,184,665 – $14,050 = $1,170,615
- Total return = $1,170,615 ÷ initial investment of $14,050 = $83.32 for each $1 invested, or 8,332% ROI over 5 years, which is an annualized yield of 1,666%

Scenario Two. Let us suppose that new chairs will increase productivity 1% and decrease losses 10%.

- 1% increase in productivity = 446,495 × 0.01 = 4,465 additional PITAs = $44,650 added revenue
- 10% decrease in losses = $116,667 × 0.10 = $11,667
- Combined net gain = $44,650 + 11,667 = $56,317 = $2,253/whomee/year
- Time to payback (ratio of chair costs to net gain per employee) = $562 ÷ $2,253 = 0.25 years = 91.25 production days
- Total gain on investment (assuming chairs last 5 years) = ($56,317 × 5) – cost of chairs (25 × $562) = $281,585 – $14,050 = $267,535
- Return = $267,535 ÷ initial investment of $14,050 = $19.04 for each $1 invested, or 1,904% ROI over 5 years, which is an annualized yield of 381%

Scenario Three. Let us suppose that new chairs will increase productivity 0.315% but will not decrease losses.

- 0.315% increase in productivity = 446,495 × 0.00315 = 1,405 additional PITAs = $14,050 added revenue
- 0% decrease in losses = $0

- Combined net gain = $14,050 + $0 = $14,050 = $562/whomee/year
- Time to payback (ratio of chair costs to net gain per employee) = $562 ÷ $562 = 1.0 year
- Total gain on investment (assuming chairs last 5 years) = ($14,050 × 5) – (1,405 PITAs × $10) = $70,250 – $14,050 (cost of initial investment in chairs) = $56,200
- Return = $56,200 ÷ cost of initial investment ($14,050) = $4 for each $1 invested, or 400% ROI over 5 years, which is an annualized yield of 80%

Economic Analysis of Interest in Ergonomic Chairs

Why Management Does or Does Not Care About Ergonomics. Five bosses worked an average of 2,400 hours per year per boss in 1993, for a total of 12,000 hours. This yields 2,232.5 PITAs per hour worked per boss (26,789,700 ÷ 12,000). If we assume that Somebody Else's Business is anticipating that scenario three will prevail, 1,405 PITAs will require an additional 0.62 hours (1,405 ÷ 2,232), or 37.2 minutes, of the bosses' time to the break-even point of a pilot program. The bosses' average annual salary is $1,156,900.

One hundred supervisors work an average of 2,000 hours per year per supervisor, for a total of 200,000 hours annually. This yields 133.95 PITAs per hour worked per supervisor (26,789,700 ÷ 200,000). Again, if we assume that Somebody Else's Business is anticipating that scenario three will prevail, 1,405 PITAs will require an additional 10.4 hours of the supervisors' time (1,405 ÷ 133.95) to the break-even point of a pilot program.

Why Should Management Do This? For every $0.01 saved in operating expenses per PITA, there is an additional $0.01 in profits, so for 26,789,700 units each boss earns an additional $267,897/2 (i.e., half the gain in profit), or $133,948.50, per year and each supervisor earns an additional $669.74 (i.e., one-fourth the additional profit divided among 100 supervisors) per year. Note that if chairs are not responsible for losses or decreased productivity, loss will be $14,050 (1,405 units × $10/unit) minus the savings due from the tax write-off of depreciation.

Case 2: Revising Manual Handling Tasks to Decrease Risk and Increase Productivity

Calculating the Recommended Weight Limit (RWL) and the Lifting Index (LI) for Modifications on PITA Breadline

In 1993, PITA Breadline had nine OSHA-reportable ergonomic injuries costing $55,177. URN Corporation entered a bid on March 24, 1994, to implement method 2, the ergonomically preferred approach, for a cost of $10,000 per machine.

Task: Lifting Full Magazines to Load and Unload URN, Method 1

$RWL = 51 \text{ lb} \times 10/H \times [1 - (0.0075 \times |V_{o/d} - 30|)] \times (0.82 + 1.8/D) \times [1 - (0.0032 \times A)] \times (FM) \times (CM)$; (where H = horizontal distance from midpoint of feet to midpoint of hands; V = distance from floor to hands at start of lift; D = distance from handgrip at beginning of lift to handgrip at end of lift; F = Frequency of lifting expressed in number of times per minute task is performed under actual working conditions; A = angle of asymmetry from the sagittal plane; and C = coupling modifier. (NIOSH 1994)

$RWL = 51 \times 10/20 \times [1 - (0.0075 \times |25 - 30|)] \times (0.82 + 1.8/25) \times [1 - (0.0032 \times 40)] \times (1.0) \times (0.95)$

$RWL = 51 \times 0.5 \times 0.9625 \times 0.892 \times 0.872 \times 1.0 \times 0.95 = 18.14$

LI = actual weight of object lifted/RWL (calculated to specific conditions) = $40 \div 18.14 = 2.2$

This is 2.2 times greater than the recommended safe risk level.

Lifting Empty Magazines, Method 2

$RWL = 51 \text{ lb} \times 10/H \times [1 - (0.0075 \times |V_{o/d} - 30|)] \times (0.82 + 1.8/D) \times [1 - (0.0032 \times A)] \times (FM) \times (CM)$

$RWL = 51 \times 10/11 \times [1 - (0.0075 \times |50 - 30|)] \times (0.82 + 1.8/25) \times [1 - (0.0032 \times 40)] \times (0.85) \times (1.0)$

$RWL = 51 \times 0.91 \times 0.85 \times 0.892 \times 0.872 \times 1.0 \times 0.95 = 29.15$

LI = actual weight of object lifted/RWL (calculated to specific conditions) = weight of empty magazine (15) $\div 29.14 = 0.51$

This is approximately half the permissible risk level for this task.

Decision Analysis

The cost to implement this modification would have been approximately $90,000 for the nine PITA production areas that needed this change. With an estimated 80% reduction in risk based on the National Institute for Occupational Safety and Health formula given earlier, the predicted 1-year savings of injury costs would be estimated at $44,150 ($55,177 × 0.80), and the projected payback period to justify this expense would be 2 years and 13 days.

The actual solution that was implemented resulted in the conversion of all nine production units and was done during normal working hours by an engineer and technician, thereby resulting in no overtime costs and no expenses for parts and supplies, for a total estimated cost of $0. Great ingenuity was applied to convert machines from method 1 to method 2 by rewiring and reversing switches to make the elevators carry full magazines (40 lb each) upward; operators then simply had to return the empty magazines (15 lb each) to the lower machine track. The estimated payback period was less than 1 day, and the estimated gain was a first-year savings of approximately $40,000.

References

Anderson DR, Sweeney DJ, & Williams TA (1989). *Quantitative Methods for Business* (4th ed). St Paul: West Publishing.

Berliner D & Cahen L (1973). Trait-treatment interaction and learning. In F Kerlinger (Ed). *Review of Research in Education*. Itasca, IL: Peacock.

Borg WR & Gall MD (1983). *Educational Research: An Introduction* (4th ed). New York: Longman.

Borich GD (1990). *Review Notes for Evaluation Models and Techniques*. Austin: The University of Texas.

Borich GD & Jemelka RP (1982). *Programs and Systems: An Evaluation Perspective*. New York: Academic.

Cascio WF (1991). *Costing Human Resources: The Financial Impact of Behavior in Organizations*. Boston: PWS-Kent Publishing.

Equal Opportunity Employment Commission (1993). 29 CFR, Chapter 14, part 1630: *The Regulations to Implement the*

Equal Employment Provisions of the Americans with Disabilities Act and, from the Appendix to Part 1630: *Interpretive Guidance on Title I of the Americans with Disabilities Act* (pp. 391–424). Washington, DC: US Government Printing Office.

Hayes WL (1988). *Statistics*. New York: Holt, Rinehart & Winston.

Mehr RI (1983). Risk management and risk analysis. In *Fundamentals of Insurance*. Homewood, IL: Richard D. Irwin.

National Institute of Occupational Safety and Health (1994). *Applications Manual for the Revised NIOSH Lifting Equation*. Cincinnati, OH: U.S. Department of Health and Human Services, Center for Disease Control and Prevention.

Schwartz RK (1994). Why ergonomics is good economics. In T Harkins (Ed). *Workers Compensation Update 1994*. Walnut Creek, CA: Council on Education in Management.

Schwartz RK (1995). OSHA's pending ergonomic rules. In M Fox (Ed). *Personnel Law Update*. Walnut Creek, CA: Council on Education in Management.

Tax Management, Inc. (1992). *Tax Management Portfolios: Section 501(c)(9) and Self-Funded Employee Benefits*. Washington, DC: Bureau of National Affairs, Inc.

Appendix 17.1

Sample Ergonomic Recommendations Action Sheet

Employee(s): _____

Area: _____

Supervisor: _____

Date of survey: _____
Time of survey: _____
Date of report: _____
Survey team: _____

Please complete this form as recommendations are implemented and return to occupational health nurse (F. Nightingale) when complete.

Recommendation 1: Ima Heurtin (and others using the same workstation) would benefit from having an adjustable-height (essential feature) chair with padded desk arms (essential feature), appropriate lumbar support (highly desirable), and a built-in footrest (highly desirable).

Action taken:_____

_____

_____

Date:_____ Person responsible: _____

Recommendation 2: Parts storage drawers should be arranged so that the heaviest or largest ones are nearest waist height, the lightest and smallest are above the shoulders and below the knees, and intermediate weights and sizes are between the knees or shoulders and the waist.

Action taken:_____

_____

_____

Date:_____ Person responsible: _____

Recommendation 3: If the UMM machine were elevated to between 75 degrees and 90 degrees from the table and the operator faced the machine, it could be loaded with the assistance of gravity and the handle (lever) could be actuated by movements of the elbow or shoulder.

Action taken: _____

_____

_____

Date: _____ Person responsible: _____

Recommendation 4: If there were a slot in the table through which the paper could feed, then the trash barrel could be placed under the front of the worktable and the paper would feed continuously into the barrel without requiring the operator's assistance.

Action taken: _____

_____

_____

Date: _____ Person responsible: _____

Recommendation 5: If the JLD machine were placed on a stand at a 45- to 60-degree angle from the horizontal plane, gravity would assist the fitting motion while work was being performed, and work against gravity would be required only for lifting the handle.

Action taken: _____

_____

_____

Date: _____ Person responsible: _____

Copies: Safety and Environmental Manager
                 Occupational Health Nurse

Index